Lost Eye

Lost Eye

◆

Coping with Monocular Vision after Enucleation or Eye Loss from Cancer, Accident, or Disease

Jay D. Adkisson

iUniverse, Inc.
New York Lincoln Shanghai

Lost Eye
Coping with Monocular Vision after Enucleation or Eye Loss from Cancer, Accident, or Disease

Copyright © 2006 by Jay D. Adkisson

All rights reserved. No part of this book may be used or reproduced by any means, graphic, electronic, or mechanical, including photocopying, recording, taping or by any information storage retrieval system without the written permission of the publisher except in the case of brief quotations embodied in critical articles and reviews.

iUniverse books may be ordered through booksellers or by contacting:

iUniverse
2021 Pine Lake Road, Suite 100
Lincoln, NE 68512
www.iuniverse.com
1-800-Authors (1-800-288-4677)

ISBN-13: 978-0-595-39264-3 (pbk)
ISBN-13: 978-0-595-83660-4 (ebk)
ISBN-10: 0-595-39264-4 (pbk)
ISBN-10: 0-595-83660-7 (ebk)

Printed in the United States of America

Contents

Foreword..vii

Part I   SURGERY AND EYE HEALTH
Chapter 1   Enucleation Surgery..........................3
Chapter 2   Appearance Surgery..........................34
Chapter 3   Eye Exams and Floaters......................45

Part II   PROTHESIS
Chapter 4   The Ocularist's View........................61
Chapter 5   General Considerations......................68
Chapter 6   Fitting Your New Eye........................72
Chapter 7   Prosthesis Movement and Solutions...........92
Chapter 8   Removal and Cleaning of Your New Eye.......112

Part III   IMPLANTS, SHELLS AND PATCHES
Chapter 9   Issues with Implants.......................135
Chapter 10   Scleral Shells.............................150
Chapter 11   Patches and Eye Coverings..................162

Part IV   CAUSES
Chapter 12   Choroidal Melanoma.........................181

CHAPTER 13	Other Cancers	210
CHAPTER 14	Disease	218
CHAPTER 15	Accidents	232

Part V COPING

CHAPTER 16	Introduction to Coping	259
CHAPTER 17	Coping With Depth Perception Issues	273
CHAPTER 18	Coping With Jobs And Careers	279
CHAPTER 19	Coping With Activities	288
CHAPTER 20	Coping with Driving	296
CHAPTER 21	Protecting Your Good Eye	310

Part VI PERSONAL ISSUES

| CHAPTER 22 | Mental And Emotional Issues | 317 |
| CHAPTER 23 | Children's Issues | 345 |

Foreword

The Good Lord has been good to me. After being diagnosed with deadly eye cancer in January of 2000 and having my eye removed, I have lived a very good life which has included two appearances before the Senate Finance Committee as an expert witness, publishing a book that has become the best seller within its category, and obtaining my private pilot's license. I have also learned that the most important thing in life is to help others as best possible.

Soon after I lost my eye, I created http://www.losteye.com that has since become the leading website to offer information and support to those who have lost an eye to whatever cause. Later, I added an online discussion forum to the website, and have been blessed to have attracted a number of regular participants who respond to questions and offer information to those in need of it.

Although my losteye.com website has been very popular, I know that there are many people who have or will soon lose an eye who do not use the internet but could be benefited by this information. This book was also created to create a tangible support resource for physicians and counselors to give to those who are being forced to cope with the loss of an eye. Hopefully, it will give comfort to those who are faced with enucleation surgery or have suddenly lost their eye, and do not know what to expect.

This book is a collection of the letters and e-mails that I have received from readers, plus message threads by those who participate on our discussion forum. I have included these, instead of writing a book in traditional form, because they represent "real life". Although I have edited many of these messages for brevity, I have been careful to leave the substance of the messages intact. In many cases, I have purposefully left spelling and grammatical errors as found in the original message.

Initial thanks as always to Karen and my mother Lereta for putting up with me during the writing of this book. Special thanks go to Dr. Robert Engstrom and the staff at UCLA's Jules Stein Eye Institute for the great professionalism they displayed in handling my case. Special thanks also to Dr. Paul Finger of the Eye Cancer Network at eyecancer.com and his thoughtful suggestions to me during my time of dealing with choroidal melanoma.

Many thanks go to my father, Ron Adkisson, who served tirelessly as my editor, helping me to edit messages and much other needed assistance. Many thanks must also to go my own ocularist, John Kennedy, who contributed a section found within on ocularistry and the making and fitting of an ocular prosthesis. Finally, thanks go to my most long time supporter and grandmother, Marie Rainwater, who also lost an eye to a botched cataract surgery, but was fortunate to regain her sight years later.

This book is dedicated to Chris, Alicia, Elizabeth, Jarrod, Barry, Ya'ara, and many others who over the years have participated on the LostEye.com discussion forum and have helped to answer the questions and concerns of those who were as distressed as I was when I first learned that I had eye cancer and was reaching out for help. God bless you all.

PART I
SURGERY AND EYE HEALTH

1

Enucleation Surgery

Some people lose an eye to accidents, and don't have any choice but to have it immediately removed. Others, like me, start off with an eye which seems perfectly healthy, but because of cancer or other disease must be removed to protect the rest of the body.

In my case, my cancerous tumor was relatively small, but it was so close to the optic nerve that any kind of radiation therapy would have destroyed the sight in my eye anyway. It would have saved the eye, but the eye would be blind and there would always be a chance of future re-growth of the cancer. So, to give myself the best chances of survival, I elected to forego the radiation therapy and have the cancer completely removed from my body. I had about a week between the time I made this decision and the time it was finally removed.

The first problem you will face, even before you get to the operating table is stress. In my case, I dealt with stress by:

1) continuing to work, which took my mind off the upcoming surgery;

2) taking time to do some really fun things, which took my mind off the upcoming surgery;

3) rationalizing that the loss of an eye for my survival (knock on wood) against cancer was a pretty good trade; and, most important,

4) realizing that my life would not be significantly different with only one eye

If you do as I did and repeatedly covered your bad eye to see what the world looks like with only one eye, you will see that it looks pretty much the same. In fact, in the days before my surgery I purchased several eyepatches and wore them around to see what it would be like. Conclusion: Not much difference.

As for the surgery itself, I'm not a doctor, and I don't have any medical training or experience whatsoever. In fact, I get queasy at the sight of blood. However, I'm going to give you some thoughts on removal surgery, what the docs refer to as "enucleation" (a really crappy Latin name that the medical profession should abandon).

In some ways, enucleation surgery is pretty significant. You get general anesthesia and are completely unconscious during the surgery. They are, after all, removing an organ.

On the other hand, enucleation is pretty quick and basic and doesn't do much harm to your body. They gas you out, disconnect a couple of muscles from your eye and that's about it. In fact, you may have the option of having the surgery performed on an out patient basis—it can be as little as five or six hours from the time you first lay down on the operating table to you are up and walking around the hospital. In my case I had surgery in the morning and stayed the night so that I could be examined the next morning, but you might be more comfortable in your own bed if you live close to the surgical center.

From the patient standpoint, it goes like this. You lay on the operating table, they wheel you into surgery, and they give you anesthesia through an IV. You pass out very quickly, and a couple of hours later you wake up groggy. There is a big pressure patch over your eyelid, and it might be a little sore (but probably not much because of the local anesthesia which is applied after the eye is removed). It takes about an hour for the general anesthesia to wear off, and then you are fine except that your stomach may be a little queasy and you feel the pressure patch on your eyelid.

During your surgery, the anesthesiologist will snake a breathing tube down your throat. You will neither know or feel this, since it will happen after you are totally unconscious. However, when you wake up your throat will probably be a little sore (like you just had "strep throat") and that is why.

If your eye or throat or anything else is sore after your surgery, please say something to the nurse immediately—not because there is necessarily anything wrong, but because they can give you stuff to make the pain go away.

You can expect to have some slight soreness in your eye for about five days. It will only really hurt when you jerk your good eye to one side or another (this causes the muscles for your lost eye to similarly react), so keep your eye movements slow. For me, Tylenol did the trick better than the drugs my surgeon gave me (don't use aspirin or aspirin-based painkillers as it will thin the blood).

What you learn is that although you don't have an eye, your eye muscles continue to move as if your eye was still there. So, if you glance from side-to-side you will feel pain for several days until those muscles heal.

In my case, when I was released I didn't have any discoloration around my cheek. After a couple of days, a small area turned black-and-blue and it looked like I had earned a "shiner" in a fight. From days four through ten, the area turned slightly yellowish and the eyelids swelled a little bit, but after about ten days the eyelid and cheek returned to normal.

What does your face look like after your eye has been removed? Keep in mind that your eyeball helped keep the eyelid up. So, when the eye is removed the eyelid simply stays shut as if you are winking. The effect is simply that you walk around with one eye closed. This will not cause you any discomfort, although you will probably be self-conscious about it. I overcame this by wearing fashionable dark wraparound sunglasses.

After your release from the hospital you will probably be given (1) a healing gel to be applied to your eye socket and (2) a saline type of "flush" for your eye socket.

Psychologically, it is difficult to confront your empty eye socket. To administer the gel, you have to pull down on the lower eyelid and leave a line of gel inside. It is psychologically difficult because you don't know what to expect to see. Truth is, when you finally get the courage to pull down the lower eyelid you will realize that it looks exactly like it did before, you just don't see the white of your eye anymore. It is NOT like you have a huge empty space where your eye once was—your muscles and other tissues kind of fill this area up so that what you see is just pink.

The flush is easy because you don't have to look at anything. Just hold your eyelid down, and without looking, squirt some of the saline inside.

About seven days after the surgery, you will probably have a post-surgery checkup. After this, you can probably consider yourself more-or-less healed from the surgery, except that you should not attempt to lift heavy objects or engage in strenuous activity for about four weeks after the surgery. My surgeon told me, for example, that I should not return to surfing until approximately six weeks after the surgery, but after that time I should be perfectly fine doing about whatever I wanted to do.

Patient Tip: *I will tell you that before my surgery I had concerns about having the wrong eye removed. I discussed this in advance with my surgeon, and he described to me the great lengths to which his staff goes to ensure that it is the diseased eye which is removed, such as dilating the eye, having two surgeons independently examine the diseased eye and locate the tumor and match it up against photographs of the tumor before removing the eye. It made me feel good to hear him say this, and you should definitely ask your surgeon about this risk.*

Still, before the surgery I had somebody write on my forehead with a big magic marker the words "Healthy" and "Cancer" over each of my eyes so that there could be no doubt which one to remove. This was probably overkill on my part, but it certainly alleviated one of my worries. After the surgery, I attempted to apologize to my surgeon for doing this, but he stopped me and said "Removing the wrong eye is our worst nightmare too—I've known surgeons who operated on the wrong kidney or something, and were so upset about it that they later committed suicide. So anything you do to help us get the correct eye is OK by me." Thus, although probably unnecessary, I strongly recommend that you do this, if nothing else for your own peace of mind.

Post-Surgery Depression: It is reasonable to expect immediate post-surgery depression, and also long-term depression from the loss of a significant part of the anatomy. Two thoughts:

1) I suggest that your best defense against depression is to get up and get around and see (with one eye) for yourself that your life will probably not be that much different than before. So get out of the house, go walk around the mall, go out to dinner, go visit some friends.

2) It can't possibly hurt to go see a qualified mental health professional, and I'll bet that your eye surgeon will be able to recommend to you someone who is familiar with these types of cases. There are now some great drugs available for depression and anxiety; a qualified psychiatrist can prescribe these for you. As I found out some years later, prolonged stress can cause chemical imbalances in the brain which can be immediately and effectively treated with certain prescription drugs. Don't wait, get help!

Post-Surgery Waiting Period. A few weeks after your surgery you will visit an ocularist and be fitted with a new eye. In the interim, you will have your choice of a plastic cup, an eye patch, or wrap around dark sunglasses.

With me, the plastic cup lasted a couple of days, and the eye patch lasted a couple of days. After that, and for about the six weeks until I got my new eye, I wore wrap around dark sunglasses. What does it look like when you've lost your eye? Mostly, it looks like your eye is permanently closed and for the first couple of weeks the slight post-surgical swelling will keep your eye looking normal. After a couple of weeks, the swelling will go down and your eye muscles will recede, and then your socket will slowly start looking kind of depressed (though your eye will still be closed).

Wear dark sunglasses and nobody will know.

LETTERS AND E-MAILS

I had my right eye removed due to melanoma in March, 2000, and actually came across your site after the surgery and right before my visit to the ocularist. I found it extremely helpful in several areas and gave the web address to my ocularist as a resource for her patients. Being a nurse, I know that mistakes are made in the OR, and the first thing I said the morning of surgery to the nurses was, "RIGHT eye, not left…RIGHT eye, not left" being an eye hospital, they marked my right eye with a black marker after asking me which one it was (to be sure we agreed). That was my worst anxiety, that my "better" eye would be removed accidentally and I would end up with no vision. Of course that did not happen.

Your section for driving with monocular vision was also very helpful. Right now I'm experiencing some additional challenges as I had to receive 6 weeks of radiation treatments prophylactically for extension of the tumor. I have very dry eye, yet it weeps all the time, no eyebrow, no eyelashes, a big "hole" of hair loss on the back of my head and very dry skin. Of course, I'm told the hair will all grow back eventually. But coping with the eye socket and prosthesis that is weepy at the same time it is dry drives me crazy at times. But through it all I know it could be worse many times over! Again I appreciate your site with its information.—*Mary*

Hello Jay, my son is an Endodontist. He forwarded your web page to me. I am an R.N. with a masters degree, and have considerable experience in health care. Your web site is one of the best I have encountered. You say it all and make it easy to understand. Patients who are about to undergo an Enucleation have great fear and trepidation, and I don't need to tell you that! Just recently, less than a month, a friend's son was diagnosed with melanoma of the eye. No one, not even the excellent surgeon that performed the surgery could appease his fears as your articles. I'm truly sorry you had to lose an eye. However, I do not believe in coincidences, I believe this is a very important mission that was given to you by our creator. Thank you for being there.—*Joan RN, MS*

Dear Jay: This is Sunday. I had my enucleation Friday (2 days ago) It was a horrible experience! The last 2 days have been the most painful I can ever remember. You were very smart to stay in the hospital for a day. I went home right after recovery. I had pain pills to take, but couldn't, as I vomited and wretched so bad my abs got so sore I couldn't even sit up. I don't know why you had yours done, but in my case (glaucoma), if I'd had a clue as to how awful this would be, I'd have said 'FORGET IT! You were very smart to insist on the overnight hospital stay.—*Anon*

Jay, I'm scheduled to have an enucleation on my left blind eye. I'm concerned about how the right eye will be affected after surgery. Like for example if there is a sympathetic affect that can happen such as blindness. Thanks,—*Mike*

Jay, I sent you an email about 2 weeks ago saying I was going to have to have an enucleation and I'm just letting you know how everything went. Overall, in the long run I know it was better to have the left eye removed but I have to say the pain was pretty bad at times. I was suffering from motion sickness like symptoms for about 2 days, so that coupled with the pain was very frustrating. It's been a week and I have a little swelling, bruising and a little pain but it's nothing major. My only real complaint is how the eye keeps tearing all the time but the doctors say that will go away soon. But thanks for such an informative website, it answered a lot of my questions and made me more comfortable about getting the procedure done. Sincerely,—*Mike C*

◆   ◆   ◆

I just wanted to write and thank you for your web site. I'm having my left eye removed this Friday and I have been blind in this eye for about 8 years. So the part about seeing with one eye is fine. I'm just a little freaked out about the surgery. After reading your info I feel much better. I'm usually an extremely upbeat person and am still that way-I guess the whole enucleation thing is just nerve racking.

I'm sure everything will be just fine but it really helps to have a first hand account (such as yours) about the actual surgery-thanks!

At 33 years old I never thought I'd be losing an eyeball but you are right in that life does remain pretty much the same only seeing with one eye. I guess I am thankful I do have one eye with close to perfect vision. Well I just wanted to tell you how much I appreciate the web site!—*Julie*

Well, it's done and I am back to work and feeling pretty good. I just get headaches if I read too long at one time. (I love to read). My surgeon sutured my eyelids shut for 2 weeks in order to prevent the implant from falling out. I guess this happens quite a bit!?! I look like I've been in a fight and I've joked around with some people about what happened to me. Some people can't understand how I can joke but my philosophy is LIGHTEN UP!

I appreciated reading on your web site how sore moving my seeing eye would make my eye socket. No one (doctors, nurses) told me about this and this has been one of the hardest things about recovering. The muscles in my socket get really sore. Next week I get the stitches out and a temporary eye so I can't wait for that. Thanks again for your very useful website!

Of course I wish I never had to deal with this but it's kind of exciting and things could really be a lot worse. We (people) need to look at the positive side of situations instead of dwell in the negative. Luckily this comes easy to me. Take care!—*Julie*

Hey Jay, I have my temporary eye and it's pretty cool! It doesn't fit that well though so it "slips" out sometimes if I mess with my lids. Last night I had my work party and as I was driving there it fell out in my car and I couldn't find it! oops! I finally did and just popped it back in! I thought it would be freakier looking at the inside of my socket but it is NO big deal. I am very relieved! Now that you have or have had your regular eye does it ever fall out? I'm a little paranoid about being certain places and having that happen.—*Julie*

Julie, it did for awhile—and it really bugged me—but I went back to my ocularist for a re-fitting, and he "built up" the prosthesis by adding some clear plastic around the edges. As your muscles in your socket go unused, they'll shrink. This will continue for about 6 months after your eye is removed, and then they'll stabilize. That's when you need to have the prosthesis re-fitted. But even now it shouldn't come out very easily.—*Jay*

Jay, I was just wondering how people have reacted to what you have been through? My closest friends have been really supportive as well as my family but some co-workers and people I have come in contact with have been really grossed out by the whole thing. I have an 8 yr old son who I was most concerned with and he has been really great about the whole process! Thanks to the internet we were much more prepared.

Do you tell people that you have a prosthetic eye ever? Can people tell? Right now I feel great but also feel like everyone can tell when they look at me which I have to get over! I hope you don't mind that I e-mail—I just don't know anyone who has ever been through this and it's very helpful to get input from someone who knows. Although most people are supportive and positive I feel like no one can relate.—*Julie*

◆ ◆ ◆

Hi Jay, bless you for your concern for the rest of the human race. I read some of the letters and just roared! I was going to circle the bad eye with a magic marker TOO! We all think of exactly the same things. I am happy to see so many people up-beat. Only God knows how long any of us have on this earth. I have had a pretty good life with the exception of losing my son last march, but I know he is in a better place and there is comfort in that. My wife will never get over it, I could face death much easier than I could face his loss, so no matter what happens, I can handle this. I will keep in touch. I think it is wonderful that people like you care enough about other people to put up a site like this. Best wishes to you and your family,—*John*

Hi Jay, went through the surgery Tuesday and it went well. I think I can adjust to this very easy and have no real depth perception problems so far but I did practice for this and that helps. Biggest problem is keeping the plastic cup in my eye, it keeps falling out. I am good at installing it but it just doesn't stay in. Do you have any suggestions? Thanks,—*John*

MESSAGES

I'm scheduled to have an enucleation on my left blind eye. I'm concerned about how the right eye will be affected after surgery. Like for example if there is a sympathetic affect that can happen such as blindness. Thanks, ~*Mike*

Have you asked your retinal surgeon this question? Write down all your concerns & just ask him. He's the expert, he can tell you more in detail, but no, your right eye will not cease to function! Our oldest son was diagnosed with amelanotic choroidal melanoma just over 2 yrs. ago & wound up losing his left eye, even after the tumor had responded well to the radiation because eventually, the tumor hemorrhaged and began to increase in size. He now doing really well and his right eye is just fine, so please try not to worry! God Bless You and Keep the Faith!—*Anon*

◆   ◆   ◆

My dear wife was born with an atrophic and 99% sightless left eye. She's lived with this for 52 years. I can't remember when she wasn't having to wear coke-bottle bottom glasses.

Late last year she developed pain in this eye that gradually became more severe. It was associated with occasional modest to severe nausea and vomiting. Her pressure in her right eye was around 19, but in the left eye it ranged from 27 to 71! She was seen by a glaucoma specialist who advised a series of laser treatments. (She had a retinal detachment several years ago and had to endure a retrobulbar block. This so terrified her that she immediately leaned towards the second choice: Enucleation under general anesthesia.)

Even though she has never had but the slightest light/dark sensation from her left eye, she abhors its loss. She says it seems worse to her losing an eye than to lose a limb. This has been confirmed by her ocular reconstructive surgeon. "There is something about losing an eye that is unique in and of itself. It can be a terrifying experience to contemplate". If your group has anyone that has undergone what she is facing and might have a moment to drop her an e-mail we would be ever-so appreciative.

She is a retired NP/PA and was a general nurse for 17 years. I'm a retired M.D. that practiced Family Medicine for 36 years. Even though' both of our backgrounds are deeply tied to this profession, the emotional shock of losing an eye is devastating. Any encouragement anyone might be able to give will be welcomed. God Bless.—*Dr. Don*

Dr. Don, sounds like your wife has been through a lot. Wouldn't she like the pain to stop? An enucleation IS traumatic, but what she's going through now is unbearable too. I had my enucleation nearly 30 years ago (I'm a 42 year old woman), and I still go through some changes and adjustments, but it's NOTHING compared to the pain that Becky is going through now. She'll adjust beautifully I'm SURE of it! Good luck to her, and to you. You sound like a wonderfully supportive husband!—*Chris*

Dear Dr. Don, it must be just awful, the contemplation of enucleation. But, I think, like Chris and Jay, that it will be better after. ESPECIALLY because she's having pain. My enucleation was post-trauma when I was a little kid, so it was very different. But, I was facing a possible hysterectomy two years ago and was very committed to not having that surgery, even though I don't have and don't want kids. So, I certainly understand not wanting to have a body part removed. Luckily, my Dr. was very sympathetic and only took out what was very damaged—a tube and an ovary. I've had much less pain since then, so I'm fine with the way it turned out. Please tell your Wife that we're cheering her on, whatever she decides. I am, and I imagine others who come to the website will be, willing to talk to her if she likes. Take good care,—*Alicia*

I know what she is feeling. I thought I was all ready for my surgery, but then when they woke me up I was crying and saying "Oh no, my eye is gone". I was half under anesthesia still, and you know how you say more things then. But it was a little traumatic and can put you in a self pity mode for a few days. However, with a positive attitude, you can easily adapt to your new look, and the whole thing soon seems like just another bump in the road of life. Good luck.—*Roadrunner*

◆ ◆ ◆

Hi everyone, here is my issue, I am a 22 year old male, and I lost the sight and the normality of the appearance of my right eye in a motorcycle accident with I was 15. For whatever stupid reason, the left my eye in, and it is horribly deformed, and is sightless. Everyone feeds me the bull of, it looks ok, there is nothing wrong with your eye. oh please, that's crap. When someone gets mad at you, they always have to talk about my eye. That one eyed this and that! To heck with these people! I can't even go into public with my head up, so I have decided to get a prosthesis, the kind with the coral implant and peg. My surgery is in two days, the mobility in my eye is good, not quite as good as my other, but I think that is due to the fact that it is looking at and upward gaze all the time. I just want some reassurance about this operation and will people not notice it? And has there ever been a case where there is no noticeable way to tell that anything is wrong with the eye? I saw a video recently of a patient who had this done, it moved exactly with the other eye. Thanx guys I hope someone can help.—*Jarrod*

First of all—I hope your surgery goes well. My prosthetic is a shell and most of the time you can't tell the difference between that and my other eye—maybe it doesn't move as fast but its hardly noticeable. My eye is quite deformed underneath too, I lost it when I was 2 and I ran in front of a swing, the movement in it is still pretty good though. Personally I think getting a prosthetic will do you the world of good—and you know one day you will be able to hold your head up high, and that will not just be because you are wearing a prosthetic. I would like to think of myself as attractive, eye or no eye.—*Tracy*

Hi! Glad you found this site. My experience is different from yours, but I have a feeling things will be better after your surgery. I'm having surgery next Wednesday, so we can recover together! The people here very nice, and I just know you'll find support and advice to help you. Best—*Alicia*

Hello all, it is now the day after my surgery, and I'm in a little pain, but not to bad thanks to some telex. The doctor said something about attaching the four usual muscles to the coral implant, and that really has confused me. The reason it has confused me is. I thought there were six muscles around the eye, does anyone know anything about this? He also said that one of my muscles was damaged, from an implant from a previous surgery, I wonder if it will get better? I'm so worried my eye is not going to have natural movement. . Can anyone reassure me on this issue? Thanx.—*Jarrod*

Hope all is going well with you post surgery. I haven't had my eye "done" yet, I am still not quite ready. I am also worried about movement and if it makes you feel any better I was advised by my Dr that the coral implant with the peg definitely gives the best movement. The implant itself is supposed to be so good that many people don't go ahead and have the peg put in. Keep thinking and feeling positive. All the best,—*Penny*

◆ ◆ ◆

Four years after the initial trauma (almost to the day) and after four surgeries to try to save the eye (2 vitrectomies, a scleral buckle & a cornea transplant) it has now gotten to the point where my eye is beyond saving. I have been very sensitive to humidity and barometric pressure (both rising and falling) causing major eye pain and headaches. At the beginning of this past summer I became very light sensitive and my damaged eye started "crying" all of the time.

I am now scheduled for enucleation. My doctor is planning to use a medpore implant which will be implanted at the same time that my eye is removed. He has told me that the first week after surgery I will experience "some discomfort" but after that my pain "should be relieved". I'm not sure what to expect but I can not imagine that the pain can be worse than when I had my rotator cuff repaired (that made labor seem like a walk in the park). I know everyone is different but the recovery from this surgery is what is scaring me. I have been wearing a scleral shell (at least I did until my eye became too sensitive to tolerate it) so I am familiar with that part of the process.

It is the week immediately after the surgery that I would like to be better prepared for. If there is anything I can do, ask for, or purchase to make this time easier I would really appreciate anyone letting me know. The fear of the unknown is what I am having a hard time dealing with. I would hate to be lying in bed after the fact saying to myself "if I had only known about this or that I could have prepared for it". Any and all recommendations/advice would be greatly appreciated. Thanks for taking the time to read my story. Hope you can give me some insight (pardon the pun).—*Heidi*

Well that must of been pretty traumatic for you! I lost my eye to hockey puck and they too tried to save my eye to no avail! After experiencing so much pain and then finding out that my eye was losing pressure I too had to have it removed. I was so scared at first, I am a big chicken and after the going through the initial surgery and stuff I was even more petrified! But. I had the eye removed and even though I had pain for about a week I realized that it was the best thing I could of done. The pain was not nearly as bad as before. The one thing I learned though is that you have to take some pain killers for a few days and had to watch what I ate! I had a turkey dinner and that combined with Tylenol 3 was the worst thing for me! Being constipated combined with my eye surgery was a night mare. Senna leaves and unsalted sunflower seeds were my best friend. But to be honest with you, after all was said and done, it was pretty uneventful (except for my emotions) and all though I had some headaches and some drainage from my eye the pain was almost 80 percent less than before!—*Ski*

Dear Ski, Thanks for the advice about diet (anesthesia will do that to a person). Since I am no stranger to constipation in my everyday life, I have a few favorite "home remedies". I will be sure to have them close at hand. Senna leaves is one I have never heard of before but will check it out. My original doctor told me (4 years ago) that this could be the eventual outcome. I too have very low eye pressure (2) which is why they are saying I am having pain. I guess that is a commonality among trauma cases like us. It seems like such a shame to have to waste a perfectly good cornea transplant but there really isn't a choice here. How long ago did you have enucleation? Did you also get the medpore implant? My doctor says there is always a slight chance of rejection—but I'm not up to worrying about that yet. First, I have to get past the initial week after the surgery.—*Heidi*

Heidi, well I had my enucleation 5 years ago! A day I will never forget. I have a coral implant, I have not heard of a medpore implant. My doctor warned me of the rejection thing too and I worried about it for a while. NO problems so far except I have a lot of discharge from my eye, sort of like I have a cold in my eye all the time and I used to have huge headaches but now they only happen occasionally, usually when I do a lot of reading and computer work. The thing that works for me the most is getting a massage at least once a month with her concentrating mostly on my neck and shoulder area and my scalp. Seems to relieve the stress and the eye pain! Take care and good luck, all will be fine! Let us know how things go!—*Ski*

Hi Heidi, I had my enucleation 13years ago when I was 15yo. At that time the doctor did not put any implant. This year I decided to have an implant and 3 month ago I went to the hospital. I've got an coral implant but the doctors were telling me that medpor and coral implant are pretty much the same, the only difference is that the coral is sort of natural as it is made of sea coral and medpor is artificial. Everyone was telling me that in terms of safety etc both are good. So I wouldn't be worried if it's coral or medpor.

Re: recovery. I woke up with a pain but it is not that terrible. They will give you pain killers and you will be fine. Actually for the whole time in my case I needed only 1 injection. I had panadol which helped. I know that it depends on person, some people said it was very painful. For me it was not that bad. Anyway if you will be in pain the nurses will definitely give you something so do not worry And I am sure you will be sleeping for the first day—that was in my case, I was just tired. And you will probably feel some pain when you will be moving your eye. But again, strong or not it depends on the person.

Re: appearance after the surgery. Well, it doesn't look nice but do not worry it will all gone. Give it some time and do not panic. It is red, swollen but after a week, 2 you will see the difference. Believe me. All the best Heidi and in case of any doubts ask. Cheers.—*Anna*

Dear Anna, thanks for the strong words of encouragement and the information. As I have said before, I guess it is just the fear of the unknown that has me a little nervous. I am not one of those people who subscribe to the "School of

Ostrich". I like to know what I am in for. Putting my head in the ground and hoping that I don't get kicked in my butt has never been my way of dealing with important issues. I was never one for surprises. I am finding that the information I have been able to glean from everyone else's experiences is helping me to stay calm and become better prepared for what lays ahead.

My eye is so very uncomfortable (painful) today due to the fact that there is a storm on the way—I'm in New York—and ever since the initial trauma the weather has always affected me negatively (rising or falling barometric pressure—especially low barometric pressure and humidity) I'm becoming more optimistic that I will be able to deal with whatever I have to post-Operatively. I am not a big fan of meds, but if I need them, I will ask. I feel somewhat better now, knowing what to expect during the first week or so post-op.—*Heidi*

Hi Heidi, I have just read your message. I had my left eye removed in2002.i had cancer in the eye so really didn't have much of a choice. This all happened very quickly so I hadn't a lot of time to worry about it. The op went well and the pain wasn't too bad and it doesn't last very long. My problem was when the eye went for postmortem the cancer had escaped into the socket. The implant I had in was removed because I had to have radiotherapy treatment so I had 2 ops in three weeks once again the pain was bearable as I'm sure it will be for you. Hope this has been of some help to you all best wishes for you,—*Anne*

I had my enucleation 3 months ago due to cancer. I found that as long as I trusted the doctors and the ocularist I had less fear. It turned out that the only pain initially was when I had any eye movement, Guess what that taught me? Turn your head to look at someone or something, not my eyes. The pain was bearable, not excruciating. I took the prescribed medicine as needed also. Within a few days, I had no pain.—*Rich*

Heidi, Hi. Good luck with your upcoming surgery. I have read all the replies. I agree with Rich, the worst thing for me was moving my eye. Although I think he may have toned down the pain level. For me it was excruciating (don't mean to scare you). But I think there are stitches under your eyelid after the enucleation, and for me I couldn't even move my eye like a millimeter to the left or right. It hurt to even watch TV. I couldn't follow any movement, the best thing was just to close my eyes. It was so painful. I remember my lovely 8 year old daughter helped me do everything for about 48 hours and I can never thank her enough. She sorted laundry and poured shampoo in my hand in the shower so I wouldn't have to move my eyes to look for things. The best thing is that having a prosthetic isn't really that bad. To others, it seems terrible and they are sympathetic ("Oh Cathy your so brave", "I don't know how you stay positive", etc., etc."), but I usually just find it a small inconvenience. Take Care,—*Cathy*

Dear Cathy, thanks for the heads up about the shampoo in the shower. It serves to underscores the inability to move your good eye. I was also glad to hear that it is ("just?") the first 48-hours after the surgery that are the worst. I had no idea what the window of "major pain" would be. Last summer I had my rotator cuff repaired and was unable to sleep for the first 48 hours post-op due to the pain and positioning requirement. (Even with meds) I guess if I did it once, I can deal with it again. (sigh—but not looking forward to it) There is a saying that the lord doesn't give you more than he/she trusts you can handle. And of course the answer to that is "I wish he/she didn't trust me so much" (LOL)

I'm not too concerned about the prosthetic as I have been wearing a scleral shell (its was actually my favorite fashion accessory) until my eye started to act up again at the beginning of the summer. I think it is a wonderful thing that you can wear a prosthetic and avoid all of the stares from the stupid people out there. I was once out shopping with my daughter (16 years-old) and she, all of a sudden, started screaming at a group of kids (about her own age) because they were staring, winking and making crude comments about my appearance (lack of an eye). It really wasn't repulsive or anything, just that my damaged eye atrophied so much that my lid stayed closed. My older daughter (27 years-old) is getting married in July and I am hoping to be healed enough by then to again be wearing a prosthetic so I don't mess up her pictures (that's my vanity talking). Thanks for the info & encouragement. Blessings, Hugs and Gratitude to all,—*Heidi*

◆   ◆   ◆

Hello all! Thanks to all who responded to my last post with their support. I've been out of commission for awhile, since my enucleation surgery was last Monday, but I'm happy to say it wasn't nearly as scary as I'd imagined it would be! I've had hardly any pain at all—Looking at myself in the mirror is a little more difficult, but I'm trying to stay positive. I can't wait to get my new eye! I had my post-op exam yesterday and the dr. said everything's going very well. Some discharge still, but he says that there may always be (it's the body's way of "rejecting" the implant) but that there are drops I can take that will help with this. Is anyone taking these drops and do they help?

As for my ocularist, I am going to see a guy who is supposed to be very good. I've been told he uses lots of little "tricks" to give a more natural appearance. Not cheap though. $2,790. And sadly, my dumb insurance company doesn't cover very much. Oh well, I'll be poor, but my eye will hopefully look good. Whoohoo! Hope everyone is well!—*Marsey*

Marsey, glad to see everything went well. I lost my eye to cancer last September. I continue to have a slight discharge even today. The only drops I use are drops for lubrication. I just live with it. As for my prosthesis, I got mine 2 months after my operation. Personally I wouldn't rush it until the eye is healed. Take care & God bless.—*Rich*

◆ ◆ ◆

Hello, I am new to this site, and I find it very interesting. I am having an evisceration March 1. I lost the sight in my eye when I was 6 months old. I had a very bad cold and my parents took me to the hospital. While in the hospital I got spinal meningitis and lost the sight of my right eye. I am 62 years old. My eye has always been ugly, but in last few years I have been getting terrible pains, No medicine has helped me at all. The Dr. said the pain will just get worse and worse, so he said I should have the evisceration done. I am so scared of having it done. Has anyone in here had that done? Does anyone know anything about evisceration? Thanks for listening.—*Anon*

Evisceration is removal of the contents of they eye. Enucleation is the removal of the eye structure itself. If your eye has been troublesome, this process is intended to provide relief from pain. My eye was damaged and removed through enucleation, so my experience is different. I'm sure there are people on here who've had eviscerations and can give you their experience. Take care and don't be scared. Please let us know how you're doing.—*Alicia*

◆ ◆ ◆

Hey guys and girls. I've been reading around this forums for months now. Only now am I more comfortable to post. I have a dying left eye and the time has come for me to have surgery. I have to finally book that appointment next Monday. I've been stalling for three years. I'm twenty years old and have studied three years in University with one good seeing eye. All this time I've had to carry a red, lazy, and dying eye. I'm terrified at the changes that will come about with this new artificial eye. Below are some questions I have, and hopefully you guys and girls can help a terrified brother out. Thanks in advance and please forgive my ignorance.

1) I'm very terrified with the surgery. I've read around and the common answer I got was that the doctor(s) put you half asleep when performing surgery. What exactly does that mean? I don't want to be able to be aware of them sticking instruments in my eye, nor do I want to feel a thing.

2) Does the artificial eye move at all? My mom told me that a resident in a retirement home has an artificial eye that moves along with the "good" eye when she is talking to someone. Now, I personally believe that my mom is lying just so my feelings won't get hurt. Somebody please shed some light on this.

3) I'm very physically active. I'm a bodybuilder, I play basketball, and I train in mixed martial arts. Will I still be able to do all three activities? I'm scared that when I run around the court playing basketball my prosthetic eye will fall out or when I'm grappling with an opponent on the ground my prosthetic will fall out.

4) Can I book an appointment for a prosthetic eye and have it made before I get my left eye removed? I'd rather have it ready than wait for awhile, but I don't know how it works.

5) How long will it take after surgery until I can get back on my feet again? I'm an avid bodybuilder and the thought of rehabbing for months makes me think of all the muscle I might lose.

Thanks again.—*Mike*

Mike, first of all, welcome. I hope that you get some information, answers and support here, as we all do! I'll try to answer some of your questions to the best of my ability. I had my eye enucleated over 30 years ago (due to a bb gun accident), so the same rules don't apply, but maybe it could be of some help. I'll answer your questions in this format:

1) I'm very terrified with the surgery. Answer: I was TOTALLY knocked out for the initial enucleation, as I'm sure most people are! Can't imagine it any other way, since it's a serious operation!

2) Does the artificial eye move at all? Answer: This depends on many variables. *I* have ZERO movement, but this is due to the type of trauma I have incurred. If the muscles are okay, you'll most likely get movement. There are implants with pegs now (other people can tell you about them) that give you a lot of movement.

3) I still be able to do all three activities? Answer: I've always been VERY physically active. I still am (for a 43 year old woman!). I've played all kinds of sports, swam, danced, lifted weights, etc., and it NEVER fell out. If someone poked me in the eye, there's a chance it might fall out, but that's never happened in the 30-years I've had it.

4) Can I book an appointment for a prosthetic eye and have it made before I get my left eye removed? Answer: I guess you can at least CHOOSE your ocularist, but they can't properly even fit you until you are healed. They will have to take an impression of your socket and create your prosthesis from that (it's not as painful as it sounds). It shouldn't take too many visits from start to finish, so you'll have to just wait until you're healed to start that process.

5) How long will it take after surgery until I can get back on my feet again? Answer: Guess it totally depends on how you heal. Someone here on the board just had a new implant and he was back on his feet, exercising right away. It shouldn't take TOO long to heal. You'll be lifting again soon after the surgery!

Hope that helps. I'm sure if you hear from others here, it'll give you an even clearer picture. Good luck with the surgery and recovery. We'll be here to answer questions and cheer you on!—*Chris*

Mike, Hi. I am sorry to read about your eye. The surgery itself is not usually very painful, but the recovery can vary from person to person. I was in quite a bit of pain (last year), but it did only last about 3 days. I was never quite as physically active as you (I do a little running and swimming), but I do a lot of water activities with my kids, and am still too scared to go on some water park rides with my prosthetic. I think the force of the water may cause it to come out. So I stick with the more quiet and calm rides now. It is all about making an adjustment to your life. I think martial arts would be pretty safe. It sounds like your physical activity is well rounded, but maybe if you find after the surgery that basketball isn't working for you, you could develop some new sports interest that you feel more comfortable with. I hope your surgery goes well. Good luck.—*Cathy*

Hi Mike, sorry to hear about your eye, I will tell you a little of my history, I lost my eye 2 years ago through cancer. I found the surgery not too bad and I was totally asleep and felt nothing. I was home the next day and pottering around very quickly. The discomfort only lasted 2 or 3 days at the most. my eye has no movement but that is because I had radiation treatment which killed the muscles in my socket. But I believe lots of people have movement. I go swimming and have never had any trouble with the eye falling out in fact it has never fell out. I think with basketball as you are so young you may cope. I hope this has been of some help to you and let us know how you get on.—*Anne*

Hi Mike, welcome to the board, just sorry it's under these circumstances. I'll just confirm what everyone else has said in their responses to you. I was totally out for my surgery, only had a couple days of discomfort and was back to the gym in about a week. You do have to be careful about heavy lifting, though. I have excellent movement of the prosthesis (I have a peg) and you should have too if your muscles are okay.

One thing I will add. You didn't mention if you have any vision in your eye now. If you do, you will go thru an adjustment period while your other eye adapts and you will gradually lose your depth perception. If you can't see with that eye, well, you're ahead of the game!

I don't think you have to worry about the prosthesis falling out due to exertion or physical activity. As long as you get a good fit, it shouldn't be a problem. And please be patient. The healing process takes a few weeks, so don't expect everything to be perfect right after surgery. I wish the best for you. Please keep us posted on how things are going. We're all here to support you thru this.—*Nancy*

Thanks for all the support everyone! To clarify things, I lost complete vision in my left eye in April 2001. I saw many doctors and they all said that it would be best not to operate on it; basically I would have to get my left eye removed because of the severity of the situation. So I went through three years of University with monocular vision and a dying left eye. Now I must get it removed because one, the color of the eye is different, and two the eye is already shrunken and is drooping. I've held out all this time because of my fear of surgery and now I finally have to face it. I hope the prosthesis doesn't fall out especially when I'm grappling. I roll a lot on the mat with other guys doing arm bars, chokes, leg locks etc. Thanks again folks, I'll keep you updated.—*Mike*

◆   ◆   ◆

Hi Guys! I'm scheduled to have my left eye removed in late July and I'm wondering if you think I'll be feeling well enough to return to school in late August. I'm kind of worried because I'm in a course of study that is vision intensive. I'm an artist, a painter. Thanks,—*Sleepy*

Hi Sleepy, sounds like you will have a good month to recover from the surgery. It's been many years since my eye was removed, but I remember that I went back to the gym while I still had a gauze patch covering it. Then again, I'm one of those people that refused to be held down by anything. I had my lower spine fused and was in a back brace for three months. As soon as I was allowed to drive after the surgery (about 4-6 wks) I was in the gym in my brace.

Do you have any vision in that eye now? If not, you won't have to make the adjustment to monocular vision, which I found took several months to get used to. I don't remember that there was much pain associated with the surgery, just some discomfort. Are you getting an implant? I'll never forget what my doctor said to me when we were discussing the surgery. She referred to it as "minor," as in not a big deal. It was pretty major to me, though! Good luck with your surgery. Please keep us updated on how you're doing. Best wishes,—*Nancy*

Hey Sleepy! I just wanted to wish you good luck with the surgery! I, too, had my enucleation done 30 years ago, so I'm of no help to you, but I *do* remember that I was patched up and in pain for a little while. I don't think I got my first prosthesis for a couple of weeks after the initial enucleation. My suggestion is that you ask your doctor what would be a reasonable recovery period and then take it from there. I ran into MANY complications (rejected implants, etc), but I think it normally takes a few weeks for recovery. Good luck, and let us know how you're doing! We'll all be praying for you & wish you a speedy recovery. Remember there will be some pain involved, as it IS major surgery, so give yourself time to heal.—*Chris*

Hi Sleepy. Best of luck with your surgery. I had my left eye out in '97. It was done as outpatient. I spent 23 hours there from start to finish. Had the coral implant put it during the surgery. Wore a comforter for about 6 weeks then got my first eye. Had some trouble adjusting to monovision, but I would say it wasn't that bad. Had much support and love from family and friends. All told I was out of work for about 10 weeks. Scariest part was not knowing what I was about to go through, plus the cancer fears. Didn't know about this site then. There are lots of wonderful people and information and support. Let us know how your surgery turns out. We're here for you if you need us.—*Ron*

I lost all vision in the eye in '97 so I won't have monocular adaptation problems. I've been told that the surgery will be done out-patient, and I'll be home that evening. I'm wondering why you were there 23 hours, is that usual? The other thing I'm wondering about is the length of time I should wait before being fitted for a prosthesis. Is it better to wait longer so the fit will be better, sort of like being fitted for false teeth? I don't mind going without an eye. I was shot with an arrow when I was a toddler, my eye has been messed up all my life, so having a messed up eye doesn't bother me that much anymore. Actually, I'm thinking I'm going to ask for a cat's eye prosthesis, have a little fun with it for once in my life. Best,—*Sleepy*

Sleepy, I was in the hospital for 23 hours because of the damn HMO. I think they(Hospital) wanted me for at least overnight because I was over 8 hours from home. HMO only authorized 23 hour stay. I was told to wait for at least six weeks by my doctor for the eye to get a better fit. Best of Luck.—*Ron*

Although my eye was removed when I was kid, I did go through two whopping surgeries and one small one last summer and fall, starting just about this time, btw. The surgeries were to replace my implant, so in a way comparable to the removal of your non-seeing eye. I was pretty much up and around a week after the first one, and I was home in the evening after the surgery. It was a silicone implant to replace a very small and old one, but it slid out of place, so I had to have a do-over. The second, though, was a lot tougher. I got sick from dehydration during the surgery—after not eating or drinking anything for about 20 hours!—and they sutured old 34-year dormant muscles to the porous implant. To be perfectly honest, it was horrible. I was admitted over the weekend and was in hospital for three days. But, again, once that was over, I was up and around pretty quickly.

Since you're already dealing with monovision, you're cool there. The main thing I tried to avoid was getting my head lower than my heart because it caused huge pounding in my healing eye area. As long as I was upright, I could lift and strain without worrying about it too much. Pay attention to what your body and your Dr. tell you. Be sure to ask the Anesthesiologist for fluids so you don't get dehydrated. And don't be afraid to give yourself a break, you know, to let yourself heal. Take care and best wishes. Love—*Alicia*

◆ ◆ ◆

Hi Everyone, I joined a few days ago and wrote a couple of posts, but I wanted to officially say hi. I won't go into my whole story, but basically I am 22 years old and I was born blind in my right eye and experienced problems throughout my whole life. Last year I underwent a surgery called Gunderson flap to try to save the eye but attach a membrane over the iris as a protective layer and then wear a shell over that. Unfortunately it didn't work and I had to have an enucleation this May. I must say, it was the best thing that I ever did. However, I only learned about this site a couple of days ago. If I had known about it prior to my surgery it would have been a huge help. I have read through a majority of the posts and I must say that you all are quite amazing. It is so nice to know that there are other people out there just like me. I have never met anyone who has shared the same experience as me so it is finally nice to be a part of a community that can relate to my same problems. I want to thank you all for all of the advice and love that you share with others that are in our shoes.

As I said before, I was blind in my eye from birth so I really give all of you who have had to give up their eye and readjust to monocular vision a lot of credit. You all really inspire me and allow me to know that everything is going to be ok. I just got my prosthesis last Wednesday so I am getting used to it, but I don't think that I have ever been happier in my life. Anyway, sorry to make this so long, but I really just wanted to say hi and thank you for give me a place to share what and how I am feeling and to finally feel like I have a place to fit in because you all understand what I have and am going through. Love Always,—*Jodi*

It is so nice to be a part of this community and be able to discuss issues that affect us all. For all of my life I always felt alone and misunderstood, and now that I have found all of you, I finally feel like I am not that different and I do have a place to resort to when I am feeling alone. So, thank you all for becoming a part of my life and showing me that I am not the only one dealing with this burden on a daily basis.

Penny, you had asked me what kind of prosthesis I had. Before my enucleation, I had a shell that I was wearing over my sick eye. It was made of acrylic just like a normal prosthesis, but the shell was much thinner and needed to be taken out and cleaned everyday. I was never able to find a shell that fit me properly and didn't cause pain to my sick eye. So, after a lot of trying, I finally decided to enucleate. After 8 weeks of healing, I started again with my ocularist to make a prosthesis in July. I received my acrylic prosthesis last Wed and haven't taken it out since! Its amazing. People who have seen me for the past year behind dark glasses cant believe what they are looking at now! They say that they cant even tell which is the fake eye! I have never felt better about myself! Love always,—*Jodi*

Hi Jody, congratulations and best wishes with the new prosthesis, it is wonderful to hear about your experience and how pleased you are at the outcome. I've had a sick eye most of my life, since I was 2 years old. It went blind in '97 and has been getting worse physically since then. Other surgery has failed and I decided to have an enucleation this summer. Unfortunately I developed some other medical problems that needed attention and might have to wait until next May for the eye removal. I wanted to ask you, since you've just been through the procedure and your eye history seems a tiny bit similar to mine, how long did it take you to resume normal activity after the enucleation? I'm thinking I may be able to have the surgery done in the four weeks we have off during winter break, but I wonder if that's enough time for recovery. I'll need to be pretty active when I return. Wishing you the best of all that's possible,—*Sleepy*

Sleepy, Thank you so much for all of your well wishes. It means so much to me. I am so sorry to hear that you are having other medical issues beyond that of your eye. I know how much energy it takes to deal with a sick eye and so another ailment on top of that is unreal. I hope that this passes soon and that you will be feeling much better before you know it.

As far as your question goes, in my case, four weeks was not enough time. My doctor told me that I couldn't go to my ocularist until it was 6 weeks after my surgery. It takes time to heal from the enucleation. In my case I found that I was experiencing a lot of headaches on top of the discomfort from the surgery. Also, I got light headed a lot. I really couldn't resume my normal exercise routine until about two months later. Your muscles in the eye need time to heal and you will find that they will be hurting when you pull the implant with the muscles. I know that you wanted to get it done over your winter break, but I think that you shouldn't cut yourself short and then have to go back to school feeling any discomfort. This is just my opinion based on my experience. I hope that I have helped. Let me know if there is anything else I can do. Best of luck and get better soon! Love Always,—*Jodi*

Hey Jodi, Thanks so much! That tells me I should really try to wait until after the school year and that is what I'll try to do. It is so good to hear from someone who is pleased with the results of surgery and a new prosthesis, that is very encouraging to me. I'm not looking forward to the enucleation, but your words help me deal with something that is swiftly approaching and with which I can maybe feel hopeful. Thank you for that. Thank everyone here, it's hard to be alone with these decisions. Best,—*Sleepy*

Hi guys, I mentioned in an earlier message I was having my eye removed at the end of July so I wanted to post an update. I was scheduled for surgery on July 21st but had to cancel because I started having trouble breathing on July 19th, went to the hospital where doctors found my throat was swelling shut from some kind of fast infection and I had an emergency tracheotomy. The infection is gone now but they left the trach while they did a biopsy. Now I'm waiting for the biopsy results and the site to heal, then the trach can be reversed. It's been stressful and I start back at school in two weeks, so I don't have time to reschedule the eye surgery until Xmas break.

I want to thank everyone for their support, I'll let you know when I get the enucleation. If I can, I will put it off until the end of the school year. So, everything is pretty much up in the air, but I'll let you know what's happening. Thanks to everyone,—Sleepy (who is having a pretty hard time sleeping with this tube in my neck. Boy will I be glad to get rid of it!) Love Always,—*Jodi*

◆ ◆ ◆

Due to an accident when I was 2 (I'm now 32) my right eye became blind (Frisbees should be banned but that's another mission!). Anyhow, three years ago

I went to my eye doc because my blind eye had a pool of blood in the iris area. I had never really had any problems with it before, just a quick surgery to tighten the muscle to get it moving better at age 16. Functioning with one eye has never been a problem because I was so young when it happened I don't remember seeing with two. (I still think 2 eyed people must see double!)

My eye doc said the blind eye was degenerating which is apparently normal for blind eyes like mine although no doc had ever mentioned that before. He said that I would need to have it enucleated and an implant put in and he would leave it up to me when to book the surgery. The doc said that my eye would become really painful and start to look bad and when I'd had enough he'd remove it.

SO. I have held off for a few years now, the eye is sometimes quite painful, rather like a migraine (pressure normally hovering around 65—70) but it doesn't look too bad, just red sometimes and a bit smaller than the other. I just can't seem to gather the courage to book the surgery. I think the longer I wait the harder it is. My HUGEST fear is that they will take out the wrong eye and I will be blind so I know that's one thing holding me back. Also, I'm worried about upkeep for an implant/cosmetically how it'll look etc. Basically just looking for some courage/support etc. I am so glad I found this site. Thank you!—*Star*

Hi. My situation created the need for my eye to be removed right away. I was a victim of an assault. They gave me no choice pretty much at all. They talked to me about a sympathetic eye, and claimed I could go blind in the other eye because of the trauma. They put it to me this way. Better 50% than none at all. I had these poor people sitting around for an hour, because I wouldn't sign the paper. If it wasn't for this one doctor who took the time, while the others were getting impatient. She sat for quite a while with me, and cried with me. She explained all my alternatives, and what might happen if I didn't. But of course there were none. This person saved my life. Because without her, I would have only wanted to expire. Sometimes you have to do what is good for the majority. Meaning the rest of your body, to live out the rest of your life healthy. You will make the right choice. I put aside everything else in my life, and went forward. Because sometimes you just can't turn back. Doesn't change anything. Good Luck,—*Michael*

Hi Star, I had my eye removed little over a year ago and I too was scared they would remove the good eye. I made a deal with my eye doctor and the nurses. They taped a plastic cap over my good eye and wrote on the tape: HANDS OFF! I recovered really quickly from surgery and the removed eye (and the prosthesis) doesn't bother me at all. You have to decide for yourself but I just wanted to share my experience with you. Good luck with whatever you decide to do.—*Willeke*

I'm on my fourth day of recovery from having my bad eye enucleated. I too had the same problem as you. I had a degeneration in my left eye that I battled for almost four years. I suggest that you have that eye enucleated: it's the only solution. You'll have to get it removed later on anyway. I waited until the very last moment and I was in severe pain. My eye was so small, always red and people noticed it. Also, it blurs your vision: you'll realize that when you have it enucleated, your vision will be sharper. This is because there are no more blurry signals the bad eye is giving your brain.

Right now I feel great. I'm just waiting for my prosthesis. No more constant headaches and no more trying to balance my bad eye with my good eye. I found it that when I tried to balance the bad eye with the good eye, the good eye ended up looking weird. Now my good eye is fully open. Your eyes have to work as a team. I feel better now knowing my appearance will look better as well as my vision. It's like the weight of the world is off my shoulders and I can get on with my life. Bottom line, get the surgery and you'll feel so much better. Take care and good luck with your decision.—*Mike*

◆ ◆ ◆

I was wondering what everyone's experiences were in terms of recovery time after enucleation? I work 2 full time jobs, one is a desk job, no biggie but the other is rather strenuous working with physically challenged kids, lifting, toileting etc. I was wondering what I will be looking at for time off? My eye doc did not really give me a straight answer when I asked so I could use the input! Thanks.—*Star*

Anyway, I only have a desk job and that's the same type of job I had when I had my eye enucleated. As I recall, surgery was a same-day deal on a Wednesday, and I was back at work the following Monday. It may be longer for you to go back to the physically taxing job, though.—*DJ*

◆ ◆ ◆

Hi, after posting here occasionally and living with one seeing eye and one blind eye for two years I'll be having enucleation done on Monday morning in San Francisco. I started this journey with a large choroidal melanoma too close to the optical nerve for plaque therapy and my only option was proton beam or enucleation. Well, I was still reeling from the cancer diagnosis, when I thought I only needed glasses and took the option of proton beam radiation. My eye has been damaged so badly that the pressure is up to 65 even after pressure lowering drops and for three weeks, I've been having severe migraines and it is affecting my whole life. After talking with the doctor, I decided to have the eye taken out. It looks ugly anyway and I've lived for two years without any vision out of it. Any words of wisdom for recovery after the surgery? I'm a little nervous about the surgery itself, but all my physical tests have come back and I'm healthy except for the eye. I'm 44 and really want to get on with all the wonderful things life has to offer and it's been very debilitating with the migraines I've been having.

Another question, how long before you could go back to work? My doctor said about a week. Also, does anyone know of some nice professional looking eye patches? Thanks again for all your help,—*Sherri*

Yes, I'm still a little nervous for the surgery, but feel a lot more capable after reading the homepage of this site and everyone's well wishes. I'm an artist so sight is so important and I've been stubborn for way too long! The pain, since August has really started interfering with all the wonderful things happening in my life right now. It's time to move forward and quit being stubborn and just get on with everything I need and want to do. Thanks so much for putting all this together, You're the best! Hugs,—*Sherri*

Hey everyone! Just wanted to let you know that my surgery went well and besides one day (Thanksgiving) of excruciating pain, I'm doing well. I did get two shiners and was going to start work on Friday and decided to postpone working until Monday. The eye is not as scary looking as I thought it may be. Jay was right, that I look like I'm winking:) I did have a couple of minor questions though, 1. After the pressure patch comes off, how long did you continue to patch the eye with the heavy duty patch material? 2. How long before the swelling subsides? My doctor didn't send me home with any info. 3. Anything abnormal that I should watch for? 4. Now this is really important:) Any suggestions on how to wash my hair? I was thinking of using goggles and using the white tape to tape them to my face, so water doesn't get in, do you think that would work? Suggestions are greatly appreciated. Thanks again for such a wonderful site! Hugs,—*Sherri*

◆ ◆ ◆

Hi! I got the full pathology report today from my recent enucleation surgery. It's good that I had the surgery done. My tumor, although it had been shrinking slowly and nicely had sent shoots of tumor cells out to other parts of my eye. During the dissection they found many epithelliol cells behind the lens of my eye. They had not formed another tumor, per se, but the cells were active and it was only a matter of time. There was also an invasion of the Bruch's membrane, in which, I was told there was not. My question is this was never found in the ultrasound and the original tumor kept shrinking. Why was it not noticed on the scans or any of the scans I have had. I'm assuming it was still too small to be detected. Another issue, is that my specialist basically dropped me once the eye was removed. His response was that he doesn't follow up on enucleation patients. So, I'm back to square one finding a specialist. In fact, my specialist had my local ophthalmologist read the results to me today. Which I'm sure I handled much better because my local ophthalmologist is a very kind and caring doctor.

I've been extremely optimistic dealing with the enucleation and going out in public to all my children's events and even joking with people that ask about it. We live in a small town, so the news traveled like wildfire and in reality I would just love to blend in. Not a chance:) Would love to hear any thoughts about this. Today shook me a little, but I have so many other things to look forward to, like my new prosthesis on Jan. 22nd that I can't be down for long and also knowing I made the right decision the have the eye removed even when I was very stubborn about it. I wish everyone the best! Hugs,—*Sherri*

◆ ◆ ◆

Had my enucleation done in November. Surgery was about 10,000, the anesthesia was about 1,500 and pathology was about 250. My surgeon participates with my insurance company which will pay about half the billed amounts. This doesn't include office visits. My ocularist does not participate with my insurance. The prosthesis will cost 2,350. They estimate the insurance will pay all but 700 which I had to pay up front. Hope this helps.—*Shaggy*

Hi, my insurance was billed $14,000 for the enucleation and they covered all of it. I was very lucky. My prosthesis is $2400, and I only had to pay out of pocket $100.00. Hope this helps,—*Sherri*

Oh my gosh! What some of you must have had to pay is absolutely insane. Here in Canada the surgery and specialists visits are free (as in covered by the government in full) and my prosthetic is covered half by the government and the other half by my employee benefits at work. My out of pocket expense so far has been $2.00 for a dispensing fee for my eye drops and that's it.—*Star*

◆ ◆ ◆

My Jacob is 3 1/2, he was 3 when he had his accident and we made the decision to have his eye removed now. His injured eye was shrinking and so he would have needed a cosmetic prosthesis anyway. He had his eye removed and things have been great. His accident was 6 months ago, yesterday. Our biggest challenge is getting him not to remove the prosthesis. There are challenges, yes, but its not the end of the world. My son has adapted beautifully.—*Bethy*

◆ ◆ ◆

I am going to have to have my left eye removed and I am terrified. I took a bad fall 4 weeks ago while on a cruise ship and had emergency surgery in San Andres, Columbia, a third world country. I have had more surgery back in the U.S. I still have the eye, but do not have any sight and it will never return. I have been told the eye needs to come out, but just the thought of it makes me a basket case with uncontrollable crying and throwing up. I am so scared. I have a lot of pain in the eye. Everyone says just have it taken out, but that is easy for everyone to say because it isn't their eye. Please, if there is anyone who will talk to me about this I would be very grateful. Thank you,—*Ruth*

Ruth, I know it is harder on a woman, than a man to deal with a situation like this. But, I for one am not afraid to admit that I went through the same feelings. I was told that if my eye was not removed immediately after the injury, that I would have sympathetic eye. You can die from that. I was given the choice to live or die. It took a couple of hours for me to make my choice. I know now that I did the right thing. Yes. life is a little different for me now, but I know in time it will seem normal to me. This has definitely put me on the roller coaster ride, and I can't wait to get off! Right now I am 50% there. My injury is new. Please remember that you are not ALONE. You should also look into talking with a professional about it, because you might be feeling [PTS] Post Traumatic Shock. I know your feeling the loss now of just the vision, and now you are facing the #2 punch. It's really a shame this is a 2 for 1 deal. Good Luck! and God Bless. Regards,—*Michael*

I wouldn't agree that you can die from Sympathetic Ophthalmia Michael. You can end up blind in your other eye as a result of it yeah, but death isn't really a factor. Just thought I would clarify that one.—*Elizabeth*

Hi Ruth, I really feel for you. When my doc told me four years ago that my eye had to come out, I was a mess. It took me four years of increasing pain to finally go to him and say okay, it's time to take it. It was an agonizing decision and you're right, no one else can really tell you what to do because it isn't their eye. I will tell you that the last 5 weeks since I had my right eye enucleated have been really hard for me but I do NOT regret having had the surgery. The transition time until I get my prosthetic is the hard part and the questions that come from wearing a patch/sunglasses etc. I truly wish you all the best with your situation. If you have any questions at all, please write, this forum is an incredible wealth of support, use it. Yours,—*Starr*

◆ ◆ ◆

Hi everyone, I had my left eye enucleation due to glaucoma and got coral implant. After 13 years of struggling with the pain in the left eye, the moment I woke after anesthesia was great. As I felt there was no eye and no pain. Yeah.

But after 2 weeks conjunctiva broke and I had 2 additional operations to stick conjunctiva together. After that it went wrong again and doctor told me I had implant infected with my own bacteria and that's why I had problems with healing the wound. I spent additional 3 weeks in hospital as doctors tried to get rid of the bacteria from the implant mainly with the help of strong gentamecine eye drops—gel, oral antibiotics and vain antibiotics injections. Then I had my 4th operation as doctors decided to try to close conjunctiva again as they thought there was no bacteria anymore.

Now, 30 days after the 4th surgery, my eye socket is irritated again and I feel there is something wrong happening again with the eye socket or implant. I am afraid doctors will decide to reject the implant (which moves GREAT). Had anyone similar problems with infections in implant after enucleation or have some ideas how to fight with it? Please help!—*Bartek*

◆ ◆ ◆

After a real confusing Monday at the hospital, I had a biopsy on the melanoma in my right eye. The results are not 100% conclusive, but my doctors will remove the right eye in another week June 20th. I was prepared as I could be for the enucleation to happen on the 13th of June, but they wanted their analysis to be more definitive. So another week of pins and needles. I have read the Singular View and Hope—both very helpful to me. And I want to thank you all for your support too! Any suggestions as to how I will feel the first week? Or what to bring with me to the hospital? audio tape player with tunes and relaxation tapes? Thanks,—*Lynn*

Hi there seaspray, I am pretty much in the exact place as you are. I had my right eye removed 3 weeks ago 5/27 to be exact. Just curious though how do you keep your eyelid closed? And are you getting close to getting your eye fitted for prosthesis soon. Keep us on the details, your day to day diary is very interesting and beneficial for someone who is going through the same process. I myself have an appt next Friday to start on the molding and fitting but I think I want to delay it to next-next Friday as I want to make sure the socket is 100% ready.

Btw how does one know for sure when the socket is really ready? 3 weeks now the socket is still moist during the day and excreting stuff during sleep at night. I feel kind of rushed by the ocularist to start exactly at the 4th week like it's some magic number.—*Masha*

I think there's a move to fit the prosthesis earlier nowadays. I think they're worried the socket will shrink. Get your ocularist to explain the thinking behind the magic 4 week date.—*Chil*

◆ ◆ ◆

Hi, I had my enucleation surgery this past Monday. How long does it take for the pain go away when you turn your head or move your eyes? They have me on percocet, and as long as I don't move, I'm okay, but any movement causes discomfort. I go to get the bandage off tomorrow.—*Renee*

Took me a few days, to a week. I don't remember. I did get in the habit for about the first week of closing my eyes when I turned my head. Sounds crazy, but kept my good eye from "following" things visually, and moving my sore muscles in the other. Don't worry. It goes away soon enough, and before long you wont remember that it hurt at all. This is just a step towards being able to resume a normal life. For me, there was far more pain before surgery than after. Hope all is well, and that the healing is speedy!—*Navig8r*

Well, thankfully the pain has passed. YAY! I got the bandage off Friday and they put the conformer in. Everything seems to be doing okay. I went to a concert Saturday night. That was the first time that I had been out to a BUSY public place since the surgery. It kind of freaked me out! Before the surgery, I still had peripheral vision, now, obviously there is none. I made my husband walk on my left side while holding my hand so I wouldn't run in to anyone. The whole experience made me kind of uneasy, but I got through it. I guess we'll have to practice going to busy public places so I get used to it. I drove a little bit yesterday, that didn't really seem like a big deal to me, so that's good. Well that's all for now.—*Renee*

I remember that prior to my enucleation, Advil, or other pain meds seemed like one of the food groups to me. within less than 2 days after the surgery, I was not taking ANY pain meds regularly. I always tell people that I felt better 2 days after surgery than I had in 11 months.—*Navig8r*

Good luck with your surgery on Friday. Thankfully, I wasn't in any pain before my surgery, I just had very blurry vision due to a choroidal melanoma. The only pain that I had was occasional headaches. I was told by the doctors not to take Aleve or Advil for a week before the surgery because I guess they both contain some aspirin which thins the blood, and they don't want that before your surgery. They said to only use Tylenol (acetaminophen). Maybe your doctors would let you use Tylenol for pain? Just a thought, anyway, best wishes, hope all goes well for you.—*Renee*

◆　　◆　　◆

I need to have my eye removed because I have been blind for two years due to AMD, and detached retina. The eye is now becoming painful and my ophthalmologist says I have not other treatment options. My concern is: The surgeon he recommends is just out of medical school and I'm concerned that she has had enough experience in this field. She has recommended evisceration rather than enucleation (sorry about the spelling). Am I being too concerned about a problem that does not exist? Would appreciate your opinions.—*Namie*

Hi Namie, It was interesting to see your post about evisceration. I have been thinking about having my eye enucleated for about 10 years (that's another story) today I went to the eye surgeon to discuss this with him. He told me that in USA (I am in Australia) more and more surgeons are now doing evisceration rather than enucleation. He told me that the eye movement is better as they do not disturb the muscles in the eye. He is sending me for an ultrasound of my eye to see if it is suitable for the procedure. I am not exactly sure what they are looking for but I have had lots of surgery on the eye in the past and my husband seems to think he said something about the shape of the eye. We discussed so much it is hard to remember it all! Let us know what you decide.—*Penny*

◆ ◆ ◆

I'm having my eye out on Monday. My Dr is doing the evisceration. I have other complications because I have Chronic Fatigue Syndrome and Multiple Chemical Sensitivity. In the past I've had some very bad reactions to the General Anesthetic. I'm more worried about the reaction to the anesthetic than the eye surgery. But, I'm glad I've finally made the decision and can get on with my life. I've been blind in that eye for over two years, but the pain has been minimal until now. After reading posts about how glad so many of you were to have had it done, it convinced me to take the step. I'm 69 and not in good health. I hope things go well. Thanks to all of you on this wonderful forum. I'm happy I found it. It has really helped to ease my stress. My thoughts and prayers to all of you who are going through rough times.—*Namie*

Hi Namie, I had an evisceration back in May. My blind eye was extremely painful and spent several weeks on heavy doses of pain medication. I usually have allergic reactions to general anesthesia. I break out in severe hives and slight swelling in the throat. But I was okay during this surgery. Just a few hives, but my throat was fine. The surgery was actually very quick. I went under at nine and I was out of surgery by 9:45–10:00-ish. I was on my way home at 11. I got my prosthetic in July and I'm feeling great. I had a small cyst, but its completely gone now. Keep us updated on how things are going! Best of Luck!—*Pixie*

2

Appearance Surgery

Some people who have lost an eye will require additional surgery for cosmetic reasons, to improve the movement or looks of their eye and surrounding socket. Usually, this surgery is very minor, such as thickening an eye lid or adding mass to the socket. But sometimes the condition can be significant and require multiple surgeries to correct.

Messages

My eyelid droops. The doc said that it is not actually drooping, but I lost the fat that builds up in the eyebrow area when the accident occurred. He tried adding to the prosthesis to push it up, but it did not really affect it much. Just made it more uncomfortable to wear. Any ideas on this anybody,—*j6044*

My eyelid also drooped after my eye was removed. We tried the prosthesis build up, but I wasn't happy with the result. I then had surgery on my eyelid, to remove the excess skin and tighten it up. It was a pretty simple procedure that was done in the doctor's office. Good luck to you!—*Nancy*

My eyelid doesn't droop but it doesn't close properly this is because I had radiotherapy treatment after my eye was removed, to have this done I had to have my implant removed. Because the radiation treatment killed off good cells as well as bad my eyelid is damaged and doesn't move at all well. wonder if anyone else has the same trouble? Would love to talk to someone with similar problem. Love,—*Anne*

◆ ◆ ◆

Hello all! I had my enucleation surgery Feb 16th and go for my first prosthesis fitting April 7th. I had my post-op four days after my surgery and haven't seen my dr. since. I'll see him again right before I go to get my prosthesis.

Here's my question: I have the conformer, but my eye still has a slightly sunken in appearance. I asked one of the nurses at my dr.'s office about this and she said it shouldn't look sunken in. It's has one stitch holding the eyelid closed so the conformer won't come out and it seems that it wants to open at little on the sides. I am just wondering if it will look less sunken once the prosthesis is made or if this is just the way it's going to look. Can some please give me some input on this? Thanks!—*Marsey*

Welcome to the board! I hope the information on this site has been helpful to you as you go through this process. I also had a sunken appearance after my eye was removed. My ocularist tried to remedy that by building up the prosthesis, but it wasn't enough and I wasn't satisfied. I consulted with a plastic surgeon who specializes in eyes and she recommended what she called a floor implant. What she did was, using the same material that the implant is made from (hydroxyapatite), she packed the floor of the socket, which pushed the implant forward. And voila! It was fixed!

There still may be some swelling, since your surgery was just over a month ago, so don't get concerned if it looks a little worse as time goes on and the healing process continues. As you see, there are ways to deal with it, and I'm sure you will find one that works for you. Good luck to you. Keep us posted on how you're doing!—*Nancy*

Once you get the prosthesis, it will look more filled out, mine was the same way. The conformer is much smaller than the actual prosthesis. Hope this helps.—*Jarrod*

Thanks to you both, Nancy and Jarrod. I feel better now after reading both of your responses. I've posted before, but I accidentally posted under Guest this time. This is such a scary, emotional time, waiting to see what you're going to end up looking like, and it's nice to know there are others out there who've been through the same and understand. Thanks again!—*Marsey*

◆　　◆　　◆

HI just a little update after a hospital visit today I have decided to go ahead with the plastic surgery to try to improve the size of my socket. After this heals my consultant is still talking about trying to get the man from Germany to try and make me a glass eye. I have no implant due to radiotherapy and it is hoped the surgery will improve the sunken in look which I have now. Don't know when all this will happen but I am on the waiting list. Will let you know what happens.—*Anne*

Anne, just wanted to wish you luck with the implant surgery. I'm sure it'll improve on the appearance of the socket. I didn't know that they still used glass for a prosthesis. Good luck getting that done too! I wish you the best. Let us know when you're going in for the surgery!—*Chris*

◆ ◆ ◆

I'm so happy I found this site it's extremely informative. I'm a 24 yr old grad student and I lost my eye to retinoblastoma at the age of six. Since I don't really remember seeing with two eyes it hasn't limited me at all. Matter of fact I rarely thought about it until this summer when I had a second implant surgery (Medpor). I had a few problems with my socket closing up but it's beginning to expand now and I'll be getting my new eye tomorrow.

Anna, I read that you were having some problems with your lid after you implant surgery. I'm actually experiencing the same problem. Prior to surgery I had a eye that was too small for my socket but had decent movement and my lid functioned perfectly. After the surgery, I seem to have less movement and my lid seems to be weaker. Does it (eyelid) strengthen and function properly over time? Also, for those of you who had an eyelid surgery did it prevent you from closing your eye?

Thank you all for sharing your stories it's good to know there are others out there who are going through some of the same things.—*Pearl*

Hello Pearl, nice to have you here I did have problem with my eyelid but now it looks much, much better. After my coral implant surgery I had another, upper eyelid surgery. They cut a little bit of eyelid skin and lift it. Now it looks almost OK but I am scheduled to have another surgery—the doctor has to fix my lower eyelid and then do another one small plastic operations with my upper eyelid. I had to have so many operations with my eyelid because when my eye was removed it was twice bigger so my eyelid was stretched. If your removed eye was a normal size you should not have so many problems. I am sure that your eyelid will be fine. Please, feel free to ask as many questions as you want. All the best.—*Anna*

Pearl, welcome to the site. After my second implant surgery two years ago (I had a bigger implant put in so the eye would be smaller), I had similar surgery to what Anna described. They did an eyelid lift. Everyone says it looks the same now as my good eye, but I still see the difference (it's still droopy to me) and some days I wish I had never had the lid lift done. Not so much because I still see it drooping, but because every single day, when I look in the mirror and blink, all I see is my scar glaring out at me (yes, everyone says they don't see that, either).—*Barrysdeej*

Hi, I had an eyelid lift myself with a tiny scar that is hardly noticeable. After 20 years I am starting to have the same problem as before that surgery, drooping eyelid in the evenings.—*Lucia*

Just to add that when I was reading your post barrysdeej I had a strange feeling that I was reading my own post. However with scar I can not see mine—I would say in most cases you can not see it. It is very tiny line. In my opinion—not to worry about. With dropping eye—well I can see it—but I think only because I am so sensitive about it. And I agree when I am tired, in the evening it tends to drop a little bit more than during the day. It is not that obvious, really. My partner is keep saying that there is no problem and other people are not noticing it. Probably he is right and it is more what WE see. Sometimes I think that after another 2 plastic surgeries which I am planning to have I won't be happy. Well, I guess it's more about what we are thinking than about what we see. Cheers,—*Anna*

◆ ◆ ◆

Hello all. well, it's been almost a year since my enucleation and while I am getting pretty comfortable with my prosthesis, I'm still thinking about getting the sunken in part above my upper lid fixed, because it's the only thing that really bothers me. I have some questions for those of you who have had this done and have been happy with the outcome. If you don't mind, could you say who your doctors were and if there were any complications from the surgery. Nancy, I think I read that you've had this done. Also, my ocularist told me that if I have this done, I'd have to have a new eye made. Do you have to wait a whole 6 to 7 weeks again between the surgery and the new eye?! Thanks for your thoughts!—*Marsey*

I had plastic surgery done last week and go back to hospital today for a check up. I have had skin fro my mouth grafted into my bottom lid to try to make room for a bigger eye. I will keep you informed how everything is going. I have to say that there was a lot of pain in my socket and in my mouth and if his hasn't had the desired effect I will certainly not be having any more done I think I am getting too old for all this. Yes you are right about having to have new eye made but couldn't say how long this will take I am from the UK and not sure where you from so there could be difference in time. Hope this helps.—*Anne*

Hi Marsey, yeah, I did have this done, about 4 months after my enucleation. My upper eyelid was very sunken in and I hated the way I looked. Fortunately, I had a great ocular plastic surgeon.She did a floor implant, using the same material as the implant, hydroxyapatite, but crumbled up so that she could reshape the floor of my socket. The effect of doing this was to kind of push the implant up and out and it worked like a charm. I still needed to get both eyelids done, to even them out, but once this was all done, I once again looked like the old me.

Recovery time from the floor implant wasn't too long, nor do I remember it being difficult at all (hard to remember all of the details now, this was in 1992!) After the usual wait of 6 weeks for the swelling to go away, I went back to the ocularist and had my prosthesis adjusted, I did not have to get a new one. I always tell people that Dr. did more to save my life than anyone else back then because she made it possible for me to start feeling better about myself. If it weren't for her, I don't know where I'd be today. Best of luck to you,—*Nancy*

◆ ◆ ◆

Well, the Fourth Attempt to Rebuild my Socket has happened. Scheduled for 1:30 on Friday, they got to me at 6. I was very sick all night from the anesthesia, but when the puking stopped at about 8 am on Saturday, I started feeling quite well.

I can already feel that it's a better fit. This implant is 17mm, replacing the 22mm one from two summers ago. There was enough room to put my prosthesis back to in act as a conformer, so it feels "full" which is a total relief. They un-did the medial canthalplasty, tried some plastic surgery to repair the appearance of the inner corner and took off a blob of plaque on my inner upper eyelid.

So, now it's just waiting to get the pressure bandage off and trying to take it easy without going crazy. My friend Rachel is here with me for the week, which is great for me and it helps John not worry. Keep your fingers crossed—this could be the end of it! Love,—*Alicia*

Alicia, I'm SO happy for you that its going well, and that it seems to have done the job. It's really important that after all you've been through, its time to find surgery that works! Lots of hugs and TLC to you my friend (With a little spare for John too!). I really hope things continue to improve, Do keep us informed, Love n Hugs,—*Elizabeth*

◆ ◆ ◆

I have been wearing a prosthesis since I was 2. I am now 30 and have developed a really droopy upper eyelid. And most recently a bit of a droopy lower eyelid. I was excited to get my newest prosthesis, thinking it would open up my lid, however the lid seems to be unchanged. Have any long-time wearers had this problem and if so what can be done to correct it? Thanks,—*Sid*

Hi Sid, I agree with Alicia, please see a ocuplastic surgeon. I had my lower lid pulled up last spring. It took 20 minutes as an office procedure at Wills Eye hospital and my HMO covered it completely! Why did I wait so many years to admit to my family doctor that it bothered me? The surgeon will also help me with my upper lid in the future. It was great getting all my eye lid questions answered. It made me feel a lot better. I hope your experience is as positive!—*Amy*

◆   ◆   ◆

Hi guys! I have had my eye gone now for about a year and a half. I really can't stand the fact that between my lower eyelid and upper eyelid I have that sunken in look. My surgeon said it is not safe to have the surgery that pushes up your eye socket to fill that in more. I was wondering if any of you have had this surgery, and what were the results? Thanks!—*Mindy*

Hey, Mindy, first of all, welcome to the board. You'll find invaluable information here. I'm a 40-something year old woman, and have had a prosthesis for over 30 years. My lower and upper eyelids had some skin grafted onto them (a surgery done about 20 years after the initial enucleation), but other than that, nothing was done to make the socket look less "sunken in". I notice that on some days when my allergies/sinuses are bothering me, my eye looks more "sunken in". Whenever I have a bad headache, it shows also.

I've never heard of any surgery to build up your socket so that the sunken in look doesn't happen. Maybe there's only so much that they could build in a socket. Are you happy with your prosthesis? Does your ocularist think that the socket is too sunken in? If not, you probably just have to get used to the fact that your eye isn't going to look exactly like your "healthy" one. Hope that helps!—*Chris*

Hi Mindy, I had the same problem when my eye was removed 11 yrs ago. I got a coral implant (you didn't mention what type of implant you got.) About 4 months after the enucleation, I had a 'floor' implant done to correct the sunken look. The plastic surgeon used the same coral material to do it. The material was ground up and the Dr. packed it on the floor of my socket to push the implant forward. I had an excellent result. Feel free to contact me directly if you have any other questions about this. Best wishes,—*Nancy*

Thanks for the info! I am not sure exactly what kind my implant is, it is the kind that moves on the base attached to your muscles. My ocularist already re-did it once to try and make it bigger to fill in the sunken look.—*Mindy*

◆ ◆ ◆

Hello, I had my surgery and coral implant about 14 weeks ago. I've got a conformer at the moment. Today I've visited my ocularist. He told me that he will make a new prosthesis for me but it will be only for 1-2 months as my top eyelid is half closed, half open and he suggested a plastic surgery for my top eyelid. He said that after the surgery when my eyelid will be in the correct position than he will make a new one/a proper one. As in the past my—now removed—eye stretched my eye lid, it is much bigger than it should be. He said that during the plastic surgery they will cut it and it will move up my top eyelid approx 4-5 mm. Then he suggested my lower eyelid to be done as well. I know that my eyelids are stretched because my natural eye used to be twice bigger but my concern is: Maybe it is better to wait for my top eyelid to move up naturally? And if I decide to have it done that is mean I will have to do this kind of procedures/plastic surgeries more often? Does anyone had a similar experience? Does anyone had an eyelid plastic surgery? Please help.—*Anna*

Anna, I had eyelid surgery about 20 years ago (10 years into my enucleation). My eye was too "wide open" and looked wrong. They needed to add more to my top eyelid. They used the skin from behind my ear and grafted it onto my lid. It was successful (which is amazing for me and my medical history!). I haven't needed any additional eyelid surgery since then, so I'm hoping that you'll be in the same boat. Good luck and let us know what they decide and how you're doing with it!—*Chris*

Hey, Anna: I've just had my first lid surgery. The lower lid was stretched because of the weight of the large prosthetics I've always had. Dr. D the surgeon pulled the lower part of the lid tendon toward my nose and fastened it there. Right now I've got two, maybe three stitches in the inside corner. I don't know if those pieces are going to heal together, or if the sutures are just to hold the tendon in place while it heals.

I don't know about your top lid. it may just never regain the smaller size it had before, and you may need a series of lid surgeries. For me, last Friday, the lid surgery was a walk in the park compared to the two implant rebuilds, especially the second one, which was so incredibly painful. I have been at work all week, and I'm starting to have some pain now, like the skin is pulling against the sutures, but they're coming out on Monday. And, I may get my eye two weeks after that! MAY is the operant word. There will be no counting the prosthetic eyes before they're hatched. I'm off to apply a warm compress—my new best friend. Take care—*Alicia*

Hi Anna, I ended up having both of my upper eyelids done within about a year of my enucleation. I lost my right eye, and that was the one done first, because the upper lid wasn't opening all of the way. I think it was just a few weeks later that the other one was done, to make them look symmetrical. Mine were done in the doctor's office, under local anesthesia. It only took about a half hour. The doctor made an incision in the crease of my eyelid and removed the excess skin. I never felt a thing, but it was kind of creepy when the left eye was done, because I could see what was happening!

This was done about 10 years ago, and it still looks perfect. The doctor told me that I would probably have to have something done to my lower lids at some point in time, but I haven't seen any need for it yet. Of all of the procedures that I went through in that first year, this was the easiest one. I would encourage you to go ahead with it. Best wishes, and good luck,—*Nancy*

Hello, it's Anna again. I've got some doubts and I was wondering whether you could help me. As I mentioned in my previous posts after the coral implant surgery my eyelid is drooping and I need a top eyelid surgery. It doesn't open enough. Do you know if there are possibilities of complication after the surgery? Is it possible to do more damage than good? Are they cutting your muscles or it is only eyelid skin? I am not sure what to expect. I've got doubts cause before my coral implant surgery I did not that there is a possibility that there will be something wrong with my eye lid. Of course I will ask my doctor questions but I was wondering what do YOU think? Appreciate any reply. Thank you,—*Anna*

◆ ◆ ◆

It all started Friday night and my socket was very sore so I took my eye out overnight, big mistake when I tried to get it back in on Saturday morning it wouldn't fit. When I had a good look in the socket I found a small lump and with my track record immediately panicked and thought cancer. I managed to get an appointment with my general practitioner who said I had an infection and gave me some antibiotic cream to use and he told me if I couldn't get the eye in by Monday to ring the eye hospital I attend. I did this and went to see my nurse 7 pm Monday and she couldn't get it back in either. This was because the swelling was right on where the eye sits in my lower lid. I have to go back on Friday and if the eye still won't go in I may be looking at plastic surgery as the lower lid is shrinking with the eye being out. They will try and make the pocket a little bit bigger so my eye will go in. was just wondering if this has happened to anyone else in here and what is the operation like. I have had 2 ops on my eye so I am not too worried about it thanking you,—*Anne*

Hi Anne, I hope your eye will get better soon. I had my enucleation over 1 year ago, and my doctor prescribed 1 drop of gentamicin a day for my bad eye. He said many patients develop infections and he has found this to be effective. It has worked for me and maybe something you could use in the future. Good luck,—*Cathy*

Just to let you all know what is happening. I went to hospital on Friday and ended up having a small operation under local anesthetic as my socket has shrunk even more. I was told this is because of the radiotherapy treatment I had. The consultant inserted a plastic conformer and then fastened my eyelids together to keep it in place. I have to go back Friday for a check up and then the week after to have that removed and a larger one put in to try and stretch the socket further. Apparently it wasn't an infection I had but was the eye rubbing on my bottom lid and the small lump which formed will take a long time to go away, so they are going to remove this in 3 or 4 weeks and at the same time are going to do some plastic surgery. Am really not looking forward to this as I thought that once I had my eye fitted all my problems would be gone but how wrong I was. I feel as far back as I ever was and everything is going to take ages to be put right the only good thing is hurray for our national health service because I don't think I would be able to have this done if I had to pay for it. Will keep you all informed see you soon,—*Anne*

Well this has me a little worried. Noah has gone through 3 prosthetic eyes and 6 buildups since December. Being as he is still a toddler who weighs about 30 lbs, his face changes quite a bit and will continue to until he is 9 years old when he slows down. We can't always keep up with the demand of purchasing a new eye right away and opt instead for a conformer. Noah also has learned how to take out his eye and hide it. So thanks for this piece of advice.—*Niccole*

I'd just like to thank you guys for being there for me. My visit to the hospital went very well. the doc removed the stitches and the conformer stayed in place, but he couldn't get a larger one in to try and stretch the socket a little more. When I got home I tried my artificial eye in and it went in like a dream as if I had never had any problems with it. The doc is quite hopeful that I may not need another operation after all. He was telling me about a man in Germany who makes artificial eyes and the hospital is trying to arrange a visit to England for him. He specializes in making eyes for problem people like me who have no implants in. Wonder if anyone in here knows about him,—*Anne*

◆　　◆　　◆

Aloha! Well, today was supposed to be day one of Making My New Eye. It turned into I Need to Have Another Surgery. Sigh. I'm bummed and disappointed. I'm worried about work—I don't have any days off until Thanksgiving. I so don't want to wait that long. Boo hoo hoo. Poor me.

Luckily, this surgery won't be cutting into my head again, it will be removing a strip of skin from the roof of my mouth and grafting it to my lower lid. So it's more like patching an inner tube. Ow. I felt so smug at the drugstore the other day, blithely walking past the eye patch, gauze and tape section with out getting any. That'll teach me! Hope all is well. Love,—*Alicia*

Hey, Alicia! I had a similar surgery YEARS ago. They took the skin from behind my ear and used it for my upper lid. It was a pretty simple procedure (even for ME!). Hope it all goes well and FAST! When will you be "up and running" and ready for the new prosthesis?—*Chris*

Hey, All. Thank you for all the support and well-wishes. My lower lid, esp. the inside corner won't hold the eye in. Dr. C said that "everyone who's had a prosthesis for 25 years or more needs eyelid surgery." I'm calling Dr. D tomorrow as soon as it's decent to do so. Hope all is well with everybody! Love,—*Alicia*

Aloha! So, I went to see the surgeon yesterday. long to short—we're going to hold off on more surgery to see how the eye fits with the lids "as is." My surgeon Dr. D had another doctor, Dr G come it to take a look at me. He was very snotty, trying to make me feel crazy for not liking his suggestion. Grrr. He suggested pulling up the lower tendon toward the nose, virtually closing off the inner corner of the eye. I told him that such further disfigurement was unacceptable to me. He got all passive aggressive on me, saying things like, "Well, other people do it all the time, because they want a more natural appearance" "If you're going to focus on just that area, nothing we do will make you happy," "Short of turning back the clock, we have limited options," etc etc. He insinuated that I had psychological issues that kept me from seeing how great his idea was. My issue is more like sewing my eye shut will certainly keep the prosthesis in there, but defeats the entire purpose of trying to make it look "normal." To demonstrate, he put a dab of super glue in the corner of my eye without even asking if he could or letting me know he was going to do it. He asks—"How does that feel." I say, "Like some idiot put super glue in my eye."

Sheesh. I wish when he said he does it to people all the time I would have said, "And they let you get away with that?" So, Dr. D and my husband and I decided to go ahead and have the eye made and see what happens. It may work out fine. If it needs tweaking, we can do little things. I'm meeting with Dr. C on Sat at 1:30 to get started. So, that's my story. I am interested in stories of lower eyelid tightening and how it went, what worked best, etc. Love and hugs to all—*Alicia*

Aloha! So, here's the thing. I'm going in for a lower-lid-tendon-tightening on Friday. I'm VERY concerned that it will essentially close the inner corner of my eye. Does anyone have experience with this? Feelings of "I never should have started this" are ebbing, and mostly flowing. I went into this with an 8 on a scale of 1—10 with 10 being unnoticeable. If I have the inner corner of my eye sewn shut on Friday, I'm seeing that as a serious step backward. It has been presented to me as my only option.

I cannot figure out why my lower lid was fine before and now it isn't. Is it possible it might just be super-hydrated from being covered? Ack. I've also got a wicked bad cold and may not be able to do it on Friday because of that. Think I can whine just a little more? Hope everyone is well! Any updates to share? It's been very quiet. Hopefully—*Alicia*

Alicia, Never think of all your concerns as whining. You deserve to ask questions and get answers. My left eye is getting droopy. It could be over the years of wearing a prosthesis. I have mine for 35 years. I'm 49 now. I have the original one from 1968. Time for a new one. Well, I just wanted you to know that I'm praying all goes well with you and the doctor. Looking forward to hearing your update.—*Lucia*

3

Eye Exams and Floaters

After people lose an eye, they have legitimate concerns about the health of their remaining eye. Most of us see an eye specialist every six months for a checkup and to catch any eye problems early. But some people face a psychological hurdle when going for an eye exam because they fear the worst.

When a person only has one eye, the things that go on with that eye are more noticeable than if there were two eyes. This is especially the case with so-called "floaters" that naturally occur to some degree in every eye. A person with two eyes may never notice them, or notice them rarely, but for a person with only one eye they notice them constantly. Fortunately, one gets used to them over time and they are typically not a cause for panic.

MESSAGES

Hi all, well, I started my anatomy class for this semester, and have used a microscope in it. I originally thought I would have trouble seeing the 3D in it, but I haven't. Everything has went fine so far. I just wanted to say thanks to those who replied to my post on the subject.

I'm also going to my ophthalmologist for my yearly check-up Monday. I'm hoping for a good visit. I have Posterior Lenticonus in my left eye (childhood cataract, and lens malformation) and am praying there has been no change w/that. I'm also praying I don't have to get a stronger glasses prescription! It seem to get worse every year! Well take care all, and have a nice week. I also want to say hi to all of the new members. Bye!—*tanunson628*

Hey, T! Just wanted to say "hi". Glad you're doing okay. Good to hear your progress. I have my yearly visit with the eye doctor in a week. I'm TWO YEARS overdue! How'd that happen? I made the appt b/c I've been so scared, getting too many migraines. I'll see where this leads me. Hopefully I'm not opening a whole can of worms. Good to see you around. Take care!—*Chris*

Hey Chris, sorry to hear you had such a gloomy visit. I know how you feel though. Since I'm clinically blind in the left eye due to a rare congenital disease called Posterior Lenticonus, anytime I'm at the eye doctor I always get treated like a freak. One eye doctor was so amazed by it, that he took pictures w/a special camera that eye doctors use. Looking at me you can't tell anything is wrong w/ me, but inside my eye is a cataract and my lens is shaped abnormal. So anyway, doctors that see it always say "wow, I've never seen this in real life, only in text books, and blah, blah, blah". It really hurts my feelings though, and makes me want to say, "it's all fun and games till you get your own eye put out doc!" So anyway, going to the eye doctor usually bugs me too, but I recently found a new eye doctor that I like, and he seems more caring, and doesn't treat me like a freak. But anyway, I hope your next visits go great and wish you much luck & health in the future. Take care.—*tanunson628*

Messages About Eye Floaters

I have some strange condition, and I have had it for about 7 years now, around the time when I lost my eye. What it is, is I see a flickering of glowing spots and things all over my visual field, but the one that kills me is there is one in the middle of my vision! It is a glowing yellow and purple translucent spot that goes in and out of sight. The doctors say my eye is fine, and just recently have given me and explanation. They say, it is coming from my brain, and that signals from where I used to have vision in one part of my brain from my eye, is now bleeding over into where my remaining eye sees. About a year ago, I had new symptoms along with the usual. like waking up in the morning and seeing a black flickering spot, in my central vision, and then, I started seeing faces within this spot, and animated things, like an evil smoky the bear with fangs! But sometimes, there would be a butterflies or little airplanes, just moving around within this spot! That particular thing is known as Charles Bonet syndrome. That has almost vanished, but the original spot remains, does anyone else have this? It drives me crazy!—*Jarrod*

Glad you're continually getting it checked out (you ARE, right?). I, myself, have the occasional "floaters", but found out that they could come from an imbalance of fluid in your eye (?), and that it comes with older age! (I'm 43). You've just reminded me that I'm WAY overdue for my yearly eye exam. LOL. Hope these spots stop bothering you! Take care.—*Chris*

♦ ♦ ♦

Hi Guys, I have been experiencing this really weird pixilated vision since Tuesday night. It happens all the time but is more emphasized when I look at homogenized things such as walls of one color. It is hard to describe, Its like a white wall will look like white but a lot of dots and white floating lights as well. in addition to this I have a headache and am extremely tired. I went to a retinal specialist and a neuralopthamologist and they don't know what it is. I had one of my eyes removed in may but I never had sight in it to begin with. I just thought maybe someone could offer a suggestion. They are ruled out migraines as well because the vision is continuous and in a migraine it only would last 30-60minutes. I'm hoping that someone will know what this is. Thank you. Love,—*Jodi*

Hi, Jodi. Hmmm. I don't know what this is. I know that our eyes "want" to see the opposite color of what they are actually seeing. That's why, for example, when you stare at a picture of a red apple for a long time, then look at a blank white wall you see an image of a green one kind of floating. One of my lighting design colleagues calls it "complimentary color fatigue." Is your vision sharp when not looking at a homogeneous surface?

I deal with migraines and the weird vision things go on way longer than an hour if I don't get my Imitrex and have a lie-down. Sometimes I have the weird vision stuff and no headache, and the neurologist said that it's called "migraine with neurological accompaniment." There are other things too. extreme fatigue, numbness in one side of my body and/or extremities. It totally sucks. I take a low dose of Elavil daily to prevent migraine and take Imitrex, Compazine and Vicodin when one hits and I've let it go too long. I can just use the Imitrex if I catch it soon enough, before the nausea takes over.—*Alicia*

Thank everyone for your responses and concern. However, I think that it is something other than gas or a migraine because my symptoms have lasted and have not changed in any way for two weeks now. I am going to get an EEG today and I have a call in to my Ocular Surgeon so that I can tell him about what's been going on and hopefully have him assure me that it is not related to the enucleated eye at all. Thanks for taking the time to offer suggestions and tell me your experiences. This website has made my life so much easier in the matter of 5 months! Thanks again Love always,—*Jodi*

◆ ◆ ◆

Hello all, it's been 2. 5 years since I lost vision in my right eye due to a retinal stroke. While driving home last Friday evening, I started to get a headache. I soon realized the headlights coming at me were blurred, and I had lost vision in the center of my "good" eye. I had it checked out. it lasted only 20 minutes, and then my vision returned to normal. My ophthalmologist said it was a retinal migraine.

I have a history of migraines, without the "aura". since age 8 until present (3. I get them 4-5 x/month, but have never had a visual disturbance. I was terrified. like I'm sure we all are. of losing vision in my good eye. Has anyone experienced something similar? Please let me know. I have a full work up on my "good" eye 2x per year. Thanks,—*Jessie*

Hi Jessie, Sound just like what I have occasionally, I used to have cluster headaches (a rarer type of headache but a vascular headache of more severe but shorter duration). From what I've read it occurs in the brain so the brain is causing the symptom. Annoying, yes but I think you are on the right track with regular eye checks.—*Jeff*

◆ ◆ ◆

Since losing the vision in my left eye I have experienced problems adapting to dim light. I used to have good night vision and now I have practically none. I'm scared to drive at night and can't see well enough to find a seat in a movie theater. I'd like to know how many of you have the same problem. Also, when you started having the problem, and if it has improved over time. I'd appreciate as many replies as possible. Thanks, this is a wonderful forum.—*Sleepy*

Hey Sleepy, I find it difficult to drive at night time, and I have a somewhat hard time adjusting to darkness. I find myself just being more cautious and careful when I have to adjust to darkness (like in a movie theatre). I don't know if this has anything to do with only having vision in one eye, since I've had my enucleation about 30 years ago (when I was 13). All I know is that I'm very cautious in the dark.—*Chris*

Hi Chris, Thanks so much for your reply. I'm a graduate student, which is why I'm "sleepy" because I study 7 days a week, sometimes 16 hours a day. I'm trying to explain how I see as part of my MFA thesis. I've asked a number of doctors about my remaining eye's inability to adapt to dim light but they tell me that is not their area of expertise. Some of them do not believe that having one eye causes the problem. I believe it does because I've spoken to a number other people who have lost an eye who complain of the same condition.

I finally found a specialist who seems interested in the subject but he is skeptical and wants more evidence that people with vision in only one eye have a common problem with light adaptation. I'm hoping people in this forum will share their experiences (whether OR NOT they have trouble) seeing at night, in dim rooms, or in other diminished light situations, and that they will give me permission to forward their replies to the vision specialist.

The specialist is at a vision research facility and I'm hoping he will become interested enough to find some answers for us. Thanks again for your reply. Do I have your permission to quote you to the vision guy? Best,—*Sleepy*

Sleepy, of course you could use my response in gathering your information to give to your doctor. I just wanted to add that my mom has always said that she has "night blindness" and I assumed I inherited it from her. I have 5 siblings and none of them really suffer from night blindness. My mom is nearly blind in one eye, so maybe your theory holds true. This is so interesting to me! I NEVER gave it a second thought! I'll be interested to see any further responses here. Thanks!—*Chris*

Hi Sleepy, I have been blind in my right eye since birth so I suppose I am just used to seeing what I see as I have never known any difference. I have always found it difficult reading in poor light and do not like it when I go in rooms that have the dimmer switch low, I always turn it up to get maximum light. I can drive at night with no problems, but as I said I have never known what it would be like to see with two eyes. I certainly do feel though that my vision is not as good as other peoples in dim or dark rooms.

I seem to be going through the same problem as you at the moment. I am having lots of pain and high pressure in my blind eye(due to surgery I had on it as a child). I get blisters and ulcers on my cornea that are very painful they suddenly pop and it feels like someone has thrown a handful of grit in my eye. This lasts for either a few hours or a couple of days then goes away and my eye can feel ok with no pain at all. Is your problem anything like this? I am also looking into enucleation but am worried that I may get more problems from a prosthesis than from my bad eye, so I have decided to wait until I get more bad days than good. I find that Xalatan drops are keeping the pressure under control at the moment. Hope your thesis goes ok and you have my permission to quote me.—*Penny*

Thanks guys! I'm going to forward your replies tonight, I hope more people write about their experiences coping with diminished light situations. I feel very much as you, Penny. My eye is going to get worse and there's no chance it will recover, but I'll wait as long as I can before I undergo another surgery. I'm terrified just thinking about it, the last one was no walk in the park. Sometimes a cortizone shot in the eyeball helps when things are really bad. It is very good to realize there are experienced people here who will help me through things when the time comes. (Thanks Chris!). Best to you both,—*Sleepy*

The specialist is interested to know at what age the vision was lost and which eye, and when you realized your one-eyed vision was different. Also, if possible, any specific instances where light is sufficient for people with two eyes to see, but where you have problems.

For example, my left eye went completely blind 5 years ago and I noticed the difference when I recovered from the surgery. Before that, I had excellent twilight vision. Now, if I have to leave a lecture and the room is darkened to show slides, I can't see to safely leave the room. I have started carrying a small flashlight at school. Thanks again,—*Sleepy*

Sleepy. Oh to be in college again! Enjoy! I have numerous little flashlights in various drawers and cupboards where I need to locate things. Usually there is one very close, for I have so many scattered around. Finding things in my purse presented a problem, so I have a key chain with a tiny flashlight beam attached. I hadn't considered that the problem was from losing vision in an eye (five years ago) but that makes sense. My good eye is 20/20 but certainly I feel like I'm in a cave in dim light. Thanks for helping me realize the cause.—*Bejay*

Hi Sleepy, I have had a melanoma removed from my eye with thermal laser therapy and I am 4/200 in that eye. I have a lot of problems with what is supposed to be my good eye. I wear a patch to block the distorted vision on the eye that had the cancer removed, and when I take the patch off I am absolutely certain I often notice I suddenly see less light in what is supposed to be my good eye. I think you mentioned a lot of doctors telling you the problems you mentioned was not their field of expertise, I have had similar problems for over three years, it seems to me that in Americas current medical system if you have a complicated medical problem it is often hard to find a doctor who has the time in their schedule to resolve the problem. It took me over three years to finally find an Ophthalmic Neurologist to diagnose the Nystagmus I have in what is supposed to be my good eye, and I was very fortunate to be referred to this Doctor/professor at Vanderbilt University who diagnosed me.

I am very interested in finding people who have had loss of vision or cancer in one eye and then started having problems in what is supposed to be there good eye. I have very limited typing abilities but would be very interested in anyone who has information they can share regarding the problems they might have with the remaining eye. Y'all take care and thanks to everyone who is a part of the LostEye family. I am very happy I have found this website!—*Barry*

Barry. I think I have the same symptoms. When my eye was removed, I was still seeing light through the side that was gone. This was causing glare to the good eye. I am still seeing that light and glare after 5 months. The eye surgeon and my therapist all say it is psychosomatic, and that it would go away after a while. When I cover my missing eye, the light and glare goes away from the good eye. When I uncover it, the light and glare are back. A week ago I was just going to sleep. When I closed my eyes, all of a sudden on my bad side. It looked like a snowy color TV set. For a second or two, and then went away. Of course after that, I was not able to sleep. It's strange how the mind is so strong that it plays tricks on you. Regards,—*Michael*

Michael, Thanks so much for your message. I have many things happen like the snowy color TV set and many other things that I see that aren't really there. This has been going on for over three years and I believe there may be a lot of things that doctors can't explain because vision is so complicated and involves the brain too. In your case I am hopeful that with time your problems will go away, it sort of reminds me of the phantom feelings that I have heard happens when people lose and arm or leg and still have feeling in the area that isn't there. I think there also may be a separate issue with you in the fact that covering your missing eye makes the light and glare go away from your good eye. That certainly sounds like there is something left in the area of the missing eye that is recognizing light. I am very hopeful for you that in time the problems you mentioned will go away.

I still have the eye that had cancer in it and after the thermal laser surgery to remove the cancer you can't tell there is a problem in the eye except it may look a little sleepy, because I patch it or wear glasses with an ocluder to block the distorted vision in the eye. I have no central vision in that eye and am rated at 4/200 which is way beyond legally blind in that eye. I think it is interesting that when I patch the eye and also put my hand over the patch I still see light and glare that merges in with the vision in my good eye and causes problems. Believe it or not I have asked the doctors if they can remove the eye but they don't want to do that unless they have to. I have so many problems in seeing with my good eye my life is very difficult. The more I type and read the worse it gets and I often type and read a lot longer than I should because I am pretty much struggling to resolve my problems and survive.

I have just found the tremendous website of the Neuro-Optometric Rehabilitation Association that has detailed information about the loss of one eye and the effects it can have on vision even after the loss of the eye. It also has a topic called visual hallucinations that covers things like what you mentioned, and many more topics that I think many people will find very beneficial. The website is http://www.nora.cc/index.html In the middle of the home page you will see links to many topics that are very helpful for people with vision problems. Thanks again for taking time to post your comment Michael, and best regards!—*Barry*

Hello Sleepy, YES YES YES! I lost my eye in summer of 2003 due to an eye tumor. I do have trouble seeing in dim lighting. It is now winter in Holland and I work fulltime. So I drive to work in the nearly dark and get home in the nearly dark. It does take a little more effort to drive. You need to concentrate. Yesterday it was really foggy besides just being dark and I drove home really slow. A few weeks ago I was in the Zoo and went to the underwater aquaria which were in a dark cave and the aquaria were brightly lighted. I had to hold on to mom not to bump in to the wall (and the other visitors). The problem was that the cave was dark, but every time you passed an aquarium you had to adjust to the very bright light again. I was going nuts and glad to get out again. Hope your doc will get the answers as to why this occurs. Before the loss of my eye I never had this, so I do not believe that it has nothing to do with my lost eye.—*Willeke*

◆ ◆ ◆

I was reading some of the past threads last night and saw some talk of people seeing odd things. I have a theory that just as people with amputated limbs feel phantom pain, that I have phantom vision. Having talked to a couple of blind people who have the same idea, we discovered that what we see resembles the last thing we saw with that eye.

For me, the last thing that eye saw before removal was the grey and reddish swirls of internal bleeding and that's what I now see when I'm tired or anxious. One blind friend said that just prior to going totally blind, she was using bubble wrap to wrap some stuff before moving house and she now sees bubble wrap type shapes.

Another friend says that she sees what she thinks of as bright red head scarves being waved. She lost her sight when she was shot in the face and the last thing she saw was blood pouring down her face. Anyone else have similar experience?—*Marmalade*

Thankfully, I've "seen" nothing. It doesn't sound good. I wonder if talk therapy can help with phantom images the way it can help with recurring thoughts. It would only make sense that the trauma of losing your eye, however it was lost, would manifest in some neurological/psychological ways. The research on the hippocampus (spelling!?) being published is fascinating and can, I imagine, explain so much about the way we process what has happened to us.

The book I'm thinking about in particular is called "Against Depression." I do not believe that there is a "mind" and a "body" that are separate. Saying something is "all in your head" is unkind and counter-productive. Has anyone been actively in therapy to deal with eye issues and is able to share some of the process? Love,—*Alicia*

Marmalade, Thanks for sharing the experiences you have had with Phantom vision. This is of great interest to me and I am actively involved in providing information to doctors so they will understand that there are some people who have a variety of visual problems that occur at about the same time they lose the other eye. I will also let you know a little about what I have learned about stress. This may not be of interest to most people but I thought I would post it because some of us share similar things. Resolving visual problems and resolving problems with corruption in our government and problems with our health care system in the U. S. is my life now so if this is TMI (too much information) I hope everyone will skip past this and read the next persons post

I think it's really interesting and I really appreciate what Alicia wrote when she said, "I do not believe that there is a 'mind' and a 'body' that are separate." I hope that is very helpful in thinking about and understanding the Phantom images that you experience Marmalade. What you mentioned about seeing the same phantom image provides great food for thought in trying to understand what is causing some of my personal visual distortions in my non cancerous eye.

I have a wide variety of unusual occurrences and have seen others post on the site who have the same things happen. I have seen people post about having Pixelizations, phasing images, and many more kinds of distortions in their remaining eye. I think a large majority of mine are caused by my physical medical eye conditions and using my vision to focus for extended periods of time. There are also occasions when I see things that aren't really there and it may be because my brain is interpreting some of my flashes of double vision, and my brains interpretation might make me think that the object that rapidly becomes doubled is actually something that it is not. When I am outside walking in a wooded area sometimes for a moment I think a large crow has flown by, when actually it was the shadows of the trees being distorted by my visual changes.

I realize this is not exactly the same as your condition but I think it may have some relationship because our brain has very important functions in vision.

You mentioned that stress seems to cause you to have an increase in symptoms so I will tell you about some of my experiences regarding that. I always have visual problems but I think my visual problems may increase as my stress does. I have been diagnosed with post traumatic stress caused by being fired when I got eye cancer. I was fired for performance even though I had a commendable performance evaluation and a raise 4 months before I was fired. I accepted the eye cancer but the company I worked for has lied repeatedly in court and that has caused great difficulties regarding my medical coverage and benefits. I have learned this is a common occurrence in the U. S. because companies don't want their insurance rates to go up.

As mentioned, what Alicia said about the mind and body not being separate is also very helpful in thinking about what may cause some of the visual things we experience. Doctors have told me that stress can add greatly to visual problems. I have recently had some improvement in my vision and there may be two things involved, the first one is physical and I think maybe my patch from L'Enfante may have helped because it cuts down on the amount of reflected light that other patches allow into my eye that has 4/200 vision.

While I have been blessed with some good doctors I have also had some who were not so good and seemed to me to be in the business to make easy money. My eye conditions are not easy and cannot be addressed in the 10 minutes that most of my doctors in the U. S. allow per visit. Some of my doctor's have added greatly to my stress. One Ophthalmic Neurologist in Nashville even became very angry because I was concerned about taking a blood thinning medication that he said could make me feel faint or pass out. I tried it for my visual problem of Nystagmus as he suggested and did almost pass out twice and quit taking it and I quit seeing Dr. Bond too. I appreciate and respect good doctors', at the same time I feel certain there are certain complications that some people have with the brain and vision that doctor's do not understand. I would like to say that I hope and pray everyone is able to find a good doctor, and it is very important that when you find a good one that you do what they say. The great news is that it seems like the majority of people who post on this website have conditions that are being successfully treated by their doctors, and I am happy that most people are not having the complications that some of us live with.

I believe it is Michael who has also had a very stressful time regarding the loss of his eye. He might have some very interesting information to share regarding stress and vision. Anyway, sorry this was so long and had so much info, I just thought I would share in case it was of interest. Thank you Marmalade and Alicia for what you wrote, it has helped give me additional information to think about. Best Wishes,—*Barry*

You are so right Barry. Just passed a year for me, and I am still having major difficulties. The traumatic way I lost my vision is affecting me. it was getting a little better for a while, but now it's ramping up. My case is coming up in court soon which is causing more stress. Take care, Barry. I know you're having a hard time as well. My prayers go out to you, and everyone on this site that needs them. Regards,—*Michael*

Hi everyone, I have posted about a pixelated vision that I have been having since October. I had my right eye (which I never had vision in) enucleated a year ago in May. Three doctors that I have seen recently have brought up the possibility of phantom vision. They say that it is a very far fetch theory, but they believe that the enucleation could have caused my right optic nerve to send signals to the left eye. I will be having a specialized MRI on Tuesday that will allow better viewing of my orbits. They have mentioned the possibility of having an anesthetic block performed on my right eye. My surgeon will inject a local anesthetic into the eye to see if this will improve the vision in my left eye and make it clear and crisp as it was once. This is only temporary though and again, very far fetched. I'm up for anything though. I don't know what will happen if that shot does work. It might be that I have to just deal with this vision for the rest of my life and that reality scares me because it makes me feel light headed and uncomfortable. I'm hoping that something comes of my MRI and that they can solve my ongoing struggle. I will let you all know what comes from this MRI and if I will be having the shot. All the best to all of you. Love,—*Jodi*

Well I know that phantom vision exists so it isn't too far fetched. I have also found that it decreases over time and is not nearly as much of a problem for me as it once was. So maybe yours will be the same and decrease as time goes on. Let us know how you get on.—*Marmalade*

I have had artificial eye fro 16 years (I am 35 now) and have developed lots of floaters in the last 2 years. The Doctors say this is very normal and my eye is healthy and normal. This being the case I am very anxious and very conscience of my only eye with lots of floaters (very annoying). Does anyone else have this happen to them?—*Spiros*

Spiros, It's normal and good to be protective of your only "good" eye. I get the reminder every time I go to my ophthalmologist to protect my "good" eye; to remember to keep my glasses on in order to protect it, etc. I'm 42 and have had floaters when I was about your age. They went away. I think that I remember my ophthalmologist telling me that it was due to the pressure in my eye and it had something to do with my age. Anyway, I rarely get them now. Hope that you check it out further if you have more concerns. We all should be very protective of our "good" eye—go get regular eye exams and be careful. It's all we could do to maintain good, healthy eyesight at this point. Good luck and let us know how you're doing!—*Chris*

Yes! I've had tons of them! I am blind since birth, after a doctor screwed up my eye (did ropey to reattach a retina that may or may not have been detaching—long story) I got floaters the day after he did this procedure. It bothered me in the beginning (I was 18) but I've learned to ignore them. Usually they are a sign of a detached retina, but this is a normal occurrence.—*Christine*

◆   ◆   ◆

Hi, my name is Spiros and I am 33 and lost my left eye when I was fifteen. Now that I am getting older I am really concerned about losing my other eye. I also have floaters in my right eye. The Doctors tell me this is normal and I am healthy but I have this underling fear something may happen. I visit the Doctors every 12 months without fail. I have never received any support or counseling regarding my lost eye and it is now really affecting me.

Have you researched nutrients for eye, medications or vitamins to take or not to take, or other preventative stuff?—*Spiros*

◆   ◆   ◆

Hi, I've been seeing quite a lot of spots in my vision field during almost a year now, especially when looking at a bright background. Sometimes I've seen this spots before also, but not so many and not for so long time. It's two kind of spots, mostly round in shape but also other formations which floats around. Then there is small "light spots" who "dances" around very quickly, this light spots I only see if the background is really bright. I'm a bit worried about this cause I've only got vision in this eye. I talked with the eye clinic about it but they said it was normal and that they normally don't examine people with these symptoms. Maybe I should insist to get an eye examination anyway, just to be sure?—*Daniel*

Hi Daniel, My suggestion to you is book the eye exam. You'll feel better when you know for sure. I have problems with floaters in my good eye as well and the doc told me that it was due to separation of a viscous layer or something, I don't recall exactly what he said, all I focused on was that he said it was normal and I was OK! But it's always best to know for sure, especially for those of us who only have the one eye, any change can be scary. All the best,—*Starr*

Daniel, Go ahead and book an exam. it's your eye and if you are worried, don't let anyone dissuade you from taking care of it! I, too, experienced increased floaters in my "good" eye and went immediately to an eye doc. There wasn't anything wrong and I'm very glad I went. He told me ANYTIME I get scared that something is wrong with the good one, come in and see him. Better safe than sorry. Go for it, friend!—*Molly*

Part II
PROTHESIS

4

The Ocularist's View

✦

By John Kennedy, BCO

Ocularistry is a unique and somewhat obscure profession devoted to the fitting and manufacturing of custom ophthalmic prosthetics including artificial eyes, scleral shells, orbital prostheses and other related appliances.

Most of the population is unaware of our profession, although the roots of this specialty and artificial eyes can be traced back for many hundreds, if not thousands, of years. A historical record dates back to ancient Egypt and the days of the Pharaohs. As mummies have been recovered it has been noted upon examination the presence of crude artificial eyes in their eye sockets. Later, during the Roman Empire there were terms in the Roman vocabulary differentiating between eye surgeons (medicus ocularis) and eye makers (faber ocularis).

In these early civilizations, artificial eyes were used more frequently in religious and funeral ceremonies and in statuary. Various researchers have also found passages in ancient texts referring to people wearing artificial eyes.

By the fifteenth century, glass eyes were being fabricated for individuals who had suffered an eye loss. Glass eyes continued to be made and improved upon and were in general use throughout most of the world until World War II when the development of custom plastic artificial eyes and modern fitting techniques were introduced. Between the 1950s and 1960s, plastic eyes had largely replaced glass eyes in North America.

Today, ocularists have developed standardized techniques for the manufacture and fitting of custom ocular prosthetics. Plastic eyes are now universally accepted although glass eyes are still available, mostly in some regions of Europe.

Plastic eyes are made from a type of plastic or acrylic resin called methylmethacrylate. In addition to plastic eyes, this material has long been used in dentistry for the making of dentures and other removable dental appliances.

Ocularists first came to the United States in 1851 from Europe and settled in New York City. From there they traveled to other cities fitting glass eyes. More European glass eye makers were brought over and eventually offices opened up in many large cities across the nation. Even today, descendants from some of these early ocularists are still carrying on their family business of providing custom artificial eye services. It would seem that for many ocularists their profession has become a family business and it is common to see younger family members or another relative being trained in this specialized field.

It is interesting to note that it is not unusual for someone working in this field to also be wearing an artificial eye. Apparently, they became interested in ocularistry as a direct result of their own experience as a patient.

In the late 1950s, a group of ocularists from across the country came together and eventually formed the American Society of Ocularists (ASO). The directive of the Society was to train and educate ocularists, and to provide an opportunity for research and presentation of ideas to the ocularist profession. Over the years, the group has developed and published many of the techniques and standards presently used in this field. The Society has also created and refined an ongoing 5-year educational program to train and keep members current with new techniques.

Most ocularists in North America, particularly the U.S. and Canada, are members of the ASO. But the membership also has numerous ocularists from other countries.

The American Society of Ocularists developed a program to qualify the knowledge and skills of ocularists. This program gave rise to a separate organization, the National Examining Board of Ocularists, or NEBO. NEBO then developed a series of standardized written examinations that tests the knowledge and proficiency of an ocularist. The exams also include a demonstration of the manufacturing of various ophthalmic prosthetics. Upon passing all of the exams, the ocularist then becomes a Board Certified Ocularist, or BCO.

About Eye Loss

The reasons for eye loss are numerous. An accident or injury might result in a damaged eye that will need to be surgically removed. This procedure is referred to as enucleation. In addition to ocular injuries, eye loss can also occur from medical conditions including diseases such as glaucoma and diabetes. Tumors occurring within the eye may also result in an enucleation.

Retinoblastoma is a tumor found in the eye of an infant or toddler, and will usually require the affected eye to be removed. Although rare, a child may be born with the absence of one or both eyes (congenital anophthalmia) or unusually small eyes (microphthamlia) requiring immediate attention from an ocularist with the fitting of small therapeutic appliances to prepare the socket for the prosthesis and encourage socket and eye lid growth. A child born prematurely may also develop an eye condition known as Retinopathy of Prematurity (ROP), which can result in a small, blind eye that usually does not need to be removed but may still require an ocular prosthesis.

As parents, we have probably all had the occasion to remind our children not to play with scissors, or run with sticks or sharp objects. Sadly, these situations have resulted in eye injuries requiring surgery and occasionally enucleation.

When an eye injury has occurred it is not always necessary to enucleate and the surgeon may elect to save the outer portion of the eye but still remove the inner contents. The end result in appearance will resemble an enucleation but, most significantly, the muscles attached to the globe which are responsible for eye movement have not been severed. This procedure is referred to as an evisceration.

Another occurrence resulting from a severe eye injury is sympathetic ophthalmia. This is a rare condition that, following an eye injury, may cause blindness in the other uninjured healthy eye. Sympathetic ophthalmia has occurred many years after the initial injury and although very rare, surgeons may choose to enucleate the injured eye for this reason.

Some injuries to an eye may cause blindness, though the eye may appear to be healthy and normal for years to come. However, occasionally, the appearance of the eye will change and the eye can actually begin to shrink in size. At some point, this may become obvious to the individual. This is referred to as Phtisis Bulbi "shriveled eye". It is usually not necessary to surgically remove a phthisical eye. A very natural appearing prosthesis can be made to fit over this type of eye.

Some blind eyes may be disfigured in appearance only; possibly there was damage to the cornea and it may have a milky white appearance. This can be corrected by the use of a soft cosmetic contact lense fitted over the cornea by an optometrist. This does require the cornea to be fairly normal in size and contour. If there are abnormalities to the normal shape along with slight shrinkage in actual globe size, a contact lense may not be recommended but a scleral lense may be more appropriate. A scleral lense is usually a thin type of a custom artificial eye fit and made by an ocularist.

An eye in such a phthisical condition may lose most of its normal sensitivity and the wearing of a prosthesis is more comfortable. On occasion though, the remaining cornea can still retain enough sensitivity to make it quite difficult to wear a prosthesis. This can be corrected by the surgeon placing a thin graft of conjunctival tissue on the cornea, thus eliminating the corneal sensitivity. This is a surgical procedure.

Patients come to the decision to have their eye removed with varying emotional responses. Some may not have had a choice in the matter, possibly due to a sudden injury where the eye has been irreparably destroyed. Other patients may have dealt with uncontrolled pain possibly for years or dealt with continued problems and failed surgical repairs and the decision to have their eye removed has been easier to accept, if not a great relief. While many are philosophical about the situation, others may feel a sense of loss for years.

The Ocularist

Some patients experience more post-surgical pain. Other patients might require longer healing time. But usually after about six weeks from surgery the patient is well healed and will be ready to visit the ocularist. During this time period, some patients will have been gathering information about artificial eyes but it is typical for many to have little, if any, knowledge in this area. Often times, the referring doctor will prefer their patients to obtain information directly from an ocularist.

So, your first visit may be more of a consultation appointment where you will have questions answered and possibly see photographs of prosthetic results. Many ocularists will have their own brochures printed which they can send to you prior to your first visit. Of course, you should ask to see final results, and hopefully you will see a range of pictures showing their best work, but also results that were more compromised.

How long does it take to make an eye? How many appointments are needed? Does it hurt? (Usually, fitting a prosthesis is painless.) How much does it cost? What will I look like? Does it move? These are typical questions that should be asked.

Equally important is your ocularist listening to you. Is your ocularist patient and does he/she answer your questions in a manner that you understand? Many patients who find an ocularist they like return to this same individual for cleanings and checkups for many years to come.

In many ocularist offices the consultation appointment may be concurrent with the fitting procedure and possibly may include the entire process of making the eye all in one day. This is possible, but will depend on how scheduling of the appointments are done. Some ocularists prefer making an eye in a day while others will schedule multiple appointments to complete the prosthesis. Usually, though, it requires one to three appointments to finish an the fitting. After you have your prosthesis, there will be future appointments for cleaning and polishing or resurfacing of the artificial eye.

Manufacturing and Fitting

The manufacturing and fitting of an artificial eye has become fairly standardized as have the materials and components that comprise the parts of the prosthesis. There are variations to these methods and each ocularist may favor one technique over another and, in addition, may further modify a procedure to suit a particular patient's needs.

Generally, an impression is made of the eye socket using a gel type material called alginate. From the impression, a plaster cast is formed creating a model of the eye socket. The ocularist can then sculpt a wax pattern forming a shape that will become an appropriate fit within the socket. The wax pattern is usually a curved hemisphere shape with much of the final size and thickness fashioned to open the eye lids and, in particular, provide support to the upper lid. The ocularist will also observe the shape, size and contours of the opposite eye and lid anatomy to help determine the final shape.

Once the wax shape has been completed, it will be converted into the actual plastic eye using a casting process similar to the lost wax techniques used in Dentistry and jewelry making. With the completed plastic shape in hand, and with the patient present, the artwork or the replicating of the iris and scleral colors along with the veining and other features unique to each patient can then be applied. Typically, this is accomplished with paint or pigments. Photographic and digital imaging has also been used in conjunction with painting. Whatever method or combination is used, the final coloring should match closely with the patient's natural eye.

The final step is to add a clear plastic layer or cap to the painted surface. The eye is then highly polished, cleaned and inserted into the patient's eye socket. If required, slight adjustments can still be made to improve the fit, comfort and movement of the prosthesis.

Ocular Implants

The majority of patients who undergo an enucleation or evisceration will also receive an ocular implant during the latter half of the surgery. An ocular implant is a device usually spherical in shape that is placed posteriorly within the socket underneath the conjunctiva. The purpose of the implant is to replace some of the volume lost when the eye was removed. Also, the implant can help aid in movement of the artificial eye. Some more recently developed implants are designed to greatly improve prosthetic eye movement. These implants usually incorporate a small titanium peg that couples the implant and artificial eye together, thereby enhancing eye movement.

The first implants made over one hundred years ago were hollow glass spheres. Various metal alloys have been used in the past, including gold. Since the late 1940s, plastic implants were developed and are still widely used today. The ease of molding plastic allowed for an evolution of non-spherical shapes to be created for the enhancement of artificial eye movement. Soft silicone spheres have also been used successfully. Beginning in the late 1980s, implants made from a type of coral have become very popular. The use of coral introduced new interest and research into implant design and materials. Today, there are any number of implants available to benefit the patient including different sizes, shapes, and materials. Your surgeon will select the most appropriate one for you.

Fees

The fees for custom artificial eyes and scleral shells will vary based on a number of factors. Scleral shells are usually more expensive than a conventional eye because there is usually more time required to fit a shell.

Many health insurance policies will pay for a portion of the prosthesis. Usually, the policy will include a deductible amount and a co-pay. The deductible is often expressed as a percentage of the total allowed by the insurance policy. The patient may also be required to pay the difference between the allowed amount and the provider's fee. Federal and state insurance programs such as Medicare and Medicaid will partially pay for prosthetics although usually with a greatly reduced reimbursement to the provider.

Fees may also vary within regional areas. Because of this, identifying an "average" fee is difficult. So how much does an eye cost? Between two and three thousand dollars might be a good place to start. But one could also pay at least twice this average or more. Keep in mind that paying an unusually high fee does not in any way suggest that the patient is getting a better prosthesis. Price alone should not be the only factor but rather the reputation, skills and talent of the ocularist should weigh most heavily in making this very important decision.

Your new prosthesis can last a long time if it maintained properly. To prevent tear secretions and protein deposits from collecting on the surface, routine cleaning and polishing once or twice a year should be provided by your ocularist. This will help to maintain a healthy socket. During these appointments the ocularist will also examine the condition and fit of the prosthesis. The shape of the prosthesis can be modified to some extent to address small changes that can occur within the socket.

Eventually, a new prosthesis will become necessary due to gradual but significant facial changes resulting over time from the aging process. An average life span for an artificial eye is probably five to seven years.

To find a qualified ocularist in your area, ask your ophthalmologist, surgeon, or eye care professional for a referral, or visit the website of the American Society of Ocularists and consult their online directory of members for an ocularist near you.

John Kennedy is a Board Certified Ocularist. He began his career as an ocularist in 1990 and in 1997 opened his own practice, Eye Design Ocular Prosthetics, located in Orange County in the City of Tustin, California. Mr. Kennedy can be reached at 714-508-8565. His office address is Eye Design Ocular Prosthetics, 145 W Main Street, Suite 120, Tustin, California 92780.

5

General Considerations

The people who will make your artificial eye are known as "Ocularists" (pronounced: "Ock-You-Lair-Ists") and are engaged in the practice of "Ocularisty". There is an American Society of Ocularists, and their research of new techniques and product development is published in the Society's annual Journal of Ophthalmic Prosthetics.

Although the first artificial eyes were made of glass (thus, "glass eye"), for about the last fifty years most artificial eyes have been made out of plastic, typically Methyl Methacrylate. These plastic eyes are typically molded by the Ocularists to provide you with the greatest possible level of comfort. With proper care and cleaning, they can last as long as a decade.

You will wear your first artificial eye only for about six months. The reason for this is that the muscles and tissues in your eye socket will slowly adapt to the new eye. After six months, your Ocularist will fit you with your permanent eye.

For days after I first learned of my cancer, I worried about having to take my artificial eye out and clean it every night before I went to bed, and of leaving it out when I slept. These fears were completely unjustifiable. Modern artificial eyes are meant to be left in as much as possible, and slept in. In fact, you are only supposed to take the eye out every so often for cleaning (some people do this every couple of weeks, others may do this only every few months!), and you are supposed to put it back in as quickly as possible to protect it.

You should visit your ocularist at least once a year (more like every six months) to have your new eye cleaned and checked by your ocularist, and to do any modifications that you believe will make your new eye more comfortable.

Message Threads

I was in a pub one time sipping my beer after long day's work. Under those circumstances one often feels a little out of focus, the mind idling. So my mind was idling and without any thought began rubbing my eye as it felt itchy. And oops, it happened, my eye fell out off the socket onto the bar top jumping in there until settled. The girls on the other side of the bar got the shock of their lives. I just quietly put my eye back to the socket and continued sipping my beer to avoid any further attention.

Lucky the eye did not drop on the floor or the other side of the bar top, that certainly had caused some confusion when people start finding my eye.—*JPH*

My Sr. year of college, I was sitting at a table in the front of my art history classroom. My professor was giving a lecture on some slides. She was talking about a particular mural, though it escapes me now which one it was. Just as she switched to a close-up of the mural and was talking about all of its intricate detail, for instance, how many pieces made up the eye of the figure, I reached up to scratch my cheek and my eye (which apparently wasn't fitting too well at that point) popped out and hit the table. My professor caught it on the first bounce and handed it back to me without even so much as a pause in her lecture. I had to leave the classroom to put it back in because I was I was trying not to laugh and failing miserably. Myself, the professor, and my friend sitting next to me all had a good laugh about it after class.

Other things I have done: Lost a (clear) conformer in a pile of leaves in the back yard. Sat up in the middle of the night after apparently rubbing my eye in my sleep only to hear it go bouncing across the hardwood floor to who knows where. Intentionally taken it out and held it up to something to "get a closer look at it" just to freak out various people. Pop it out and started playing with it when waiting in long lines or during instances of being ignored by whoever it is I need to talk to—they tend to give you a little more attention and faster service then.—*Kelli*

◆ ◆ ◆

I wanted to give a warning about the beach though, before I forget. I went to the beach today, and went into the ocean. I usually only go in knee-deep. My sister and a few friends encouraged me to go deeper, where they were, citing that they'd be right next to me (I have a RESPECT of the ocean!). I went in, and when I realized how rough it was, I turned around and headed out, only I didn't see the HUGE wave that was about to crash over me! It sent me flying! I tumbled THREE times, unable to get up. My prescription sunglasses were ripped from my head and sent somewhere out in the ocean. Even my hair elastic was sent flying! I eventually got up and was wobbly. I looked all over for the glasses, but they were gone. $300 down the drain! I realized then and there, how lucky I was that my prosthesis didn't go flying out there too! So, now I have even more respect for the ocean, and I'll remain only knee-deep! Has anyone else had scares like this?—*Chris*

Yeah, I have them about 20 times a day, three times a week when I go surfing with my prosthesis in. I wear some goggles to protect my good eye from accidents and also from the sun (I've often wondered whether my eye cancer was the result of being in the sun so much without so much as sunglasses). Anyhow, the goggles are tethered to my suit because sometimes they go flying in really big waves. What I have learned to do is to close my eyes tight when I start to spill, and my prosthesis has never gotten close to popping out (knock on wood).—*Jay*

It happened to me AGAIN yesterday! I got knocked down by a wave at the ocean, and I was only in knee-deep this time! Argh! I'm thinking of buying goggles just so I could dip in the water! I feel like such a dodo bird, being so sturdy, yet able to be knocked over by the water like a feather!—*Chris*

My fear is going swimming in the pool, and having my lens fall out into the water. The horror of it floating on top of the water across the pool is too much for me to fathom.—*Michael*

That's NEVER happened to me in a swimming pool! Anyone else? I think it's pretty safe to swim in a pool, and you can easily wear goggles. Don't let it stop you!—*Chris*

I think I posted a couple years ago about having my eye come out during a fancy-diving lesson with my older cousin's hot friend from college. I was 15 and I really had to think hard to decide whether to drown myself or swim to the edge and tell him my eye was heading for the big drain. But I lived.—*Alicia*

Alicia, I nearly knocked myself out walking into a door jamb in front of the incredibly adorable PR guy who worked for one of our implementing partners last year. That must be why he's not dating me. that, or maybe the fact that his taste in women has proven to run to the "thin but busty blonde bimbo who wore a bra and an unbuttoned blazer to dinner the last time we all went out" side. Pooey on thin blondes,—*Ya'ara*

Hi, I found your site very interesting. I lost my left eye in '96 & due to the nature of enucleation, cannot fit a prosthesis. So I've worn an eye patch ever since which generally is OK, you sort of get use to it. However, has anyone heard of the following or will it always be just a dream of mine. Mirror glasses that don't allow people to see in but you can see out clearly, including at nighttime. The night vision is critical as sunglasses are no good in the dark for people like us. Leave that to the rock stars. If such glasses were possible, then I could do away with the patch which has two main drawbacks: 1. Kids always stare & either become frightened or bombard you with pirate queries/jokes; & 2. Patches tend to sweat

& become uncomfortable in a working environment. Anyway, any advice is much appreciated & thanks for the site. It's great! Regards,—*Julian*

6

Fitting Your New Eye

Your real eye had muscles attached all around it that kept your eye in the socket and moved it around. When your eye is removed, the surgeon inserts what amounts to a small ping-pong ball sized insert into your eye, and ties the muscles up around and in it. So, what you have in your eye is a small ball which is surrounded by muscle tissue. Your muscles continue to move around this ball, similar to how they moved when your real eye was there.

Your new eye will NOT be—contrary to popular expectations—round like your real eye. Instead, it will be sort of in the shape of a bottle cap (although very smooth) and will fit OVER the ball of muscle with the ping-pong sized insert inside.

The making of your new eye takes about a day to accomplish, and can either be done in one session or in several depending on the preferences of your ocularist. My ocularist (whose article appears in Chapter 4 above) generally gets the job done the same day—although it is certainly a full-day affair.

Your new eye will be created in a multi-step process. It is not painful, though it is tiring and towards the end you will probably be worn out (I was) and your eye socket slightly irritated.

When going to the ocularist, your greatest fear will be that you ma experience severe pain in the fitting of your new eye. This will not happen, although you will get some very weird (though not painful) sensations. The problem is that psychologically you are not accustomed to somebody sticking something into your eye socket. You've gone your whole life protecting the eye in the socket, and your mind and body is geared to reject anything near the socket.

You can—and must—overcome these fears simply by reminding yourself that there is nothing in the socket that can be harmed. You have to psych yourself up that it will feel weird, but that there will be no pain.

The first step is that your ocularist will place a "plunger" into your eye socket. The plunger looks very much like those suction-cup arrows that shoot out of a child's toy.

You really will not feel the plunger in your eye, but you will get a weird sensation because of your eyelids resting on the portion that it sticking out.

This doesn't hurt, but psychologically it feels very weird. It takes a few seconds to get used to, but you will do so as quickly as you realize that it doesn't hurt, it just feels weird.

Next, your ocularist will insert some plastic-like materials through the plunger into your socket. This doesn't hurt either, but it also feels weird. You have to sit there for a couple of minutes while the plastic-like materials hardens. Then, when the ocularist removes it, the sensation is gone.

Psychologically, this portion is the hardest part, not because it hurts, but just because it is weird. Fortunately, this entire process only takes about 5 minutes and IT DOESN'T HURT. Again, just weird.

What the ocularist does with the plastic is to create a wax impression similar to the cavity in your eye. He will then take the wax impression and place it into your eye to see how it feels. You probably won't feel some parts of it, and other parts will cause pressure inside your socket. You will tell your ocularist which parts are causing pressure, and he will take it out and smooth it as needed, and then reinsert it.

Your ocularist will primarily be smoothing and reshaping the wax so that the impression is the right shape for your eyelids to rest properly when your eye is open, and then to close properly when you blink. He will also be trying to shape the wax so that it fills out certain areas around your socket to give your eye a natural look.

The ocularist will insert and take out the wax impression several times during this process. It is not painful, although your eye socket may get a little irritated. My eyelids in particular got irritated, but not by the wax but by one of the lubricants the ocularist was using. When he switched to a heavy silicon lubricant, the irritation went away (so don't hesitate to tell your ocularist if your socket is irritated as he can probably do something to lessen the irritation).

After the ocularist has completed your wax impression, the plastic insert will be made. This takes about an hour and you will end up with a plain white piece of plastic the same shape as the wax. The ocularist wil take this in and out of your socket several times, adjusting the shape for comfort so that the eyelids rest and close properly. The plastic is completely smooth—and tough! My ocularist probably dropped mine on the floor a half-dozen time during this process (it is slick because it is covered with lubricant) with nary a scratch or dent!

After you and the ocularist are satisfied with the shape and feel of the insert, and how your eyelids rest, the ocularist will take a few seconds to draw on the insert how the eye hole should be aligned.

The next step is for the ocularist to drill the eye hole into the plastic and insert the colored area. The ocularist actually starts with something which looks like a button which is very close to your own eye (I was a "T-17" colored insert), and fits it over and around the hole which the ocularist has drilled.

You will then sit next to the ocularist as he paints your eye, looking closely at your remaining eye for a guide. The painting process is interesting, for instance the small red veins in your eye are duplicated by taking small strands of fabric and carefully placing them on the plastic. When completed, you new eye should pretty much resemble your remaining eye.

There is a final fitting, and then you are done!

Your new eye should look and act very similar to your remaining eye, except that there will be some slight variation in how your eyelids rest, and your new eye will not have the movement of your remaining eye. If there is significant variation in how your eyelids rest, you may want to consult with your surgeon about making some slight alterations so that it blends in better.

Painful no! Weird, yes! Tiring, yes!

You should get used to your new eye in a couple of days, and probably won't think much about it after that. It will, for all practical purposes, look and be like your remaining eye—but it won't see worth a darn (I'm told they are working on that!).

After you lose your eye, many of the muscles in you eye recede, since they have nothing to do. This is fairly dramatic for the first six-to eight-weeks, which is why you should not even attempt to go for a fitting until after this period.

However, even after you are first fitted with you new eye, your muscles will continue to shrink, although much more slowly. After about two months, I found that my new eye was way too loose, and on a couple of occasions was knocked sideways when I was sleeping, and in a couple of instances was accidentally knocked out.

So, I went back to my ocularist for a "second fitting". This, I learned, is where your new eye is really made to fit your socket.

Usually, your ocularist will not make you a completely new eye, but will merely add wax (and then permanent clear plastic), until the eye fits correctly.

Now my artificial eye fits perfectly, and there is no possibility that it will be knocked out of place or out. I feel that I can even surf with this modified eye without protective goggles (though I would be foolish to do such a thing). The fit is so good that it honestly feels exactly like my other eye.

Also, while I am writing, when you go for your second fitting, get your ocularist to make a "mold" of your modified eye, in case you accidentally lose it. This will hopefully keep you from having to re-start the eye making process.

MESSAGES

Greetings, I've been viewing this sight for about a year and have decided finally to participate. This is a very important forum, I only wish I had this growing up (all those questions!). Retinoblastoma as an infant has left me monocular for this life of 32 years so far. My parents were told not to treat me any different or place any limitations on me growing up, so naturally as a young adult I was simply not aware I could not play sports. I did, in fact, excel at many of them setting a few school records. Always safety first I might add. After art school I decided to pursue a career in ocular prosthetics. That took care of all those questions and I often recommend this sight to patients. You guys really are great. Thanks for being here.—*CanDo*

Hey, CanDo, welcome to the board. It'll be kewl getting an ocularist's perspective! Very impressive that you went into that line of work! It *is* artistry! My daughter watched my ocularist paint my eye this time (a long process) and she was intrigued with it (she's 16). I've been living with monocular vision for over 30 years also.

Just wanted you to know that I posted something a while ago about retinoblastoma. It was an article in my local paper. Also, I read a book by Hunter Tylo (she was a soap opera actress). She became an advocate since her baby daughter was diagnosed with retinoblastoma. SHE discovered it when the light shone in her daughter's eyes, and it wasn't even. Now there's more testing on babies to look for this. I'm glad they're making strides. Anyway, welcome again. We look forward to your posting!—*Chris*

◆ ◆ ◆

Hi Everyone. Just a note, ocularists are not doctors. Many of us are members of the American Society of Ocularists. We become board certified in the fitting of ophthalmic prosthetics after completing 10,000 hours in fitting and fabrication of custom ocular prosthetics, and after passing a rigorous examination and proctor observation of our laboratory practices. We do not prescribe medications nor should we refer to ourselves as "doctors". Any ocularist who refers to themselves as a "doctor" should be reported to the ASO.

However there may be a few dentists out there practicing ocularistry. If they are not BCO, BADO (NEBO ASO) they are doing a disservice to the patient even though they can rightfully be called "doctor". As dentists, they have no specific training in the fitting of ocular prostheses, similarly as I have no training in the fitting of dentures.

Check the credentials of the ocularist you want to work with and look at before and after pictures, talk to other patients. Look at the cleanliness of the laboratory, if it is dirty stay away. Best Wishes,—*Lisa*

Hi Mary, I experienced the same thing. When I was 16 my first prosthesis came out—unfortunately I wasn't on my own but with other girlfriend. Thanks God, she did not say anything and I just grabbed my prosthesis from the floor and went home—crying of course. After that accident I am very careful with jumping or any movement with my head. Once I woke up with my prosthesis with changed position, since then I am always checking my prosthesis every morning. This is painful especially when I am camping and there are no mirrors around and I cannot check how my prosthesis is positioned. That's why I decided to keep a small mirror with me. Cheers,—*Anna*

Usually, this means that your socket has shrunk in mass, and therefore it is time for a refitting. This happened to me about 6 months after my prosthesis was first made. At first, the fit was tight, but then it started to get loose, and then to fall out. I simply went to my ocularist, and he built up the prosthesis with clear material, took about 30 minutes, and then it was a great fit again.—*Jay*

This is my first time using a message board so forgive me if I do it wrong. I would agree that the prosthesis should absolutely not drop out or move. If it does it is the wrong size and a new molding needs to be done. I would also suggest hard contact lense wetting solution particularly for windy weather. Here in the UK we have a new prescription medication called "oculube" which comes as a lotion or an ointment and which I find useful sometimes. Regards—*Chil*

♦ ♦ ♦

I have been trying to get an eye made now for 6 months I no longer have a lid for some odd reason when I put the eye in after waiting for 6 weeks and driving for over 2 hours it just does not work. I had surgery Nov 4 and I still do not have a workable eye. I have had an artificial eye for years and had to have a new base put in, in Nov after 33 years it broke lose now I can not get an eye to fit and I am thinking of trying to find someone else to try and see what they can do. I have always been happy that no-one could tell at first glance and I even had an eye doctor exam my artificial eye and tell me boy you really have poor vision in that eye. I was being cute and showed him the eye and I still got charged for an exam with bad vision the eye looked that good. Now it looks awful and I can not blink the lid will not come down. Please tell me where to look for another person.—*Bea*

♦ ♦ ♦

Its been six years since my eye was removed. I am now unhappy with the appearance of the implant—it appears to be sinking. Does anyone have a recommendation for an ocular plastic surgeon in the NY area? Has anyone else had similar problems. Thanks.—*Alma*

Alma, I had to have this done as my socket got loose as the base detached after many years and I had to go to an ocular plastic S. I do not know of any in New York if you want to talk about the newer versions I would be happy to reply.—*Bea*

♦ ♦ ♦

Hi I've enjoyed reading your messages here and hopefully figured out how to join and write with you I'm not a computer whiz but trainable! My eye was removed because of a malignant tumor. I have actually felt lucky in the large scope of things, this was the least, cancer contained in the eye so I have been grateful and can deal with this no problem, except my prosthesis does not want to stay in when I look certain ways—especially up and to the right does this happen to any of you, or is this repairable?—*Loralsar*

I had the same problem when I first got my prosthesis. Part of the problem was the fit, which was adjusted to help prevent that from happening. The other thing I had to learn was to move my head more to look at things, rather than my eyes. This way, I avoided the extreme angles that would cause my prosthesis to come out. It takes a little practice, but it soon becomes second nature. Good luck,—*Nancy*

Your prosthesis is too small and needs to be built up. What happens is that after surgery the muscles in your eye socket will continue to lose mass for up to a year, meaning that you should get one or more refittings beginning six months or so after it is originally fitted.—*Jay*

◆ ◆ ◆

My 69 year old mother was recently diagnosed with invasive squamous cell carcinoma, mecoepidermoid type. This resulted in the exenteration of her right eye socket on January. She was referred by her surgeon to a prosthodonist rather than an ocularist. The prosthodontist told her since she did not have any eye muscles left in her eye socket that she could not receive a prosthetic eye because it would simply roll around and not stay in place. She told her that she would have to have another surgery to remove her eyelids and after this healed she would make her a patch to wear with an eye painted on it. I was wondering if anyone else had experienced this and would be willing to share advice and experiences with us. Also, does anyone know if there are any other options for her? Thank you very much for any assistance you can provide.—*Anon*

I had my eye removed 2 years ago because of cancer. I had to have radiotherapy treatment which killed the muscles in my socket and so I do not have an implant in. But I do have an artificial eye and believe me when I say it certainly does not roll around and stays exactly where it should be. The only difference between my eye and other peoples is mine is slightly sunk in because I have no implant but it looks better than a patch with an eye painted on. I am 55 so no young thing to go through this and I hope this has been of some help to you .come back and tell me what happens.—*Anne*

Hi, and welcome to the board! It sounds like your mom, and you, are going through quite a lot with this. I'm sure you will find lots of support from the folks on the board. I would think that there are more options for your mom than a patch with an eye painted on it. I would suggest you go the web site of the American Society of Ocularists at www.ocularist.org to find one in your area. They are doing amazing things with prostheses these days, and I'll bet you can find one that could help your mom. Good luck, and keep us posted.—*Nancy*

◆ ◆ ◆

Hello! I just want to let you know that this page is great. It really helps me because I live in a small country and I actually don't know nobody else with the glass eye, so sometimes I fell like nobody can understand how I fell but this page helped me with some great stories that I've read. I only have one question, what is difference between glass eye and acrylic eye, and can I sleep with acrylic eye without taking him out during the night? Greetings from Croatia!—*Dajana*

I'm a 55 year old professional woman. My doctor recommended I wait 3 months from date of surgery to get the prosthesis fitted over my implant, and I too have the clear plastic shield in the meantime. Instead of an uncomfortable and oh-so-obvious eye patch, before I had the surgery, I had eyeglasses made in a nice trendy frame but with shaded tinting, like back in the 70's. The tint creates a shadow that hides the bad eye. I also opted for regular instead of non-glare glass. The reflection serves as a mask also. As my eye opened, showing just a blank (sort of like Night of the Living Dead), I put a very small piece of regular frosted scotch tape on the inside of the glass right where you could see my open eye. With the tinting and the reflection and the tape, unless you're really looking into my eyes, it now just looks like my glasses need cleaning. Not one person who knows nothing about my surgery has asked what's wrong with my eye. It was well worth the extra investment to feel normal. And just the other night LL Cool J was wearing glasses just like mine on Jay Leno!—*Janet*

◆ ◆ ◆

[Follow-Up Message]—I went for my consultation at the ocularist last week. I was very impressed and comfortable with him. Due to a cancellation while I was there, I am scheduled to have it made this coming Tuesday, Wednesday and Thursday. They do it in 3 appointments, 3 days in a row, and it's strictly all hand-made, no photos, etc. You can imagine how excited I am.

Also, I got to the office a little early, and while I was in the waiting room I met and spoke with 3 other women who had eyes made there. Two were relatively new and the third had hers for many years. Unless you really looked (and knew what you were looking for), you really could not tell which eye was which. The one lady who'd had hers many years said she dated her husband almost a year before he knew! And all 3 wore just regular glasses (not tinted) with non-glare which makes your eyes very clearly visible. And they looked great!

Because it's pouring and flooding here in Houston, I'm staying in and had a chance to read all the Letters from Friends on your website. I hate to feel good at the expense of others, but many of the letters made me feel so badly for them and made me wonder what I did to remain so positive through it all. (We won't discuss the hysterical tears at 3:00 am the weeks before the surgery! But that helped too; sort of a cold shower for the soul.) I wish I could help them somehow.

Thanks for being there, Jay.—*Janet*

Jay, funny thing, I am getting a new eye made, which my whole office seems to be involved in, and a co-worker asked me if I had ever surfed for false eye sites.

I had never thought about it. I'm on the net everyday and have had a false eye since 1977 but had never taken a look. Today I did.

My ocularist is making me new eye and he is really doing a great job of it. I have had 4 visits so far and at least two more to come which is a good thing. He is really working to get a good fit. I never knew the importance of a good fit in maintaining the health and integrity of the socket and conjunctiva therein. He is taking a lot of time to let the socket stretch and accept a larger eye that will hold my implant in place better. A small prosthetic has permitted my socket to "head south" for lack of a better phrase. The cavity has gotten larger in the top\rear and narrower in the front\ bottom. Something important to note.—*Christopher*

My husband was fitted with a prosthesis this spring. His story is a little different from yours in that he had to have all tissue removed from his left orbital area. His prosthesis is much different than yours—it is about the size of a large marble, has a sort of clear plastic "cap" sticking out of it, on which his upper eyelid sits, and is removed each night. He doesn't look totally "normal" with it, but it sure does beat having to deal with a large hole in his head! The purpose of my e-mail is two-fold: First, thank you for your site and the information it contains. Your site is a valuable resource for those who have lost an eye. Second, please feel free to use my site as a resource for others who might contact you about a condition similar to my husband's. We are especially interested in informing those who are facing the loss of not only the eye, but also all tissue in the orbital area, that there is a surgical option they need to know about. Mayo Clinic performs a procedure that only a handful of other institutions in the world do—that of saving the eyelids and inserting a muscle flap to enable a prosthesis to be used. Thanks for a great site!—*Bev*

Hi. Just found your website after living 30 years with an artificial eye. When I was two, a stray cat scratched my eye, and it had to be removed when my good eye began losing sight to sympathize with the blind eye. I've had three artificial eyes. The first I had from when I was 2 until I was 14. Then, I was self conscious of my drooping eyelid, so my parents took me to a plastic surgeon in Chicago who recommended that I instead take the elevator down two floors to an ocularist! Apparently, I just needed a bigger eye. This ocularist has made my last two artificial eyes, and even though I now live in New York, I will definitely return to his office in the future. They make them the old fashioned way—sculpting them by hand, and my last two are more triangular to keep the lid from drooping. Many friends and family are confused as to which eye is fake because of the fantastic work they do. In addition, the cost of the eye was considerably less expensive (I believe around $800, and that was in 2003) than other prices being mentioned on the site. Best of luck to all!—*Stacy*

Take your time and be patient. It is difficult to judge by yourself how your eye is being made. Maybe bring a friend with you to inspect the eye as it is being made and finished, a 3rd party if you will. It is difficult to judge yourself.—*Doc*

Hi there everyone, Just thought I would share this with you all, I had my prosthesis made in a day! I arrived at the ocularists office at 8:00 A.M. and had my new eye by 4:00P.M. that day. She is an awesome lady who does wonderful work and like I stated before, it only cost me $800.00 for the prosthetic here in Winnipeg, Manitoba! I had to go back a couple of times to have it shaved down and then once to actually have it built up! It has been 5 years this December that I have lost my eye and I still really think I have issues with it, I am having a really hard time accepting the fact that I cannot seem to get to the same level of pool playing that I used to be at! And boy does that get to me! I love pool and it is so frustrating and what is more frustrating is the fact that no one seems to understand how I feel! I mean shooting at a ball when I have to shoot over another ball or shooting a ball off the rail is a nightmare for me now when 5 years ago it was a routine shot! Makes me so made I broke my favorite cue last year because I missed a shot that had me in fear again!—*Ski*

◆ ◆ ◆

Hey. Does anybody have a problem with their prosthesis floating around in your socket?. mine gets twisted around and they pupil/retina moves over to the left. It looks really weird when it does that. I was hoping some of you may have some tips to prevent this?—*Pim*

I've NEVER had my prosthesis move at all! Sounds like there's too much room in the socket, or the prosthesis is too small? I'd call your doctor or your ocularist (or ask your mom to call). It shouldn't move that much.—*Chris*

◆ ◆ ◆

Yesterday, I drove nearly 3 hours to my ocularist to get my prosthesis refitted, and it turns out, he tried and tried and cut it down and reshaped it, but to no avail! I was so disappointed, he told me that he would have to make me a brand new eye. I have to drive to Nashville Tennessee in two weeks, which is about 5 hours or something like that, and he is going to make me a brand new one for half price, which is only 500 bucks! Wow, that is great isn't it! Except for the long drive! Well, I just figured I would update everyone. Take care.—*Starter*

Jarrod, that is great news! It's always good to be able to save some money! Starting over and getting a brand new prosthesis is probably the best way to go, especially with all of the work you had done. My first one had so many adjustments done to it over the course of several years, that I didn't realize how uncomfortable it was until I got a new one. Let us know how you make out in Nashville.—*Nancy*

◆ ◆ ◆

Hello everyone, I was wondering how long (how many eyes) it took before you all felt like you had The Perfect Fit for your eye? Did your ocularist make your eye right the first time you saw him? I guess I'm a little frustrated with the ocularist(s) I've been seeing b/c I feel like I'm paying them entirely too much for one try. I wore the same prosthesis for fourteen years and had a second implant surgery in May. Prior to surgery I had no problems with my lids but they are giving me some trouble now.

I've been to three different ocularist who of course came up with three totally different eyes. Each having their positive and negative points but I haven't been pleased with any. Has anyone had a similar experience? and did you finally find The Perfect Fit?—*Pearl*

Hi Pearl, welcome to the board. Sorry to hear you're unhappy with your new prosthesis. I know how frustrating that can be. I haven't had a problem exactly like yours. I did have to have a lot of adjustments made to the first prosthesis I got and didn't realize how uncomfortable it had become until I had a new one made a few years later. The new one fit felt so good, I couldn't believe it. I had that one for almost 8 years and just got another new one about 6 months ago. This one feels good also, but not as good as the last one. My ocularist wanted me to come in for a check-up around now. I just haven't made the appointment yet.

I wonder if part of your problem is that you are still healing from the surgery. Maybe it's still a bit swollen. What kind of problem are you having with your lid? Is it drooping? And I'm also curious as to why you had to get another implant. I hope you don't mind me asking you all of these questions, but I always assumed that once you had an implant, it wouldn't have to be changed, unless it got damaged or something. Anyway, I hope the best for you. Kindest regards,—*Nancy*

Thanks, for responding Nancy. I had the second implant surgery b/c my doctor recommended it—she said that the increased volume would help me gain more movement. My doctor just said that the implant I got when I was six was too small for my socket now that I'm 24—that makes sense right? I just never imagined that I could have an outcome that was worse than what I had before. In retrospect I probably shouldn't have gotten the surgery seeing as I had no problems with my old prosthesis or socket except for a little sunkeness at the top of my lids which I guess led to the ptosis (drooping) that I'm having now. I'm trying to avoid having a lid surgery so I'm hoping for an eye that can help correct it. If not then I may have to have the surgery. I'm going to get one more opinion before I decide.—*Pearl*

Pearl, Thanks for the answers! I had lid surgery on both eyes (although not at the same time!) about a year after I lost my right eye. The lids didn't match, so I had the right one done first, and then the left. The left one was done in the doctor's office, as it really isn't a big deal. I don't remember exactly when the right was done, but I think it was during another procedure I had, like when they had to re-drill for the peg. The lid surgery was probably one of the easiest things throughout the whole ordeal.—*Nancy*

◆ ◆ ◆

For about 6 weeks I have had a provisional prosthesis. This was a prosthesis the ocularist took out of 1000 other prostheses. It was a little bit smaller then my eye but it moved very well from the left to the right side, up and down. The color was a little bit darker than my eye but people told me it was almost not perceptible if one should not have known about it. Since yesterday I received my definite prosthesis. It is bigger than my previous one. Now my prosthesis does not move to the right side but it does to the left side. The background of the prosthesis is not as white as my eye. I do not feel as comfortable with this prosthesis as I felt with the other one. Question: does anyone has experience in this matter and can give me a solution for my problem? I would be very grateful receiving suggestions.—*Chrissie*

Chrissie, if you are not happy with the way that your prosthesis looks, then you need to tell your ocularist. The prosthesis that you are wearing is an example of their work and so they want it to be perfect just as you do. It is a reflection on them. I know that my ocularist only wants my prosthesis to be as close as physically possible to my eye. Don't be afraid to speak up to them because this is your eye and you have been through enough that it should be to your approval. As far as movement goes, when you get the eye enucleated, you will lose movement. It is something that we all have to deal with but it is better than being uncomfortable. I hope that I have helped you. Take care.—*Jodi*

Hello Chrissie, so sorry to hear you are not happy with your prosthesis. I totally agree with Jodi, you should tell you ocularist. When I first got my prosthetic eye it was just a little bit lighter blue than my real eye. I told him and now the coloring is just perfect. I also lost some movement, but like Jodi said I think that goes for everyone who had enucleation. Make sure you feel comfortable wearing you prosthetic eye. Good luck.—*Willeke*

◆ ◆ ◆

I've read a few different threads and most of you seem pretty enthusiastic about it, but I can seriously not stand mine. It's a huge inconvenience, gets a lot of attention from others, especially during class presentations. Girls aren't really attracted to it and it's just a big black cloud over my sunny days, so all that's left is rain. I don't understand why they haven't made any further advancements for this. Yes I understand there are a lot of muscles to attach and all that, but still there must be something other than an implant, which doesn't really add a huge difference in mobility. An eye patch is not an option. Just look at the society we live in, an eye patch is even worse than a prosthetic. What's left? Join a religion, and let God handle it all?—*Anon*

Don't give up! I'm so sorry that you do not like your prosthetic. I think you should try a new ocularist. They may be able to make you one that you are more happy with.—*mak*

Hi, just wanted to say that no you are not the only one not happy with their prosthetic. I have had mine for nearly 2 years now and it still isn't what I call right. But at last I a getting something done about it, in the next 6 weeks I am having some plastic surgery done to try and improve the damage done by the radiotherapy treatment. My eye is very sunken in and the bottom lid doesn't have enough room for the eye to sit in properly so the surgeon is going to try and rectify this. I will let you know how it all goes. So my advice is if you're not happy go see someone else. I don't know where you live and if you have to pay for surgery, I live in UK and while surgery is free the waiting list was about 6 months so I will be pleased when it is all over. I also thought about an eye patch and bought a couple on the internet but they are not easy to wear under my glasses, hope this has helped you a little.—*Anne*

◆ ◆ ◆

Hi Everyone, The continuing saga . So I got my prosthetic eye today. It took 3 and a half hours start to finish and I had my new eye. I have to say I am REALLY disappointed with it. The color is fine but it's smaller than my old eye and of course the movement is not too good. The really annoying part is (when I look at it closely) that there is a white line through my pupil area that I pointed out to the ocularist and she said that the paint separated during the curing or something? Anyhow, it's not noticeable unless you look right into the eye but I know it's there and it's really bugging me. You'd think if the paint separated that she could fix it? Apparently if it is really bothering me I can have her fix it in 6 months when I go for a cleaning. Sorry to be complaining, I just want my life back with no more EYE STUFF! It's been a long day.—*Starr*

I know I was expecting perfection where there cannot realistically be any. However in addition to the paint line in my pupil, there are also 4 small AIR BUBBLES (what is it with me and air bubbles?) in the iris of the prosthetic.—*Starr*

Hi Starr, I will be having eyelid surgery to correct the many problems from my enucleation. I did find out that it was a mixture of things. Surgery, radiation damaged tissue and the ocularist didn't do the prosthesis correctly. The ocuplastic surgeon is having them make the eye bigger and it will be done from scratch. We told her we didn't want the eye if it didn't look right and she said she wanted to do it now and then add to it later. My pupil is so much smaller than my real eye too. I will be having surgery soon on the lid problem. So, I can fill you in. So looking forward to getting on with life. Hugs,—*Sherri*

Huh? Most of the prosthesis that I have seen are indistinguishable from the natural eye, except of course for the lack of motion. The paint line and air bubbles are NOT the norm; feel free to quote me on that. To make up for the lack of movement, buy some glasses that are slightly tinted which will disguise 99% of it. You should be wearing glasses anyway to protect your good eye, whether you need them or not.—*Jay*

Thanks for the tips Jay. I do wear glasses and have a few different colored clip-ons for computer use, outdoors etc. The prosthetic is certainly not the "norm" as you say. The pupil white line and the air bubbles are quite annoying. The color of the eye is good, but sadly that is the only positive. I do have an appointment booked with the ocularist to have it fixed and to get an adjustment done as it is "pinching" at the top and is very uncomfortable. I actually prefer not to have it in. The socket is very red and inflamed from the poor fit. On another positive note the one side of my face is continually moisturized from the amount of mineral oil I am using to try to combat the discomfort! Thanks again.—*Starr*

I've worked in the field of Ocularistry for years and Jay is right, bubbles are not the norm and in fact are indications of a flawed curing process. To fix those, the bubbles need to be ground out and re-cured, which depending on her method, could take up to a few hours. Insist on correction I hope all goes well.—*Concerned Guest*

Wow, sorry you are having so much trouble. My prosthesis actually looks better than my original. It had died basically and was gray and shrinking. I do wish mine would have better movement too. I think I am too picky sometimes because I see this line that no one else seems to notice-but to me it always looks like I have a hair on my eye-drives me nuts! After 3 years I am finally getting comfortable with mine and have found for the most part I have a bigger problem dealing with it than everyone else-but then again that is just me. My ocularist appointment took about 8 hours! And my insurance said that a prosthesis was cosmetic and didn't pay for any of it Anyhow I do hope you get this problem fixed and finally have some peace. I know you have gone thru more than enough and don't need any more stress. I hope you feel better soon,—*Cyn*

It's interesting that there is so much variation in the quality of the paintings. processing, etc of our eyes. I was very disappointed by the first new eye I got here in LA—I couldn't believe how bad it was. The man was very nice, but I think he was out of his depth. Insist on getting a better fit and look. If the person can't handle it, try to find someone else. When I had my accident, my eyes were very dark brown, almost black. They've lightened over the years and it is interesting to see the old, tiny eyes from when I first started having them made. Here's hoping for a better result. Love,—*Alicia*

Hi, I just wanted to give my 2 cents. My prosthetics turned out great this time. perfect color etc., but now the oculoplastic surgeon doesn't want to complete the next round of surgery. I will never look normal, but I will keep searching. Hugs,—*Sherri*

I just got my new eye. Took all day Tuesday. I have no discomfort at all. She was not happy with it. She says the iris is 1mm too small. I can't tell, and people at the club who don't know I lost an eye can't tell. It looks real nice and the movement was better than I expected.—*Guy*

Lisa is right. My eye took almost 8 hours to make. It took me about 10 minutes to get comfortable with my eye. Not one problem since.—*Guy*

◆   ◆   ◆

Hello everyone was at eye hosp yesterday for fitting for new eye which went very well but it will take about 8 weeks to make it but I know it will be very good as my last one was and the same man is making it for me. I was talking to him about this site and how much it costs for a prosthetic in the us and he told me that if someone comes to England from abroad and wants an eye made there will be no change out of £500 I don't know how much this is in U.S. dollars. I am pleased to say that I get it for free from the National Health Service as I am now waiting for my 3rd eye due to new surgery.

In America how do they match up the color of the new eye? My man was telling me that the artificial eye service paid £5,000 for a digital camera which wasn't as good as he could do just looking at peoples eyes. He is really very good at his job and his own eyesight must be wonderful. So do they do it like this in US or have they better technology but I have to say the finished eyes can't be any better than the ones I have had.—*Anne*

Hi Anne. Painting from a photograph is not the way it should be done. I hope that they take the time and paint the iris while looking at your natural eye. Good Luck!—*Lisa*

My Ocularist did a great job with the color. He did it by eye. You can't tell one from the other. If it wasn't for the scaring on my top lid, it is hard to tell.—*Michael*

Hi folks! Wkd, so great to hear from you again! I'm sorry to hear about your eye, and I know what you mean about feeling down for a while when you get home from the hosp. Unfortunately, although the NHS is a blessing in that we don't have to pay. It often means we all have to join the queue! I really hope you get sorted soon. Good to hear about your progress too Anne, I hope all keeps on track!

Lisa, You say that digital imaging is not the way it should be done. It seems that the UK is adopting this process rather than painting eye to eye. I had digital photo's taken of my good eye to get my occlusive contact lens, and also like Wkd, it took about 8 weeks for them to come back (it actually took more, as they got lost and it ended up being nearly 12 weeks!) and then after this the prosthesis is made, so it really slows things down! Why do you think the NHS are opting for this method?—*Elizabeth*

Thanks Michael. It is a pleasure as always. Regarding the "digital camera ocularist". The fitting technique looks suspect. If the eye is looking up a bit, they can reduce the lower border so the gaze drops down (hopefully), but it should not have to come to this. The patient needs to be present during the fitting and painting process to get a good result. You can't take a picture, take a mold and suddenly come up with an artificial eye ready for delivery. This is not like making dentures.—*Lisa*

While we have a different health care system, the problem lies in the skill of the person making your artificial eye. Ocularists are not part of the health care system. There are some ASO members in your area, check out the website http://www.ocularist.org Hopefully you can find someone close to you,—*Lisa*

◆ ◆ ◆

Hi, folks. I've been reading for a bit and just wanted to introduce myself and say hello and let out something that's been bothering me a bit. I have been blind in my left eye since birth with retinopathy of prematurity and have decreased vision in my right eye. At 17, for aesthetic and pain management reasons, I had an enucleation of my left eye. I was very fortunate to have a great retinologist perform the surgery and by the next day I was in less pain than I was before the operation.

I was then also very lucky to have a great ocularist create for me a perfect eye on the first try. It looks just like my right one, fits great, and is very comfortable. I've never had a problem with it. I can't even tell it's there, never have to take it out to clean, etc. My prosthesis, however, will be 10 years old this October! I know that's a long time to go on one prosthetic, and it's definitely showing a little wear and tear. I'm losing my paint job! I have an appointment next week so that he can evaluate the prosthetic and make a recommendation to Voc. Rehab as to what to do (I'm sure he'll recommend replacing it).

I know he's good, and I know he did a great job last time, but I'm nervous. My eyesight has never really been a big deal to me. It's bad, but it's been bad all my life, so I'm used to it, and everything regarding getting my prosthesis went as smooth as silk the first time around, so I never gave it any thought. I'm just apprehensive that the new prosthesis won't fit as well or as comfortably. Logically, I know it shouldn't be a problem, but it still worries me.

I guess I have a sentimental attachment to my old worn-out prosthesis. It's like that old pair of shoes that you've worn for so long and they're so comfortable that you hate to get rid of them even though they're falling apart at the seams. I'm excited about getting a new eye that looks better and I know it needs to be done, but in a stupid sort of way, I feel a bit as if I'm losing an old friend. Pretty dumb, huh?

I'm kind of glad to hear I'm not alone. I would be really nervous if it was someone different making the eye. I just feel like the one I have now is the perfect fit, though it is starting to look pretty crummy.—*Kelli*

Your Oculist did such an excellent job the first time. I'm sure he will be as conscientious and expert the second time around, as well.—*JK*

Well, I just got back from the ocularist a few hours ago. He said he was surprised at how well the eye had held up. The finish wasn't that bad, but you could definitely see signs of the acrylic starting to break down after so many years of wear. More importantly, though, apparently the fit is all wrong now. I'd never paid much attention, as I'm not one for looking closely at myself in the mirror (don't want to damage what little eyesight I have left!) the prosthesis looks down and in. I've also noticed that my left upper lid droops more than it did and I was told this is because of the poor fit as well, I also have less movement than I did 10 years ago. The general consensus was that this thing is old and a bit too small, so I get a new eye on the 19th of next month! He's only here one day a month, so he will make the eye in one shot, like he did last time, so it will be a full day of being in and out of the office. I am excited, and I was a little disappointed that he couldn't fit me in to do it today, which he normally would have. On the other hand, I have a really bad head cold at the moment with tons of sinus pressure and messing around in the socket hurts because of it (anyone else get that?) so I guess it's a good thing. I'm sore just from them taking it in and out today, which is rare for me.—*Kelli*

Best of luck with the new prosthesis. It sounds just what you need—better fit, better appearance and an ocularist you know and trust.—*Chil*

◆   ◆   ◆

Finally! New prosthesis Thursday! After months of waiting and rescheduling, and being within 30min of the ocularist's office last month only to have to cancel because our car died a horrible death (one which made the entire vehicle worth less money than the tow bill to get it home), a new vehicle has been purchased, a new appointment made, and I get my new prosthesis on Thursday!

I am a little apprehensive, because the old one is just so darn comfy. I'm also excited, though, because the one I have now is 10yrs old and in desperate need of replacing. It's losing its finish and it doesn't fit quite right anymore.—*Kelli*

Unless you need changes, your ocularist will probably just make your new eye from a mold of your old one, so it should fit exactly the same. BTW, what are you going to do with your old one? I've thought that I would have my ocularist drill a hole in my old prosthesis so that I could keep it on my key chain just for the sheer fun of weirding people out with it.

I've had people tell me that my prosthesis looked more authentic than my real eye. Of course, these ocularists really do remarkable work!—*Jay*

Have you all read "Fried Green Tomatoes" (not the movie, the book)? The bad guy in it has an artificial eye. At one point he bets a stranger he can't guess which is real and which isn't. The stranger gets it right, and later explains, "The glass one was the only one that had a glint of humanity in it."—*Ya'ara*

◆ ◆ ◆

Hello all. We're just about ready to get in the car for the drive north to Seattle for family/friends visiting and MY NEW EYE! It's being made in six appointments on the 8th, 9th and 10th. I'll be so happy to be shut of this whole ordeal. Even the minor stuff like NO MORE EYE PATCH or CONFORMER will be a huge relief. Thank you to everyone for all the help and shoulders and support—you guys mean the world to me. Love,—*Alicia*

Well, it's now late Friday night. I've had the eye in since Wed. afternoon. We left the Seattle area this morning after a difficult and complicated week. It's a great eye—my ocularist is amazing. My doctor who did the last surgery did a great job on the implant—I even have some movement. Closed, the lids look good, and the curve of the crease and the outer corner is great. But—the inner corner is still messed up. I'm trying very hard not to be disappointed. So, I'm glad it's over, and that I can stop dodging mirrors and tearing up my skin with the eye patches. Thank you all so much for the love and caring. Love,—*Alicia*

◆ ◆ ◆

I GOT MY NEW EYE! I GOT MY NEW EYE! I went to the ocularist this past Thursday and picked up my new eye! Woo hoo! No more "evil red eye" (although I must say I really had fun grossing people out with it) It looks really good, even the little veins that he put in. Being that my eye is brown, there really isn't much detail in it. I was looking at a couple others that he made that were blue and green, and the detail was incredible! The little hints of gold and other colors that he put on them was just amazing. I wanted to see those people get their new eyes. He let me keep the molds that he used to make it too, so it kind of makes it easier to describe the whole process to people when I can show them too. My husband was really excited and amazed too. Everyone at work said it looked just like my other eye. When I try to watch it in the mirror, it looks like I'm cross-eyed or something, I guess because I'm trying to make it move while at the same time trying to watch it? I'm going to have my husband recorded me moving my eyes so I can truly see what other people see. Then I'll believe everything looks great. My husband says that you can only tell something is different when I look to the extreme left or right, then he says it doesn't follow the other eye as well. I don't know. All I know is I GOT MY NEW EYE!—*Renee*

Congratulations, Renee! It really is an awesome feeling to get your eye and see the results. It's been nearly two years since I got mine and I still sometimes look in the mirror and am amazed at the artistry and at how my eye improved my appearance. I'm so happy you're happy with it!—*Adeline*

7

Prosthesis Movement and Solutions

From an appearance standpoint, your new eye should be indistinguishable from your other eye, except that your new eye will not move very much. The reason for this is that the muscles in your eye socket aren't attached to your new eye like they were to the old one. Probably most people will not even notice this (or care), but if you are self-conscious about it there are a few possible solutions:

First, you can wear sunglasses or have your eyeglasses slightly tinted. To protect your other eye you will want to wear some sort of protective glasses anyway. This is the easiest solution.

Second, you can have installed into your eye socket a special type of implant made of a porous material to which your muscles and other tissues will slowly connect. This implant will better interface with your artificial eye, thus giving the eye more natural movement. The implant was first approved by the Food & Drug Administration in 1989, and it is claimed that over 30,000 people have had this procedure done. There is a possible downside, however, and that is that the porous materials may also make the eye socket slightly more susceptible to infection, so you will want to consult not only your ocularist but also your ophthalmologic surgeon about the benefits and risks.

Third, promising research is now being made into artificial eyes which will not require the implant, but will more closely interact with the muscles in your eye socket to provide natural movement. So, if you can wait for awhile, you might be able to take advantage of new technologies.

MESSAGES

I have recently been concerned with what kind of movement I am going to have in my eye, and what is really getting me down is this. I can see the implant through the clear plastic shield they have put in my eye socket temporarily, and it doesn't seem to have much movement at all. Does anyone have any thing they can tell me about this?—*Jarrod*

You are lucky to have a clear plastic implant. When I lost my eye back in 86 they had bright white implants with 3 drain holes that I called my Jason eye. No your implant will not have the movement your permanent one will. Your next implant will conform with your eye socket for movement.—*Nas*

Jarrod, I'm the "worst case scenario". Due to the type of accident I had (shot in the eye with a bb-gun) and the follow-up surgeries (20-something), I totally lost ALL mobility with my prosthesis. Sometimes it gets to me. You adjust. I'm sure that you'll have some mobility. Wait until you get your final prosthesis to see. Either way, as long as you're healthy, you'll adjust and be fine. If you need any more information, I'd be willing to share it with you. ~*Chris*

Movement of the prosthetic eye is a big concern for most of us, I think. I've always had a little movement, but not that much. If I closed my eyes and moved them back and forth, I could feel the eye moving under the lid, but it didn't translate to much movement. In photos, if I'm looking down, my real eye looks down, but the other one doesn't. That's what I've noticed the most. How much movement we get must depend on the nature of the accident/trauma/disease. My shrapnel wound caused a great deal of damage, and my ocularist has always said that is why I don't have a lot of movement. The main thing, as Chris said, is that you're healthy. Anything above and beyond that is just extra-good. Your prosthetic will move as much as it's going to move, whether you're depressed about it or not. That has been my big lesson: Acceptance—learned over many years.

The only thing that really mattered to me that was impacted by the lack of movement in my right eye was my work as an actor. I'm a good actor, with many roles as a "child actor" but as I got older, and looking "beautiful" became important, it became clear that the lack of movement in my eye would be an issue. I was always so concerned about the eye movement that my work became self-conscious and not very good. Luckily, I'm a theatre scholar, designer and stage director, so I've made a career as a teacher and professor, and have not missed the acting. When I was in my late 20s, after a number of years as a high school Drama teacher, I was in grad school for an MFA in Theatre Directing and I had to take acting class with all these Masters' in Acting students. It was crazy-making enough being in class with these really good actors, let alone worrying about my damned eye! Since I'd already moved beyond wanting to be an actor, I just approached the whole thing with an attitude of "what the hell!" Turns out, my work was very good, I wasn't afraid and my fellow students found ways to work around my eye. That was about 12 years ago. Now that I'm far too old to be the "ingénue" and have made peace (usually) with the whole "eye thing" I may do some work on the acting thing again.

Worrying about something you can't change just makes you worried. Acceptance is a very hard state of mind to reach. I hope you, Starter, and the rest of us too, find ways to not waste precious life driving ourselves crazy about what can't be helped. Love and hugs to all,—*Alicia*

◆   ◆   ◆

I am in need of support from others who wear a prosthesis and have learned to deal with accepting the way it looks in darker lit restaurants etc. when the pupil doesn't dilate with the other one and having the confidence to look people, especially dates, in the eyes during close up one on one conversations. This is tough! I feel so self conscious about my appearance! Please write me. Friends and family and other people who do not wear a prosthesis have no idea what this is like! I need to talk to someone who does. I know that we will see "eye to eye". LOL—*Alice*

Hey guys, after going through a suicidal mode yesterday, I feel better today! I come up with something that may sound retarded, but in theory it's sound! If you work your arms, they get bigger and stronger, this should also work with your eye muscles! Imagine not just moving it around, but looking in one direction with some strain to tax the muscle! In theory this should strengthen the muscle and therefore increase movement, at least to some degree! I am going to pioneer this theory, and if it can be done, it will be done! Sounds stupid huh, well, I know, but so is suicide! So I'm off to do this!—*Jarrod*

my ocularist did mention this some time ago but she thought that the reality of someone putting in the right amount of effort regularly enough to make a difference was unlikely. But if you're well motivated, give it a go.—*Chil*

That particular ocularist doesn't know Jarrod! I will do this, and will succeed if can be done! It's a matter of everything to me! My motivation to increase the movement of my eye exceeds that of the sex drive of an Angus bull in mating season! If this does work, I can bring hope to lots of people unsatisfied with the movement of their prosthesis! Wish me luck. I just need to figure out how often I should do this for, I will do some research.—*Jarrod*

I always wondered what would happen if you had a laser installed in the glass eye, and then you spent time trying to manipulate your muscles to try to get the laser pointer to where you wanted it to go on a wall, or to track your normal eyesight. Personally, I think that with practice you could probably teach the muscles to track the movement of your remaining eye.—*Jay*

I have been doing my eye exercises of only a few days now, and I can tell a big difference it the movement of my implant! I say it is about 80 percent as good as that guys in that link I posted in my last thread! All I do is throughout the day, look around in every direction, roll my eyes in circles, then I will look in one direction and hold it with slight strain for maybe ten to 20 seconds! I do this until all directions are covered, and I wait a few hours and do it again! I would really recommend trying this guys! It has saved me lots of heartache! I urge anyone here who desires improvement in the movement of their eye, to do so! It is moving so good now, I can hear and feel the implant raking against the bone in my socket, and it's making a grinding noise! Hell, I can lay my finger on my eye lid, and press against the implant and move my eyes, and my hand starts shooting side to side! Damn! It works! Engage in these exercises immediately! To add, I'm doing these exercises with no prosthesis!—*Jarrod*

Gosh, I am so happy for you. I guess it does not help to try it. I don't like the movement of my eye. When I look to either side I look like I am cross eyed, I hate that. I have to remember to move my head when looking side to side, that way it is a little better. And when I look up, forget it, my eye just looks straight ahead. I guess I am stuck this way, I don't really want the peg. Oh well, at least I can see. God Bless You, and good luck to you. I will try what you are talking about and get back to you in a week or so.—*Anon*

So far I have been improving the movement of my implant, and it seems to be doing quite well, of course it doesn't match the movement of my other eye, but improvement is improvement! Here is just a wild thought, I wonder if they can transplant extra ocular muscles? Imagine if you could get brand new ones implanted and they work just like your other eye, I bet if can done! I bet it has been done as well, I'm going to do some research.—*Jarrod*

Hey, Jarrod! Glad to hear you're doing well. Sounds good about the movement. I'm happy for you, especially being that I have ZERO movement and no chance of ever having any. I'm not bitter though (do I sound bitter? Lol). It would be interesting to check if there's any research being done pertaining to eye loss. I'm sure that they've come a long way, but we never hear about any miracle eye replacement surgery or even eye muscle surgery. Let us know what you discover! Take care. Glad to see you posting and feeling well! Keep up the good work!—*Chris*

◆ ◆ ◆

I was wondering if we could start a thread containing tips on improving the illusion to others. I am new at this, and it doesn't seem that it is going to work. How do you guys create the illusion so other people have a hard time knowing that one of your eyes is not real? I feel like I am punishing my good eye by not moving it. Instead I move my head from side to side, and left and right. It takes a lot of work, and my good eye becomes tired. I tried practicing in front of my web cam, but maybe it doesn't look right because I all ready know. How do you guys do it?—*Michael*

Michael, yes, we turn our heads quite a bit. Does your prosthesis move at all? I think that most people's do. Mine doesn't—at all. I also have tinted prescription eyeglasses that I wear, and that helps. Some people have commented that they didn't even know I had a prosthesis until I told them. We assume that everyone is zeroing in on our flaws, when in reality they're too busy thinking about themselves. Try not to worry so much. Many people have differences in their eyes, and it's not due to a prosthesis! Good luck!—*Anon*

Michael, I agree that head movement probably is most effective for me. I've worn a prosthesis for 18 years and when I had my second implant surgery this summer everyone though I was getting the Lasik surgery so I could where contacts—hardly any of my friends knew. However, I've had quite a few problems with the fit of my new eye.

I'm not sure if you have good lid movement but I learned to use my lids to create an 'illusion'. As far as the movement of my eye, I also have minimal movement due to the treatment of my retinoblastoma. But most people just thought my eye was a little lazy.—*Pearl*

Tips on building the illusion eh? I'm the master of that aspect of the whole monocular world! (sarcasm of course) All the ideas that everyone has offered are great, and that is what I would suggest to anyone. But, if your wondering what I do, my approach is a little different! I simply where shades so dark, no one would know anything different! No one can make fun of my eye, they may make fun of me wearing shades all the time, but who gives a rats ass. I don't even wear a prosthesis, just the mental picture of one of my eyes not looking in the correct direction angers me to the point of suicide, so this is my illusion! It's very effective if all else fails. I'm currently conducting exercises to increase the movement of my implant, it seems to be having an effect. Peace to you, and may you find comfort in whatever road you choose my friend.—*Jarrod*

One of the most important things we can do to create and maintain the "illusion" surrounding our prosthetics is to look people right in the eyes, hold your head up proudly and live without fear about it. I've been dealing with "eye issues" intensely for fourteen months, since having my implant redone. I've had my eye since I was seven and I'm now 42. I've worked with the same faculty since 1990 as their grad student and as a colleague. And I was totally amazed that almost all these people had no idea about my eye. Some were very confused when I emailed them about the possibility of missing some of the start of the semester last year. "Artificial eye?" "Implant?" "What?"

My eye has never moved more than a little bit, I've never concentrated on moving only my head. My glasses never had darkened lenses until last year, when I had to teach a semester with no eye at all, wearing a patch. People are not observant. When I take off my darkened glasses now, when someone asks to see "the new eye" hardly anyone notices that the inside corner is sewn closed. It's ALL I can see. But my dear friends who tell me the truth say they can see it, but just don't notice. I've been wearing my non-dark glasses. I've started putting on face makeup again. My "rebuild" is very easily irritated, so I rarely wear eye makeup.

I've thought for so long that when people noticed my eye they would judge me. Freak. Defective. The little kids in school were frequently cruel. What I've learned for sure is that adults for the most part either don't notice or do notice and realize something terrible happened and are sympathetic. Any adult who would mock any of us over a result of our personal tragedy can kiss my ass. I feel as if I've been hiding for over a year. I don't like it. I am not "less than." I choose to own my experience. It is hard and it is scary. There are worse things that could have happened to me, sure, but this is enough. And I will handle it. And I am choosing daily to handle it with grace. I will not hide anymore. Take good care. Be courageous. With fierce love—*Alicia*

All right, Alicia! You go, girl! I'm with you on many of the points you bring up. I'm often amazed that people don't notice any difference between my eyes. It used to really freak me out, when several months after my surgery, with my prosthesis nearly sunken into my skull, that people (even friends and family) would say they couldn't see what I was so concerned about! How could they not see this! To my mind, they weren't being kind by saying that. I needed them to validate how I felt, not dismiss it.

Even though I'm 12 years down this road, I'm still sensitive about how I look, despite the fact that I have an excellent prosthesis, and get great movement with the peg. Maybe it's our perspective, since we see the world through only one eye and have this dark hole on the other side. I can't ever forget I have only one eye, from the moment I wake up to the moment I go to sleep, my world is perceived this way. There, I've said my piece!—*Nancy*

Hi Guys. Actually I'm not sure how to act or what to think. This is all new to me. Not even three months. I am at the starting point, and of course the way I am perceived to others is important. Especially for my job. People all around work have passed the word around to everyone, and also to other people from my old jobs. I feel like I am the main attraction at the circus. I have not been back to work yet, because I am looking at more surgeries. I think I have dealt with this pretty good for only 2 ½ months. And I can relate to what Nancy said about knowing from the moment you wake up. The only sad part for me is that I dream that I am, and can use both eyes. But when I wake up. The reality sets in. Sometimes before I go to bed, I hope and pray that when I wake up this will have been a bad nightmare, or a really lousy dream. But when I do awake, I am of course reminded of it. Regards,—*Michael*

Michael, I wish their was some way to ease your pain. If I could snap my fingers and fix you, I would, along with everyone else here and myself, but technology is advancing, and maybe one day they can just grow new eyes!

I know what you mean about the dreaming, I used to do that, but after a while that goes away. We all have our methods of dealing with and blending in with everyone else, my way is the chicken shit way, hiding behind dark glasses, hell I don't even wear a glass eye anymore! Pray about it and find your best way to cope. I'm not a religious person, but I do have my own relationship with the Almighty, and I believe one day, we will all have both our eyes back! If I'm wrong, we'll simply cease to exist, and it won't matter anyway. I'm surprised that I feel God would accept me, I mean, I don't live the best, and I curse like sailor, but the God I believe in will one day fix me, whether it be here or in another existence.—*Jarrod*

After also having my prosthesis for 18 years, I, too am constantly amazed that friends and family tell me they don't see a difference and I, too often wonder if they are being kind because if I see the difference, everyone else must, also. I guess I'm wrong on that one. I guess I move my head a lot and just don't realize I'm doing it anymore and I do try to keep eye contact with whoever I'm speaking with. I do have one friend who said that they saw something different with my eyes, but thought that my left eye was just a lazy eye. It turns out that this friend worked in the optical field and was more attune to people's eyes.—*Danielle*

♦ ♦ ♦

I have had a glass eye for about 30 years. I received it at age 8. Back then eye used to move better in socket than it does now. Seems it is way more noticeable now as I get older. Certain movements makes it so obvious. Has this happened to anybody? I had the best doctor since 8, but unfortunately he passed away a couple of years ago and I have not found one to replace him. Always wondered if as you get older should the eye be replaced?—*Curious*

Hi there, I am new here. My ocularist told me that the eye should be replaced about every 5 years, and polished every year. I had had mine for just about a year now, and it is ready for a polishing. I think I need to have mine rebuilt because it does not seem to fit as well as it did when it was first put in. This is a very informative place to visit. Thanks for reading this, and have a great day.—*Emily*

MESSAGES REGARDING PEGS

Jay, Great site! I lost my right eye in late 94 at the age of 28 as the result of a childhood accident. It is good to hear others perspective. I had the coral implant put in when I lost my eye, but I never had the stud installed for complete motility. I'm considering it now, but would like others experience before I do, did you have this done or do you know anyone who did? Thanks,—*Larry*

DO any of you have the center peg? My doc says that after the peg is installed- (in a year)-that I will have about 100% mobility. Is this true?—*Anon*

I have a peg in my implant, but I wouldn't say it gives me 100% mobility. I do get a lot more movement with it, though. In fact, there is so much movement, and it looks so natural, that my doctors made a video of it to show other patients what they could expect.

One word of advice—ask your doctor about getting a sleeved peg. The first peg I got was not sleeved and after about a year it started to be pushed forward and out. It was replaced with the sleeved peg, and I haven't had any problems with it. I was one of the first patients to get the sleeve, which was new back in 1992. I would recommend the peg to anyone thinking about it. Good luck!—*Nancy*

I have an appointment next week to get the peg. It's been 1 year for me, and although I do get pretty good movement, I want the peg anyway. I will keep you posted. Thanks for the info on the "sleeve", I will definitely ask about that when I go in.—*Roadrunner*

Hey, guys, concerning that "peg", do you need a whole new implant? Is that peg attached to the coral implant? I've had the same silicone beads implant for 25 years, and I'm SURE that my doc would NEVER allow me to voluntarily opt for removing it (I reject nearly everything and I'll allergic to so much). So, any info on this peg would be GREATLY appreciated! I have ZERO movement, BTW. Thanks!—*Chris*

The way I understand, the peg is inserted into the coral implant after about a year. I guess they drill through the eye muscles that are wrapped around the implant. I've only had my implant since December, so that's about all I know about it so far. As far as the method of actually attaching it to the coral I have no idea. My question is this: Once the peg is inserted, doesn't that make it impossible to remove the prosthesis for cleaning? If anyone can shed some light on this, it would be greatly appreciated.—*j6044*

Hey guys, I hope I can shed a little more light on getting the peg, and how it works. This may be more information than you want, but it's how mine was done. I lost my eye in August of 1992. By the end of December of '92, the implant was vacularized, so I had the peg put in. I was taken to the operating room, given what I guess you could call "twilight" anesthesia, where you're not knocked out like general anesthesia, but you don't remember anything. The doctor then drilled a hole in the center of the implant and inserted the peg. Believe it or not, they used a regular power drill. The next step was to go back to the ocularist to have my prosthesis adapted for the peg. All he had to do was drill a small hole in the back of it to accommodate the peg. It's a little tricky to do, because the hole in the back must be positioned so that when the prosthesis sits on it, the eye is looking straight.

After awhile, the peg started to extrude, or be forced out. The solution was to get the sleeved peg. They tried to do it in the doctor's office (I won't tell you the details of this!) but were unsuccessful. So it was back to the operating room for another quick drill, and the new sleeve and peg were in. Having the peg makes no difference in removing your prosthesis. It pops out just as easily. The only difference is putting it back in, as you have to get it on to the peg, but it just naturally seems to do that.

Again, I have had such good results from the peg that I would really encourage anyone to consider it. My eye movement is so natural now that it fools everyone. The doctors were so pleased with the results that they took lots of pictures, and even a video, to show how good it looks. Every time I went back to Wills for follow-up, all of the residents were called in to see it.—*Nancy*

I don't have the peg, and my eye barely moves any at all, would the peg help me? Mine doesn't seem to move as good as other peoples for some reason. I try to strengthen my muscles by moving my eyes around a lot when I'm by myself, but I haven't really noticed any difference. Is there anyone else in here, who hardly had any movement to begin with, and the peg helps pretty good?—*Jarrod*

◆ ◆ ◆

I was told that the peg method caused more infections does any one have this and what do you think?—*Bea*

I was thinking about getting the peg, but my ocularist told me that it is more trouble than it is worth. So many people have a lot of trouble with it. My eye doesn't move perfectly, but I don't need anymore problems with my eye. So, I am taking his advise and forgo the peg. I just have to get used to this eye. Actually it looks much better than my ugly real eye, so no more complaining from me. At least it is the same color as my good eye.—*Anon*

Bea, I've had the peg for almost 12 yrs now. It was put in about 6 months after I lost my eye. It was pretty new back then. In fact, I was one of the first people to get the sleeved peg. The first peg I got had to be replaced because it started to push out. Since I've had the sleeved peg, I've never had a problem. I get excellent movement with the peg and, personally, couldn't imagine not having it.—*Nancy*

◆ ◆ ◆

Hey friends, when I put my finger on my eye lid, and move my eyes around, and feel the implant move, it doesn't seem to move that much. I was just wondering if I get the peg, if my eye would move more than what it feels like it moves? Maybe one of you guys could test this out for me? Thanks.—*Jarrod*

Yes, your eye will move more than it seems to be moving now, without the peg. It has something to do with the peg projecting the movement of the implant. It's physics, or something! When are you scheduled to get the peg? How have you been feeling about things in general? Hope all is well.—*Nancy*

◆ ◆ ◆

Hi everyone, I had an artificial eye put in place of my blind eye in March. I am not very happy with the movement. I was thinking of getting the peg. I don't know too much about it, but my doctor said he does not recommend it. He says it causes a lot of problems. Can I please have some feedback about the peg from people that like it and from ones that don't like it. Do you really get more movement with it, and is it worth all the trouble to get it? I should probably be happy with the movement I have now. At least I don't have the terrible pain I used to have in that eye before my operation. But, I guess I just want to look "normal" too. When I look to the right and left I look like I am crossed eyed. Makes me very self conscious, and looking up freaks me out. Thanks for listening,—*Anon*

Maybe I can help you out here. I'm currently in a similar situation, my eye didn't move very much, but my implant has decent movement. My eye is currently in a thousand pieces, due to a shotgun blast administered by yours truly, I become very angry, very fast when it comes to slacking movement in prosthetic eyes! But I figure, if your implant moves in a superior fashion to the prosthetic, then logically, the movement of the implant should be transferred to the prosthetic, increasing the movement! I'm going to get a new eye made after I get the peg, which I'm going to talk to the doctor on the 1st to set up an appointment for the procedure! I'm confident the movement will increase to the maximum amount of movement my implant has, and yours. To heck with the risks of infection, at least in my case, but if the infection concerns you, then put a lot of thought into your decision! I'm going to do it, the risks are low and I think the success will be well worth the while! I support you in whatever you decide! The others and I are here for your support!—*Jarrod*

I'm a big supporter of the peg. I got mine as soon as it was medically feasible, about six months after I lost my eye, which was 12 yrs ago. I have been extremely happy with mine and can't imagine not having it. Check out the link that Jarrod provided in another post, if you haven't already. And don't let your doctor discourage you. I think the benefits of having the peg far outweigh any of the risks. As Jarrod said, we are all here to help and support you with whatever decision you make. Good luck and best wishes to you,—*Nancy*

Hi, thank you Jarrod and Nancy for answering my post. This is a very hard decision for me to make. I have a few months before I see my doctor again. I hope I will be able to make up my mind then. It sort of sounds weird to have a metal peg in my eye, it sounds like that would be very uncomfortable. We were also told as kids to be careful not to get anything in our eyes, now I am thinking about getting a metal peg in my eye. I guess when you get used to it, it doesn't hurt anymore. I wish I knew how much movement I will get with it, and then if I didn't like it, I could get it taken back out. The insurance paid for my operation and artificial eye, but it will not pay for the peg because it is cosmetic. Well, thanks again for listening.—*Anon*

In a best case scenario, this is what will occur with the peg, but I don't know anyone that has movement this good http://www.texaseyeplastics.com/ enucleation.htm scroll to bottom of the page. Remove your prosthesis, and put your finger on your eye, and look around. You should be able to feel the movement in your eye, and get a better idea! If that isn't enough, put your finger on your eyelid of your good eye and move it around, and compare the movement of both to access the movement ratio between the two. Peace.—*Jarrod*

Just to reassure you, the peg doesn't hurt at all. You can't feel it. And there was only minimal discomfort from the procedure. I know that now they are using a titanium peg. They were just starting to do the peg when I got mine and it's plastic. My doctor was so pleased with the resulting movement that they did a video tape of me showing how well my prosthesis moves. Don't try to make a decision about it now. We will be here to support you and answer any questions that come to your mind.—*Nancy*

◆ ◆ ◆

Hello everyone! I have been reading posts on this board for some time and thought I'd finally say hi to everyone! I am scheduled to have a "modified enucleation" on Feb 16th. By modified I mean that my doctor is going to only leave the part of the eye that has the muscles attached, but the rest will be implant. He says that this will give me better movement. Needless to say, I'm very nervous.

The short version of my story is that I had a piece of roofing tile thrown into my left eye when I was six years old (I'm 31 now), cutting the cornea out. They saved it, but it is pretty scarred and, since I developed traumatic glaucoma in it shortly after, it's been painful and swollen for most of my life. I'm excited at the prospect of no longer having the pain, irritation, and constant questions from strangers, but I am also very scared. I'm used to how I look.

I am interested in getting the peg eventually, but my dr. and ocularist are both very much against it. They both tell me that risk of infection is high and that sometimes the peg causes movement to be "too good," which I guess means that the sides of the prosthetic can pop out when moving the eye side to side. I'm wondering if anyone else has been told this or has been discouraged by their doctor regarding the peg. Thanks for any advice/support!—*Marsey*

Marsey, Welcome to the board. There are many fantastic and compassionate people here. Everyone understands. I too was told, by my surgeon, not to get a peg for similar reasons. My prosthesis, without a peg, moves very well. It can't move to the extremes but I am satisfied. I recently hired a new employee and after 2 interviews, I had to tell him that I lost an eye to cancer. He never noticed. Therefore I'd say it looks natural. All will go well with your procedure. Take care & God bless.—*Rich*

I too had asked my surgeon and my ocularist about the post and they were not keen on it. My surgeon states that sometimes scar tissue can grow around it and therefore I would require further surgeries as it would become uncomfortable and not fit properly. I work in the public sector and most people do not even notice my "Fake eye". Although sometimes I get funny looks if I am looking down at a document and look up from there, my eye moves great from side to side but up and down is another story all together. I have to admit that I still don't feel real comfortable with how I look. I can count the times I have put on make up in the last 5 years. I never wore much as I always felt I only needed a little to enhance them and my ex-husband always told me I had the most beautiful eyes! After all the insurance money was gone and I paid off his student loans he found he was having much more fun with his blonde haired 2-eyed, blue eyed assistant! Am I bitter? You bet, but life goes on and I am coping! I have met someone nice and things may progress! Sorry to go on here, sometimes I just need to vent!—*Ski*

Ski, funny, right before my accident, the "coolest" girl in my school (whom I was trying to be friends with) gave me the biggest compliment. She said, "You have the most beautiful eyes. They're your best feature", then, BOOM, it happened. Sorry about your situation with your ex. Although I DOUBT his being so lame had anything to do with your eye, right? Sorry you had to experience that!

As far as makeup, I stayed away from it, figuring it would only make my eyes look more different. It took an understanding, experienced ocularist to show me how to try using eye makeup, and to this day I'm never without it! One more thing—at least your prosthesis has SOME movement. Mine does not move an inch—not left, not right, certainly not up nor down. I've learned to TRY to be conscious of it and accommodating myself by moving my head more, but then once in a while I'll see pictures of myself with my eyes looking in two different directions, or the up/down thing you said, and it makes me want to crawl away and hide. Guess it's hard to accept sometimes.—*Chris*

I don't have the peg, and my eye barely moves any at all, would the peg help me? Mine doesn't seem to move as good as other peoples for some reason. I try to strengthen my muscles by moving my eyes around a lot when I'm by myself, but I haven't really noticed any difference. Is there anyone else in here, who hardly had any movement to begin with, and the peg made a difference in there eye movement? I guess the question is, my implant does move some, and the peg would have to increase the movement, at least a little right? Someone please help.—*Jarrod*

◆　　◆　　◆

Ok, I just visited the doctor who installed the coral implant back in July. He had me look in all directions, and he said your eye movement is as good as planned. Then he had me remove my prosthesis and he said the implant moves pretty good, considering the damage done by my accident. He said the movement wasn't being transferred well from the implant to the prosthesis. He also stated the reason was my bones were broken so badly that the implant wasn't far enough forward and therefore they had to make the prosthesis really thick thus, less movement. He told me that I could have the implant moved forward and my prosthesis thinned down and ad a peg to the prosthesis, and I would get about 30 or 40 percent better movement. Should I undergo this surgery? Would any of you? He said the peg would not help me in the current situation. I wish both my eyes did this.—*Jarrod*

Jarrod, interesting questions. Would I undergo that surgery with the hopes of my eye movement improving 30-40%? Heck, yeah! I have ZERO movement now, and if the surgery wouldn't be too bad, I'd certainly sign up to do it! It all depends on how long the surgery would be; what the surgery would entail; how long recovery would be; what exactly would be involved, etc. If you're talking about a pretty quick recovery and then just getting the prosthesis re-done, yup, I'd do it!

You know what? Take your time and think about it. Think it over. Do you want to take that recovery period and go through all of that? It's totally up to you. If he's not rushing you into surgery, I'd think it over for a while! Good luck with your decision and let us know how it goes!—*Chris*

Jarrod, I am a big supporter of the peg because mine works so wonderfully. I sometimes hesitate to respond to posts like yours, because I am so pro-peg. I realize, though, that everyone has their own ideas, and I respect that. I'll borrow a phrase from Dr. Phil—"Never substitute my opinion for your own."

That being said, it sounds like your problem is very similar to mine when I first got my implant. It looked sunken into the socket, and I was very self conscious of it. The first attempt to fix it was to build up the prosthesis, like you had done, with the same result you have. I then went to a plastic surgeon who specializes in eyes and she recommended a floor implant for the socket. The implant is of the same coral material and is kind of packed on the floor of the socket and pushes the ball implant forward. It worked perfectly. I don't know what your doctor is suggesting for you, but this is what worked for me.

I then had the peg put in. I had to wait for the swelling to go down so that the peg could be correctly placed. I would also recommend the sleeved peg, because the first one I got wasn't and in time, it started to push out. Since having the sleeved peg, I have had absolutely no problems with it. And I've had it for 10 years. And the movement of my prosthesis is very natural looking. I don't think I could do anything more to improve how it looks and moves. Good luck to you,—*Nancy*

Jarrod, I just went to the eye guy this week, the same thing, wanting the post. He told me the same thing as you. He said my prosthetic was too far back, and the peg wouldn't work well. He suggested building up from the back, I think he called it a sled. But in all honesty, he didn't sound really like he was recommending this, just that these surgeries were available to me. My eye does have fair amount of movement. I left the office feeling a little down, but have decided not to have the surgery at this time. He said that in years to come, the eye could sink further back, then it might be more worth my while to get the sled thing. Good luck.—*Roadrunner*

Hey Nancy, how was the movement before you got the peg, and how is it now? The thing is, the up and down movement of my implant, isn't that good, and when I try to see the implant moving in the mirror, it doesn't seem to move that much, but it seems to move good when I place my finger on it.—*Jarrod*

Hi Jarrod, as I remember (I lost my eye 12 yrs ago and got the peg about 6 months afterward, so I didn't have a lot of time without it) the movement of my eye without the peg was so-so. It wasn't enough to satisfy me, but I was told by my ocularist and doctors that it was typical. After the peg, I'd have to say that the movement got back to about 75% of normal. In fact, whenever I go for a checkup to either the doctor or ocularist, they comment about how good it moves.—*Nancy*

◆ ◆ ◆

Hello there, I was wondering if there is anyone from Australia here who has a coral implant with a peg? I am planning to have one (peg) and would love to talk to someone how it looks, works etc. Please feel free to e-mail me on. Thanks guys.—*Anna*

I am wondering about the peg too. My movement is pretty good except when I look to the sides. Everyone told me that the peg would improve that, but my Dr. said it is not worth the trouble. He said people with the peg have problems with infections. The ocularist (spelled wrong) said the same thing. I would love better movement, but am afraid to try it since I can't go back. I wonder how bad the operation is. I wish I knew someone with it and would tell me all about it, the good and the bad. Need to hear both sides of the story.—*Anon*

I have had the peg for many years and can't imagine not having it! The movement of my prosthesis is almost "natural."—*Nancy*

Hi guys, getting the peg is only an option if you have an HA (Coral) or Med-Pore implant. And, yes, there is a much higher risk of infection/exposure associated with these types of implants, not to mention they are much more expensive (as opposed to an acrylic sphere). If they do have that type of implant, many patients opt not to get drilled for the peg simply because their movement is fine with out it. Other factors include cost (titanium pegs can cost $150.00 or so and those little buggers are easy to lose! LOL). Some people have a problem with the "clicking" sound that may happen with the peg, and don't forget that not all eyes are created equal. Some shapes simply can't allow a peg hole due to size. These are just other factors that you, your doctor, and ocularist must consider. It simply is not a solution for every prosthetic wearer. Period. Get informed for YOUR particular situation. Good luck,—*Anon*

Very well said. I agree the peg isn't for everyone as circumstances vary. Titanium pegs weren't around when I got my peg in 1992. It's plastic, and has a sleeve. The first one I got did not have a sleeve, and after about six months, it began to be pushed forward. Then I got the sleeved peg and have had not problems since. It also requires a good ocular plastic surgeon, which I had, to place the peg correctly. It's a little tricky getting it right.—*Nancy*

◆ ◆ ◆

I know it's probably a stupid question, but I wonder if there is any doctor who can perform surgery and increase eye movement? Like surgery on the muscles? There has to be, I mean doctors work on muscles all the time!—*Jarrod*

I don't think the muscles are the problem. My (removed) eye moves perfectly all the way around. Problem is that the artificial eye has edges that "bump" into obstacles it cannot rotate under (eye socket) like a real eye does and therefore won't turn further. Up and down looks great, to the left looks great but "looking" towards my nose is a lot less perfect. I am happy with my artificial eye though. I just turn my head more instead of just moving the eyes. Hugs,—*Willeke*

I did hear something about a new prosthetic eye that uses magnets behind it. When your transplant moves, the magnets complete the movement cycle. I just can't remember where I saw it though.—*Michael*

Hi, my muscles were attached the implant. I was told if I wanted more movement there is a new procedure out, but my doctor opted against it because it is a longer surgery process and in my case I had cancer and follow up appointments. It would be hard to gauge if the cancer ever came back to the socket. It's done in San Francisco and I'm sure other medical facilities. My doctor said he did it mostly on Movie Stars. I will try to find the correct name for you. If you are interested I could give you my doctor's name for a consult. Hugs,—*Sherri*

There is a way to get a little bit more movement and it is the peg. My doctor, however, suggested against it because it might complicate things in the eye. Also, the movement with the prosthesis is fair enough.—*Mike*

◆ ◆ ◆

Hi: Happy to have found this site as confusion has led to questions. Nov. 1 they will remove my left eye which has gradually gone totally blind since the radioactive plaque treatment nearly 6 years ago. But a change produced pressure headaches plus constant irritation, so I made what I hope is a good decision. The doctor says I am a good candidate for a magnetic implant which will control eye movement, if I understand correctly. I can find no info on this, so I turn to you folks with the hope that someone either knows about this or can tell me where I can learn more. Thanks much. ~*Borisa*

I haven't heard of anyone having one of those for a while but if you explore a website something like http://www.ioi.com you will see how implants in general work. With a magnetic sort a magnet is used to keep the prosthesis 'stuck' to the implant so that the eye tracks along with it. I couldn't find much about it except this. http://www.porexsurgical.com/english/surgical/sprodAttractor.asp~ *Marmalade*

◆ ◆ ◆

I know my prosthesis will never move that good, even with the peg, because I can look at the movement of me implant and from what I can tell, it only moves about half that good, but that's not bad I guess. That is just one lucky man in terms of prosthesis movement!—*Jarrod*

I wonder if there are more people out there who are reading your ongoing chats—I haven't been able to post—I guess this is another test to see if it works—saw the article about the prosthesis/movement on that man—looks good, do a lot of you have the peg? Was that an option after a certain amount of time with the prosthesis? My ocularist hasn't mentioned the peg to me. I wonder what the criteria is to get a peg?—*Loralsar*

Loralsar, I believe that your ophthalmologist would be the one to suggest the peg method. *I* am not a candidate, since I've rejected implants and I'm pretty blessed to still have the same implant for over 20 years now (finally stumbled on the right doctor with the right implant for me!). Anyway, they usually have pamphlets on the peg there. Talk it over with your doctor. I'm glad that you get something out of reading this board. There are lots of people here with helpful words of encouragement.—*Chris*

◆ ◆ ◆

Well, I have a surgery coming up the thirty-first of this month! They have to move my implant further forward and then give me the peg. The doctor said I would probably get 30 to 40 percent more movement, which is good because my eye barely moves at all now. I see people every great once in a while that have glass eyes, and I can tell because I know how to spot them, and to me it just looks horrible! They always look cross eyed or something! I hate it, and I think, do I look like that too? I hope not! Cause if I did, I would rather just be dead! It's not me, I was not born this way, and I hate it more and more each day! I look at pictures of me with to eyes, both 20/20, and very healthy, and then I just get more sad! I don't feel like me, (Jarrod) anymore, I think I am just going to change my name and be someone else, cause it is not me. Does anyone else feel this way? If I am not any more happy after this surgery, and believe I will just pray for death. I'm sick of this!—*Jarrod*

Jarrod, hang in there, buddy. Good luck with your surgery. I have a peg and I'm extremely pleased with the amount of movement I get with it. I don't know how long it's been since you lost your eye, but I can understand how you feel that it never ends. There always seems to be something you have to deal, or cope, with. And now there is this additional surgery and you're wondering "What next?" You get on this medical merry-go-round and you just want it all to stop.

This is a process you have to go through, and the only thing you can do is take it one step, one day, at a time. We are all here to help and support you. It will get better, trust me. I was in exactly the same place you are now, and I'm still here. Lean on us, Jarrod. We will get you through this.—*Nancy*

Jarrod, good luck with the surgery. Sounds exciting at the prospect of having 30-40% more movement. I have ZERO movement and no chance of it changing, but I want to tell you that you're more than the sum of your prosthesis. You'll be affected every once in a while, but hopefully you'll get past it, like we all do. We are all here to support each other through the tough times (and to share in the good times), so please don't say that life isn't worth living if your eye doesn't look good. Everything will get better, and you'll see that you are much more important than how your eye appears. Take care and let us know how you do with the surgery.—*Chris*

Thank you guys for your support, it does help me. I just hate my prosthesis so bad, I feel like slinging it far as I can or smashing it with a hammer, but it cost to much to destroy it like that. The doctor told me, I may get 30 to 40 percent better movement, but there is the small chance movement could be lost, and knowing my luck. If I get better movement, then, I believe I can abandon the suicidal thoughts, and if I lose movement, I'm just screwed I guess! I think it would be wonderful to sit and talk to someone in person that has a prosthesis, but I know not anyone personally in my life that has one. I wish we all could have a face to face conversation with each other, all of us here on the board. Maybe one day, we could arrange such a meeting, I know it would help me, and I'm sure it would help everyone else just as much. Thank you all for your support.—*Jarrod*

Greetings everyone, I'm back to this computer to let everyone know how I'm doing. Well, today is the first day I have not had to take a pain pill, which is good, and it's the first day I have came from my grandmothers (where I stay when I'm sick) to back to my own home, where this computer is. I tell you, this surgery was the worst pain I have ever experienced! Bar none! All my surgeries combined and all the pain accumulated in my entire life time doesn't add up to the pain I went though Wednesday! The doctor said he had to move around implants that were already in there, work on a few of them, put a new implant in and some screws! I know this much, if he said he could do this surgery again and give me 100% movement, I don't think I would go through the hideous torture to do it, but then again, I don't know. I had some kind of allergic reaction to a medicine they gave, that I told them I was allergic to, and I almost killed over, I threw my guts up four or five times, with this freshly worked on eye, and strained it even more, and that really hurt. So I hope this all works out good for me, cause I have went through pure hell so far. Well, I will go for now, I'll write back again soon.—*Jarrod*

8

Removal and Cleaning of Your New Eye

Do you have to take your new eye out every night? Of course not! It is recommended that you take your new eye out and wash it with regular soap and water about once every couple of weeks, though I almost never take mine out except for semi-annual cleanings at my ocularist.

The point of cleaning the prosthesis is simply to remove enzymes and such which may build up on it. At any rate, the care of your eye isn't a daily thing or even a weekly thing unless you want it to be, and (believe it or not) you'll soon almost forget that you have the darn thing in there!

Another issue that everyone with a fake eye has is that it will generate matter. So long as the matter is white, there is nothing to worry about. But if the matter turns yellow or mass amounts of it begins to be produced, it may be a sign of an infection within the socket.

LETTERS AND E-MAILS

Hi—What a neat web site—I'm sure it will be of real comfort to a bunch of people who will lose an eye in the future. I lost my left eye in 1981 (detached retina—four unsuccessful operations) and haven't looked back since. I take my ocular prosthesis out every night and wash it with soap and water once a week. After almost 20 years it's still working great.—*Patrick*

Your website is EXACTLY what I wanted to find! I have put off having the prosthesis done for many years due to doubt, but within 5 minutes of reading your site I had the answers I needed; specifically about removal and cleaning, which I was VERY uncomfortable with. I'm much reassured now. Thank you SO MUCH for the time and effort. As a long-term insulin-dependent diabetic, I have found the web and sites like yours to be the answer not only to a million questions, but also a million prayers. Thank you so much for this!—*Laurel*

Hi, I've had my fake eye now for a little over a year and I keep having a problem with it getting a film on it making it look dull. My ocularist says it's a protein that my body makes and there's not much I can do about it. He gave me a lubricant called Silo something but, that seems to make it feel even more gummy. Any ideas? I clean it with baby shampoo and polish it every once in awhile with crest toothpaste but, it comes back quickly.—*Mary*

Hi: I have had an artificial eye for about three years. It has always goosed a little but the last couple of months it has been goosing a lot more and sometimes it is tinged with pink (blood) and yesterday, definitely blood. Have you had any such problems? Do you know of any other groups that may have had this problem? Nobody talks about the goop problem and the doctor seems to largely dismiss it. Thanks,—*Cecilia*

MESSAGES

I've been reading the new posts about watery, gooey, and other wise leaky eyes. My eye goes through cycles of behaving well and behaving quite badly. I've found that there can be a correlation between estrogen levels and the tendency to become irritated. For example, (boys, put your fingers in your ears and hum now) just prior to and during menses, it is more prone to irritation. This makes sense, because, for example, you skin is more prone to tenderness and irritation from waxing during the same time. (Now back to the uni-sex discussion.)

You can make your own saline swabs to carry around with you by cutting Q-tips to fit a film canister, putting a few in there and filling it part way with saline solution. How cool is that? Just be sure you clean it out and replace regularly.

If you wear makeup, you can do the same thing with OIL FREE makeup remover, Q-tips and film canister. If your eye is misbehaving it can mess up your mascara, etc, and having the swabs ready can help you with a quick clean up. It is best, of course, to not wear makeup when your eye is already irritated, but sometimes it happens after you've already made up. Did I say OIL FREE makeup remover? OIL FREE!

Anyway—regarding the title of this post—I've been a makeup artist for a long time and have used just about every kind of everything made in the last 20 years. I've kept track of how things affect my eye. It would be so cool to have a posting section to collect and share ideas specific to skin care and makeup. I did a special event for women with prostheses called "For Our Eyes Only." It was the only time I'd ever met other women in the same situation. It was so amazing. Love and love some more,—*Alicia*

Your ideas sound great! I always carry q-tips, mostly for too much moisture in my eye. It also just wipes away excess mascara. I haven't needed to use the oil-free eye makeup remover during the day only at night. I'm allergic and/or sensitive to lots of makeup, unfortunately, so I stick to what I know is good for me. I use Mary Kay mascara (or Estee Lauder), L'Oreal eyeliner, which is soft and easy on my eye, and I use Revlon creamy eye shadows. I do have one question for you. My eye is somewhat sunken in and I cannot fit an eyelash curler in there. Is there anything else I could use to curl my lashes? I had some lashes surgically implanted a while back, due to chunks of my eyelid missing, and now sometimes the lashes grow straight out instead of curling. Any advice would be appreciated!

Great post! I'm glad to see that we can share this type of info! Believe it or not, my first ocularist (a man) suggested that I don't even try to wear makeup as it would make the prosthesis look "more obvious". I then went to a female ocularist who took the time to show me how to shade, etc., to make it look the most natural. Thanks again!—*Chris*

◆ ◆ ◆

My eye also get discharge daily (not at night though). The only thing I'd suggest is to carry q-tips with you and swab the eye when it's watery. Since I cannot close my eye, it also gets things adhered to it, and I have to check it often and keep it free of debris with the q-tips. I never thought of sleeping with the glasses on! Maybe the eye isn't getting enough circulated air and the discharge builds up at night? You should ask your doctor or ocularist about this. Good luck and let us know how you do!—*Chris*

Hello! I also have a discharge problem. My doctor gave me an antibiotic cream, but that didn't work! nights are also the worst for me! It is very irritating! I am seeing my ocularist again on Tuesday, and I will write back if he has any new suggestions!—*Mindy*

This occurs at first simply because you have an alien object in your body and it will respond by producing "matter" to attack it. This will subside over time, usually after the first year. Afterwards, you'll only get significant "matter" if the prosthesis isn't regularly (at least every 6 months) cleaned by an ocularist to remove protein build-up. Simply removing the prosthesis and washing it with soap ever few weeks will slightly help, but won't totally get rid of the protein build-up.

Otherwise, to avoid the early-morning dryness, before you go to bed squirt a lot of saline into the socket and clean any matter that comes out with a swabby. Then, as another poster suggested, carry some swabbies around and clean the corners of the eye every time you go to the bathroom. Then, when you get up in the mornings, immediately squirt some more saline in there. The only thing I use with my eye is saline. I will not use lubricants, as I think those cause the socket to generate more "matter". Hope this helps.—*Jay*

Interesting! I was told (30 years ago) ONLY to use Dacriose solution in my eye. I use it every morning to clean my prosthesis. When I use saline solution, I get an awful migraine, as if the moisture balance is totally thrown off. The Dacriose, however, is MUCH more expensive than saline (it's now about $9 a bottle, which lasts a month). Anyone else only use Dacriose?—*Chris*

◆ ◆ ◆

My doc has me putting one drop of gentamycin in my prosthetic every day. He says if I do this for the rest of my life I will have less discharge and prevent infections. I have been doing this for 4-5 months now and it does seem to cut down on mucous accumulation. Good Luck,—*Anon*

I'm curious to see how many of us could close our prosthetic eye. I guess I'm one of the worst case scenarios. I can't close it, nor do I have ANY mobility. I'm curious about everyone else though. Please feel free to comment. BTW, since I can't "blink" or close that eye while I'm sleeping, I get particles adhering to the prosthesis pretty often. I don't get a lot of discharge just water sometimes.

And as far as cleaning and taking it out, as we discussed, I have been in the habit of taking it out every morning and thoroughly cleaning it with Dacriose (a sterile solution). I know that the new studies show that the more we take it out, the greater our chances are for infection, but my body is so used to this process that even skipping one day of cleaning drives me crazy.—*Chris*

The regular cleaning issue, for one. For a long time, when I'd go on a bout of "self improvement"—making sure to floss twice a day, getting my roots done, starting an exercise program (!) I would also go on a "clean it every week" or "every day" or whatever. My eye would always get irritated, and I would abandon the cleaning regime. Followed, of course, by all the other schemes. So, for me, it's better to leave it alone. We're all kind of solo trail-blazers, it seems, in how do to this "eye thing." Until now, for me anyway. SO glad I found this site.

I have a question about all this petroleum-based ointment I'm squeezing in there twice a day. Whenever I used mineral oil or Vaseline to remove eye makeup, the surface of my prosthesis gets all "draggy" then it gets irritated. At this point my eyelids are so pickled with petrolatum I wonder how long it will take to clear it out of there once I get my holy grail, er, I mean my NEW EYE! Any experience with this? Love and hugs—*Alicia*

◆   ◆   ◆

Hi everybody! I have some questions for you, and I sincerely hope that you will give my answers. Next week I'm going to get acrylic prosthesis, now I have glass one so I want to know what are differences between them. I'm wearing prosthesis since I was 4 years old, I had acrylic one but that was long time ago when I was child, last I think 7 or 8 years I have glass one (I'm 21 now). I only remember that I couldn't sleep with my acrylic eye and I had to take it out every night, that is my biggest fear because I don't want to sleep without an eye. Do you have to take your prosthesis out at night? How often do you clean acrylic prosthesis and how?

I clean my glass eye every day, mostly just with water and then I put some eye drops in eye socket(Tears Naturale, Refresh Contacts), every few days I wash prosthesis with soap, and 1 or 2 times a month I put my prosthesis in vinegar for 10 minutes and after that It feels so clean and fresh. But I don't like the thing that I have to use drops every single day, is it possible that that is just a habit how often do you use eye drops and which one? And for the end, how does acrylic eye move? Is it moving like your other eye or is it depend on what kind of accident did you have? Because I'm very satisfied with movement of my glass eye, but I have also seen people with glass eye that doesn't move a lot. My only problem with glass eye is that last year I had a little "accident" in my bathroom and I broke it, doctors made my new one but I still feel some kind of fear so I hope that I'll have more lucky with acrylic one.—*Dany*

Hi Dany, I think you'll be great with acrylic eye. One of the advantages is that it can be molded for an exact fit so it should move better than the glass one. It's also not so fragile. We only use glass for people with an allergy to acrylic. There's no need to take it out at night in fact I think you definitely shouldn't because it maintains the shape of the socket. Here in the UK I've never been recommended to use vinegar. It must be expensive to keep using the drops. My prosthesis maker gave me hard contact lense wetting solution but I don't use it often. Let us know how you get on. Regards—*Chil*

The most uncomfortable thing up until this summer has been when my Ocularist takes out the eye to polish it—the empty socket feeling just bothered me so much. I have learned that what I could never stand for just 20 minutes I've had to learn to live with for six weeks so far.

I have a dream of starting a non-profit foundation to help people who live in areas where eye-makers are scarce get time off work and transportation to good eye makers, financial help with the eye itself, and transport back home. Best wishes to all and thank you for all the wonderful sharing and writing that makes this such an incredible resource. Love and hugs—*Alicia*

As far as cleaning it, there are many different methods. I've been taking it out and cleaning it with Dacriose (a sterile solution) for 30 years. I clean the prosthesis, and put some drops in my socket. I've NEVER cleaned it any other way (with soap and water or vinegar), and never had a problem. The new "theory" with cleaning it is to only take it out and clean it once a week, but I can't get used to that. It's no big deal to clean it every morning for me, and I feel "fresher" that way. If you're not happy with your new prosthesis after a while, I'd try to find another ocularist too. Good luck!—*Chris*

◆ ◆ ◆

I've used Dacriose eye irrigant solution practically from the day I got my first prosthesis (nearly 30 years ago). It's a little costly (about $9.00/bottle), but it lasts about a month. I take out the prosthesis every morning and irrigate it (and my socket) with the solution, and pop the prosthesis back in (much like contact lenses). I rarely have a problem with the moisture balance in my eye.

You can find Dacriose at most pharmacies. Sometimes I have to ask them to order it, but they mostly keep it in stock. It's a 4 oz. bottle and on it, it says, "Dacriose sterile eye irrigating solution". It's in a blue and white package. Hope that helps! I know that people with "normal" eyes use it sometimes for eye emergencies and for eye comfort. I don't EVER use generic irrigating solution, as this one REALLY works for me! Good luck! If I could be of any more help, let me know!

I live in NY and we have rough winters occasionally, plus I sometimes travel to Western Canada, so I've experienced dry, cold weather. My best advice is to wear sunglasses or eyeglasses when you're out in the wind or cold. That really helps keep the moisture in my eye. If it gets too dry, I put a drop or two into my eye and it's quickly relieved!—*Chris*

I have tried this and every eye drop known to man I think my eye gets very dry as the lid does not close correctly, I also use a gel drop called Tears Again it is thick then a eye drops but not a ointment they also have an ointment I use when in the cold and wind. They also have a spray it is sort of hard to aim and spray but you can do it and not take your eye out and it does not hurt the skin it burns at first at times but it is helpful. KS has cold windy winter and hot windy summers so I wear glasses and my eye still gets cold wish there was a way to not have a frozen eye feeling.—*Bea*

Hi Grammy, I have also tried Sil-Ophtho, and a lot of other things, with limited success. Usually, my prosthesis feels fine, but there are times when I need some help. My normal routine is to irrigate my eye every morning with saline solution. I also take it out occasionally to wash it.

My ocularist in Philadelphia, invented a self-lubricating prosthesis. He was still developing it when I got my first prosthesis, and he retrofitted the eye he had already made for me. We tried several solutions in the chamber, some better than others. When I got a new prosthesis, I opted not to get the self-lubricating one, only because I felt I could do all right without it, since the dryness was only an occasional problem, not a constant one.—*Nancy*

◆ ◆ ◆

Hi all my friends I wanted to thank everybody for this site and the responses When all this happened to me I didn't know how I was going to make it! I know now I will It has been 2 months since I have had my prosthesis everything is going great but I have headaches Is that normal? Also lots of mucous I have to clean Q-tips I need to buy stock in them But is all this just a part of it My sister told me the other day just think of it as a bad pink eye infection for the rest of your life I said really that is exactly what it feels like. Does anyone have any recommendations on eyewashes and lubricants Please let me know! Thanks again And God bless everyone—*starlit7777*

Hi Starlit! I, like you, feel this board has been a godsend. I have found it comforting to belong to a community that understands and shares with one another our experiences. If you have just recently lost your eye, then I believe the headaches are a normal occurrence as you adjust to monocular vision. I had headaches also, but they diminish as you get used to seeing things a new way. As for a lubricant, I have tried a number of different ones. There are a few I use, like Sil-Optho, on occasion. I think you will have to try a few to see how they work for you. Good luck, and stay in touch!—*Nancy*

◆ ◆ ◆

hi all, I have a question, I have had my prosthesis for almost a year and it still isn't comfortable, it is always full of matter(or eye buggers, whatever)and there seems to be no way to make it stop. When I wake up in the morning, it usually takes me 10 minutes to get my eye open because its crusted shut, I know this is gross but I don't know what to do and you guys always seem to be supportive. Anyway, please leave a reply. Thanks all, stay strong everyone. I love this site!—*Tyler*

Hi, I appreciate your reply, yes I am young, I just turned 21, so I guess I am pretty stupid still. Thanks for your tips, I usually clean my eye with a non-smelling soap and then rinse with saline, but this still doesn't help. its funny to hear about your little habit cause I did the same thing, except I do it to get all the matter off. I am starting to wear my eye a lot more now that its summer and I am single and its starting to get more comfortable(except mornings of course), I used to only wear it if I had to do something important like going to job interviews, weddings, etc., and then take it out immediately after I got home. this of course turned out bad. my dog really likes to chew stuff and managed to get a hold of my eye (that I set on the table all drunk one night) and ate it! $2100 down the drain. Why didn't I ever have a dog that ate my homework, instead, I have one that digs eyes, oh well, just being stupid like his dad. Oh well. And does any body know where to get cool safety glasses at? I was wondering because I think I might work up the courage to mow my grass this summer sometime. Thanks again (and no prob. about calling me stupid, I know I am!)—*Tyler*

You'll get quite a bit of matter the first year, and then less the second year, and then by the third year almost no matter except when your prosthesis needs cleaning. What happens is that in the first couple of years, your body is rejecting the prosthesis, and so your socket produces chemicals and cells to attack the prosthesis. After a while, your body gets used to it. In subsequent years, the only matter that you'll get will either be ordinary dust, or some matter when proteins have built up on your prosthesis. Personally, I've found that by dousing the prosthesis and socket with saline before I go to bed at night and then each morning, I have much fewer problems with matter during the day. I think this basically flushes it out.—*Jay*

Definitely douse, but don't remove your prosthesis! All of the germs that you get on it by touching it really help create the discharge. Even if you wash your hands, they still have bacteria. Use clean or sterile Q-tips.—*Anon*

◆   ◆   ◆

Hi Jim, thank you for sharing your story with us. You have been through so much and you manage to have a great, inspirational attitude. As far as the gooeyness goes, it will always come and go in varying amounts. When the weather is cold, dry or windy (or all three) the surface of your eye can dry out, causing the lids to become irritated, and that will generate more "matter." I've had my eye since I was seven and I'm going to be 42 at the end of the month, and after the first year or so, my mom told me, the mattering reduced enough so that I didn't wake up with my eye stuck shut. I'm going through it again, because I had a socket "rebuild" last summer. I didn't get the eye I'm wearing now until Jan 3, and I'm experiencing "stuck shut" in the mornings. My best friend is a warm washcloth. I've found that if I just kind of rub it or pick at it, it makes more irritation. Keep eye drops on my bedside stand, in my purse, in my car, on my desk at work. I've been trying out different kinds of pre-moisture wipes baby wipes, handiwipes, "personal care wipes" "makeup remover towelettes" etc to find one that will dissolve the dried matter but not leave a film on my eye, or contain a high quantity of alcohol, which is really bad for the acrylic. Hope that helps. Great to see you here. Hugs—*Alicia*

Welcome Jim! I'm sure you've read how we all use different methods of cleaning and caring for our prosthesis'. I've had mine for over 30 years, and I've been successful with only ONE type of cleaning irrigant. It's called Dacriose Eye Irrigant. I take out the prosthesis every morning, clean it with the Dacriose and a cotton ball, and pop it back in. The discharge is at a minimum. I keep a handy supply of cotton swabs in my purse to get at it if it's too weepy, but other than that it's been fine. Hope that helps!—*Chris*

You'll get a lot of discharge the first year, and then it will gradually taper off to where some days you will only have a very minimal amount. It will help if you get in the habit of regularly flushing your socket out whenever you go to the bathroom. Also, after you get your prosthesis you will know that the longer you go between polishings, the more matter that will start to appear again. After it is cleaned, the amount of matter is usually minimal for at least a couple of months.—*Jay*

I did not know I had to get regular polishings. How often is that supposed to happen? Also, I pick at the surface of the eye to remove dried "matter" Will this dull or scratch the surface of the eye? It is an acrylic one.—*Jim*

Jim, I pick off matter that adheres to my prosthesis from time to time, and it hasn't dulled the surface at all. Mine's acrylic also, and I was advised by my ocularist to TRY to come in once or twice a year for polishings and to check the fit. ANY change in your weight (adding or losing 15 lbs. or so) can change the way it looks too, so keep that in mind. (I recently lost 42 lbs. and it changed my whole prosthesis so drastically that I needed a new one!). Anyway, things are bound to adhere to the prosthesis, especially when you can't close your eye (like me!). If you're getting too much matter on it and it's weeping too much, it's time to be checked.—*Chris*

◆ ◆ ◆

I've only taken mine out maybe a half-dozen times since I got it, and for the last two years the only time it has come out has either been for the semi-annual exams with my surgeon, or for the semi-annual cleanings. Other than that, I don't touch it, and I really don't have any problems by leaving it in. Comments?—*Jay*

Jay, last year when I visited my (prominent) NYC ophthalmologist, he told me that the newest findings were that you should limit taking the prosthesis out to clean it, as you are introducing new possibilities of bacteria each time you take it out. *I* have been taking it out DAILY now for 30 years. At first my parents had to do it for me, as it was traumatic (I was only 13). I take it out every morning, douse it with Dacriose irrigating solution, douse my socket with the Dacriose, and pop it back in. No problems. I feel "clean" every morning. I tried to skip a day, but I get lots of dry matter on the prosthesis and find myself picking away at it, which isn't too good. Anyway, I take it out daily and clean it, and I have minimal discharge and minimal dryness. The balance is JUST RIGHT for me! Hope that helps! I'm curious to hear what everyone else does!—*Chris*

Hi, Jay. Through the years, I've found it's better for me, to just leave it in. Since the socket rebuild, it's been a trial to leave it in, but I have been, and it's slowly calming down. The eye I'm wearing (from my regular "eye guy" in Seattle on Jan 3) "floats" well, and it's easier to leave it alone than it was with the first one, made here in LA (which I got in mid-December.) That one would suck down onto the implant, and I'd have to pry it out to get some moisture behind it. Gack. Through the years, when I've gotten a sore throat, tonsillitis, colds, etc, my socket would get inflamed as well, causing a lot of irritation. In that case, I irrigate it all the time with buffered saline, and that helps it calm down.—*Alicia*

Jay, I take my prosthesis out about once a week and I do that mainly to look for stray eyelashes that have been caught behind it. I had been having a problem with a lot of matter coming from the eye, more than the normal amount. I happened to have an appointment with my ocularist and when he took it out, he saw about six eyelashes stuck back there. Some were almost embedded in the tissue! I never thought eyelashes could cause a problem like this, but ever since, I have become diligent in checking for them. Has anyone else had this problem?—*Nancy*

Nancy, Yup! I have about one eyelash in there a day! There's also some eye makeup that gets washed away daily in the socket. It just feels "cleaner" to me to do that daily!—*Chris*

Hello guys, I am like Nancy, once a week is enough in my case. I used to do it on daily basis but I do prefer do it once a week. My eye-socket feels much better. Cheers,—*Anna*

I was scanning through some of the posts, and I am wondering if any of you have trouble putting in or taking out your prosthetic. I have had my eye since May (almost 4 months), and I have never taken it out or put it in. I just leave it in all the time. I get real freaked out when it turns sideways and I have to massage my eye lid to get it back in place. When I go to the doctor he takes it out for me. I guess I am a pansy about this (Alicia's words, not mine), but I am scared if I take it out I will never be able to put it back in. I might be house ridden for days. Please help.—*Roadrunner*

Okay, I did it. I took it out and put it back in. My eye has been so dry lately. I have been using gallons of Visine tears, and thought it might help if I rinsed off my prosthetic. So last night I took it out using the suction cup, and it took only about 5 minutes or so to get it back in. Next time it should be a breeze. It was kind of weird looking at it though.—*Roadrunner*

Taking your new eye out and putting it back in is just a psychological hurdle you have to jump over. Don't think about it just do it. Having said that, I don't like taking mine out (feel naked without it) and so usually it just stays where it is except for cleaning visits every 6 months to the ocularist.

BTW, your new eye should not easily turn sideways. If that is happening it is too loose and you should get your ocularist to build it up for the correct, full fit. In the first six months, the muscles in your socket will atrophy (is that the correct term?) and lose mass, thus resulting in a loose fit. You should always plan on getting your new eye built up about 6 months after you first get it.—*Jay*

Hi everybody. My doctor told me once I get my prosthesis to start using mineral oil and putting drops in when needed he said you can buy it at the drugstore and just to use a dropper that I have laying around the house.—*starlit7777*

I've found that the mineral oil just causes the socket to produce white matter. Personally, I just use saline to lubricate the socket.—*Jay*

Be careful of mineral oil. It will cause drag and dull the surface. I certainly don't want to second-guess or nay-say your ocularist, but my experiences with mineral oils and my prosthesis have not been good. As Jay said, it creates more matter. My long-term ocularist strongly urged avoiding mineral oil. When ever I had on waterproof eye makeup, and had to remove it with mineral oil, my eye was dull and irritated for quite some time afterward. Just my experience. I've been using various forms of saline with lubricants throughout the years. There are some with cellulose that seem to work well.

My new ocularist said that he recommends once a month taking it out and putting it in a solution of 1 tsp baking soda and 1 cup hot water for 10 minutes. He said it removes the protein build up. I'm going to try that with my new eye. (Oh, gee! Did I mention I'm getting a new eye?) Over the years, I've had the best luck with just leaving it alone. I wear eye shadow, mascara, eye liner, and other makeup stuff pretty regularly. The things I've noticed that get on the eye are rich eye-creams they apparently go right through the skin! and the oil base for concealers. I'm always looking for a gel-based eye cream and a non-greasy concealer. Love,—*Alicia*

It is OK if you can't remove your eye, since you should have a lot less problems or infections if you leave it in. Your ocularist can clean and polish you eye once or twice a year. Otherwise, just clean the front with a Q-tip if it gets some build-up in the corners.—*Anon*

I love you guys. Thanks for the tips. I think I have conquered another fear. The day I wrote that email I was at work and my eye was bothering me SO BAD. I was scared to go in the bathroom and try to fix it because I might be in there for hours. But I was only in there about 30 minutes, and have taken my eye out 2 more times since then. I think I may need a refit though, because my eye is a little loose. Take Care.—*Roadrunner*

Today when I went to my ocularist she gave me a sort of suction cup to grab my artificial eye. It makes it a lot easier to pull out and put back in. Next time you go, ask for one. My ocularist also told me to use Vaseline and eye drops to lubricate it. She AND my optometrist both said it was the best thing to use in my situation.—*Pim*

I have no problems at all taking out and putting back my eye. And you will find that it gets easier the more you do i.e. have to remove mine quite often as I get a lot of mucus behind it which isn't very comfortable. My biggest problem is my lid doesn't close properly and this I sometimes find upsetting. My ocularist says he could alter the size of my eye but then I run the risk of it moving about which it doesn't do now. So we decided together to leave well alone as it is very comfortable most of the time.—*Anne*

◆ ◆ ◆

I have a prosthetic shell, and find I can't wear it for more than a number of hours. My eye starts to exude and just wants to be rid of that foreign body, the prosthesis. I'm allergic to the proteins that form on the shell and perhaps the fit's not perfect. One of my dreams is to have reconstructive surgery since my eye area is shrinking. Thanks for listening.—*Claudia*

It is probably not the prosthesis so much as whatever you are using as a lubricant. I would get similar discharges with a silicon-based oil, and so I just use regular saline and do not lubricate the prosthesis with anything.—*Jay*

I went to my ocular oncologist last week and he gave me a RX for Patanol. He wanted me to use the drops 4 times a day for a month. He said it would help with the discharge and itching. The retail price for it at Target was $76.00, but I don't know how much of that my insurance would cover. Before I make that investment, I thought I'd ask if anyone here has used it and what they thought of it. Thanks for your input,—*Nancy*

Hi Chris, the discharge I was talking about is the normal, everyday stuff and the itching is because I get an allergic reaction to the prosthesis. It doesn't itch all of the time, kind of comes and goes. I'm getting a new prosthesis on Tuesday, so I didn't plan on getting the RX filled, if at all, until sometime after I've worn the new one.—*Nancy*

◆ ◆ ◆

I use no lubricants, drops, etc. with any loyalty, but I am never without these eye lid scrub pads. They come individually wrapped (like moist towelette products) and are indispensable for crusty mattering/stuck eyelids. Very soothing and gentle. The box says "patented cleansing formula effectively removes desquamated skin and oil which can cause eye irritation." They leave no residue on my prosthesis, even though they are not specifically for prostheses. Must rinse off, but you do not have to remove your eye—I use the pads on both eyes (it feels so good!) and just a quick splash of water to rinse. OCuSOFT (R) Lid Scrub, For Sensitive Eyes. Any drugstore should have or be able to stock for you. Bye now,—*Anon*

I learned of those eye pads for the first time two days ago when I was at the drug store. Two older ladies who were on a layover (LAX is about a mile away) were talking, and I heard them having trouble finding what they wanted. I'm always up for lending a hand, so I asked if I could help them search. We looked and looked and found them—they are from a very cold, windy and dry part of Canada, and they said these pads are very useful. Since I've heard of them twice, in such a short time, I'm going to take that as a sign to give them a try.—*Alicia*

This product sounds very good. I wonder if they are sold in the UK will have to look out for them. At the moment I don't use anything like this but have to remove my eye pretty often to clean it Thanks for the help.—*Anne*

I also use them all the time, they are very handy to have when not at home. My doctor said they are the best pads around, and I also use the eye wash they have out too. That I use every morning to wash my eye, I just leave the eye in and put some wash in the eye. My ocularist told me to just take the eye out once a month. So far that is working just great.—*Anon*

◆ ◆ ◆

Hi Jodi, Welcome. One great way to keep a clean eye and socket is to flush with copious amounts of saline solution. Since I've started this routine, I've gone from having to remove my prosthesis daily to only monthly, if that. This usually flushes out any mucus without having to touch the eye, which of course as we all know can lead to more irritation and discharge. The mucus should subside after your body adjusts to the new eye regardless. Take care.—*CanDo*

◆ ◆ ◆

What has anyone found for the socket itching. My eye gets dry as my tear ducts do not work right, now I am having a lot of problems with the inside of the socket itching and part of it has to do with the lashes being messed up but there has to be something that can give relief hopefully.—*Bea*

The best thing I can do for myself when my eye gets dry is a shower—letting warm water flow over my eye area. Then I put in some cushioning drops. A warm washcloth can help, too. Good luck! Please share anything you find.—*Alicia*

Bea, I had a problem with dryness and itchiness, also. My doctor prescribed Patanol, which I was to use 4 times a day for a month. It didn't cure the problem, but it did help. I've also used Sil-Ophtho for when my prosthesis gets really dry. Hope you find some relief.—*Nancy*

Bea, I use Minims Artificial Tears, as my tear duct on my bad side is totally messed up due to surgeries. I don't know if Minims are marketed under the same name in the US, but they are super. They are also Preservative Free so they will not annoy your prosthesis. I hope you get sorted,—*Elizabeth*

◆ ◆ ◆

FWIW, I never take my prosthesis out and almost never even irrigate it these days. I do carry some of those plastic vial "artificial tears" things in my briefcase for the occasional "dry" days.—*Jay*

Jay, I've been SO used to taking it out every morning. When I don't do it, it feels so dirty and there's a lot of build-up on it. I guess it's what we're all used to. I've been doing this for over 30 years and it's working for me, so I won't change now. Too bad I had to change my Dacriose though!—*Chris*

Hello, when I got my final prosthesis a month ago, my ocularist told me never to touch or take it out. I can clean it but just from the outside. He told me it is not good to remove it frequently to clean because the eye produces more mucus if you do so. To my opinion it feels more like my own eye when I do not have to remove it to clean it or to sleep with. But I understand that the situation is different for each one of us. You have to do what's best for your own comfort. The only thing I use to clean or if the eye feels dry is physiological serum. It seems to be as good as all the other products which exist for prostheses and it's a lot cheaper.—*Chrissie*

I do take mine out every couple of weeks. I wash it with soap, rinse it thoroughly and then put it back in still wet. I move the prosthesis around a bit and I am ready to go. I never have a dry "eye" but because I wear eye make-up it just feels better. Every two months I put the prosthesis in warm (not hot) water with a spoon of kitchen salt. Leave it for about 10 minutes. Rinse with clean water, polish it up with a clean dry cloth and rinse again just to make it wet. Looks perfectly shining again. Just a pointer I got from my ocularist to make it shine.—*Willeke*

◆ ◆ ◆

Who takes their prosthesis out regularly? I take mine out every morning when taking my shower. I take it out because I like to wash it and the socket as well. I first take the eye out and wash it with Dettol soap, then put it aside. Next I shampoo my hair and after rinsing the hair I spray the eye socket with the shower head. Only after I have completed my shower I put the eye back to the socket.

This may sound unusual to the most, I think many use some irrigation agent and very seldom take the eye out. However, I do not feel clean if I do not wash my eye and the socket. I have told my ocularist about this, she has nothing against it, said do as you feel, but she was concerned whether it hurts to spray the socket. It does not hurt. She said, at least spray with warm water.

Other times I take my eye out is when I do not feel like wearing it. I have never gone one whole week without removing my fake eye, not even a full 24 hour day. Any opinions; could my practice have any detrimental effect on my socket or is it perfectly OK. My thinking it is better practice in cleanliness point of view. Thanks,—*JPH*

Hey JPH, I used to be like you in cleaning my eye on a regular basis for about a year and a half but it always seemed like it took hours to reseat properly and was uncomfortable during that time. I, like you, was concerned about cleanliness and I didn't want any infection or seepage forming. So for an experiment I tried leaving it in for a week. No problems. Two weeks. No problems. Then three weeks. Still no problems. Its now been almost three years since I've taken it out and I have never had an infection or any seepage whatsoever. All the articles I've read say to remove it regularly to prevent infection or seepage. All I can figure is that in my case I'm not normal. I have even got debris in my eye and I treated it just like my other eye, with eye wash. The only reason I can think of for this is that the ocularist did a fantastic fitting.

◆ ◆ ◆

Dear Star, you shouldn't have so much mucus that it seeping like that. Try rinsing with a sterile saline solution and applying an over the counter ointment, like Refresh PM to the front of the ocular, always with washed hands. In the morning, you can take a clean washcloth and wipe away the discharge and apply the ointment. Some mucus is normal, and there will be more if the prosthesis is not well lubricated. Just watch for excessive mucus, with a yellow or green coloration. This is the beginning of infection. It may be time for a polishing too. Good luck,—*Lisa*

◆ ◆ ◆

Sorry couldn't really think of a better subject title. I recently met a friend who I realized also had one eye, which is cool because we can share tips etc, much like on this forum. But I also realized that I seem to have a lot more mucus accumulation in my prosthetic eye. One difference is that his bad eye has been enucleated, while my prosthetic is actually a shell on top of my bad eye (which was a birth defect and is very small) Is anyone else in the same situation?

An ocularist mentioned to me that more mucus might be generated because the eye rubs against the prosthetic which then causes the mucus. I used the eye drops pretty often. (Switched from Dacriose to OcuSoft-I think someone was asking about other products since Dacriose was discontinued) But mucus accumulates and dries causes the appearance of the prosthetic eye to be more apparent. Does anyone have any suggestions? Thanks a lot.—*Andrew*

◆ ◆ ◆

I recently got my artificial eye, and would like to know if it is ok to use mascara and/or eye shadow. If so, is there any particular kind I should use.—*Susan*

Dear Susan, it is perfectly OK to use eye shadow and mascara. Because risk of infection is slightly greater on the side where you are wearing your artificial eye, you may want to keep a separate eye shadow and mascara just for that side only. Use new products too, and don't share with others. Sincerely,—*Lisa*

Thanks for the info, Lisa! As luck would have it, I bought 2 new mascaras, and had labeled one L for left, and the other R, for right. I wasn't thinking of infection, so I don't really know WHY I decided to get 2, and do it that way. Just a "spur of the moment" decision.

I used the mascara yesterday, and by last night, I was experiencing some MAJOR itching! I have had itching before, but only once was it this bad! I used Max Factor mascara, because that's the brand of foundation I use. I know I should probably try something else, because this was obviously an allergic reaction. Any suggestions as to which brand is more hypo-allergenic? Thanks again. If you think of anything else I should know, please send it along! I'm really new at this.—*Susan*

Dear Susan, I had major itching (and swelling) of the eyelids too, since October. I was tested and found to have a nickel allergy. The welt on my back from the test site was huge. Check to see if there is any nickel in that makeup. Also, stop using the makeup and call your doctor. You may have an allergy like me. I started using Elidel cream and it worked, but now carries a black box warning by the FDA, that it has a risk of causing cancer. So I only use a little every other day. Nothing else worked so I have to use a little. I use Maybelline mascara. Good luck!—*Lisa*

I love to experiment with eye makeup. I lost my eye when I was 5 due to a bb gun accident. I couldn't wait to wear eye makeup so I could minimize the visible differences between my two eyes. Now that I'm in my 30's (and have been wearing makeup for YEARS), I really enjoy experimenting. The only problem that I have had was that my left eye waters sometimes and washes the eye liner off. My ocularist suggested that I look into permanent tattoos. That's my next step. As with any eye makeup, you need to determine if you have any allergies to the contents. I would suggest using quality products, but try not to worry too much. Have fun experimenting with different looks.—*mchandler*

Just had to answer this. I have "permanent makeup" (eyeliner and lipliner) and I LOVE it! Mine's very subtle, so people say things to me like "With your natural coloring, you don't even need makeup." Heh, heh, heh, little do they know. I'm going back for darker eyeliner AND eye shadow next month.

Be warned that even though numbing drops are put in your eye, your eyeball still feels the vibration of the needle, and it's somewhat queasy-making. And I have no idea how they would numb an eye socket. same drops, I suppose? I have tattoos on my ankles too and found the pain of a traditional tat less unnerving than the vibrations. That said, I'm overjoyed that I had it done and can't wait to finish the job.—*Ya'ara*

◆ ◆ ◆

As far as the matter goes, carry around some saline solution and just give it a good squirt every now and then. You'll find that if you give it a good squirt in the morning that it will usually remain free of gunk the rest of the day. Also, carry around a bunch of swabbies, since those clean it in one swipe.—*Jay*

Every morning I use Bausch & Lomb Eye Wash. It cleans out everything, and makes you feel fresh as a daisy. Jeez. Now I feel like I'm doing a commercial for some feminine product.—*Michael*

I have found that my eye is totally gunk free unless it's windy or I'm in a place with air conditioning and then that irritates it and it gets sore and gunky. A woman at work likes to use a fan when it's hot but if it's anyway pointed near me I end up with a totally irritated and gunky eye.—*Marmalade*

Anti-bacterial soap and other alcohol based should be avoided.—*Anon*

I too get a lot of gunk in my eye(well conformer at the moment) and all I do is run it under warm water and I find this does the trick for me. When I had my last eye this was all I did with this too.—*Anne*

◆ ◆ ◆

Hi all, I clean mine once a week with, ok, no laughing here, Johnson's baby shampoo and warm water. Hey, you know, they were right about the no more tears thing! Lately I've been rather emotional about some stuff and crying a lot, so I've had to clean it twice a week.—*Danielle*

I also use baby shampoo as that is what my doctor told me to use. But, I only take it out once or twice a year. I just wait for him to clean and polish it once a year.—*Emily*

Clean mine whenever I feel I need to. Sometimes daily if I've been working (or playing) in dirty/dusty conditions, sometimes it stays in for a few weeks at a time. I used to use Dacriose at first, but I've become pretty comfortable with taking it out, rinsing it off, polishing it dry with a CLOTH. Not tissues or paper towels, and putting it back in. occasionally. Maybe once every 6 months or so, It will get irritated and I will take it out overnight (after cleaning it, and the socket) just to let any inflammation subside. This is rarely necessary. I was told by my ocularist that unnecessarily cleaning it too often can actually INCREASE discomfort, because you are constantly washing away the body's natural secretions, which help to lubricate the socket. I do find that it feels better after a day or so after I clean it.—*Navig8r*

I only take my prosthetic eye out once every two to three weeks. I haven't seen my cleaning tip for prosthetic eyes yet, so here it is: DISH DETERGENT. It cleans it up perfectly. Rinse carefully, dry it up with a clean dry cloth, wet the prosthetic eye again and pop the prosthesis back in.

Every two to three months I put my prosthetic eye in some warm (not hot) water, add a teaspoon of kitchen salt and let that rest for about ten minutes. Rinse carefully, dry and polish it up with a clean dry cloth, wet the prosthetic eye again and pop it back in. I got that cleaning tip from my ocularist. I have had my prosthetic eye for two years now and done this since day one. I've never had any irritation or infection. It is weird to see how everyone does it differently.—*Willeke*

I don't know what dish detergent is really but I just take my eye out in the bath every now and then and wash it in the water. It seems to work okay. We have been told that baby shampoo is a good soap but I don't buy it.—*Marmalade*

Hi Marmalade, sorry I didn't make clearer what I meant. I don't know the correct English word, but I mean the soap you use to hand wash your dishes with. My prosthetic eye gets a little greasy every now and then due to make-up and this gets it cleaned up very nicely. I think everyone should stick to what works for them. There is a big variety in products being used, it seems.—*Willeke*

Wow! I don't understand how you guys could stand any soap touching your eye! When I get a dot of shampoo in that eye (even with the prosthesis in!), it burns like hell! I'd be so hesitant to clean it with anything other than sterile eye irrigating solutions.—*Chris*

I was told by my Ocularist not to use dish washing detergent. It removes the oils in the paint, and could cause the finish to lose it's color, and coating more rapidly. I use Johnson's Baby Shampoo only. It's made to clean well, but not be harmful to the finish.—*Michael*

I'm also part of the Johnson's Baby Shampoo club! I usually end up cleaning my eye about every other week and I have found that it helps if I put a puddle of Tears Again MC (my lubrication drop) into the back side of the eye right before I pop it back in. It seems to feel better if there is a layer of lubrication between the eye and my implant and I've noticed less discharge since I've started adding it.—*Adeline*

Adeline, I haven't heard of the drops you use. I wonder if they might help with the crusty issue I have in the morning. I'm willing to try anything:) Where can you buy them at and any info would be great. Thanks,—*Sherri*

Hey, Sherri! The Tears Again MC drops are part of a line called OcuSoft. I got them from my ocularist when I first got my eye. I had trouble finding them at drug stores, but I discovered that I could get them at their website, ocusoft.com. I actually order their irrigating solution, hand soap, and eye wash pads as well. The hand soap is great because it doesn't leave a residue and that helps with both the eye and my contact lens. I'm sorry to say that I still wake up sometimes with the crusty discharge (weather, allergies, who knows), but the eye wash pads are a handy way to give my lids a good cleaning. The MC drops really just help me with dryness and when my eye starts to feel itchy. Hope this info helps!—*Adeline*

◆ ◆ ◆

Gee, I'd NEVER feel comfortable talking about this anywhere else! My prosthesis has hurt me for a few months now, since they took my eye irrigant off the market (I'm STILL crying about it!). I get a discharge, and I get that crusty stuff stuck on my inner lids and on the prosthesis itself. Doesn't help that I can't blink.

Anyway, here's my question. Sometimes there's a TON of discharge in the socket (I clean it every morning) and now it's turned a yellow color (instead of clear or white-ish). Does anyone else have the same color discharge, or could this be the start of an infection? I'd HATE to trek all the way back into Manhattan to see my nearly-retired eye doc!—*Chris*

Hmmmm, discharge. Well, we generally don't like yellow-y looking purulence, and def not any other variation i.e.—green etc. However it depends on the individual, like Anne says, with her its yellow all the time, but with you it could be the start of irritation/infection. I'd keep an eye on it, and even go see your GP/local ophthalmologist instead of having to trek back to Manhattan if you get worried about it. Take Care,—*Elizabeth*

Hey Chris, I'd get to an O.D. or an ophthalmologist ASAP. Pain with the change of discharge usually indicates infection. If you get a good antibiotic early you might nip it in the bud. My O.D. gave me a prescription that I can fill anytime I feel an infection coming on & now I've not had a bad one in years. Tobradex is wonderful. Best wishes & get it checked soon. You can even go to a Doc-in-a-box & get the Tobradex right away. They'll usually want you to see your eye doc too.—*Liz*

For whatever reason, when I was in Dublin in June I had to use eye drops like crazy and had some massive discharges. I can only speculate that it was pollen or allergies.—*Jay*

Thanks, Jay. That's what I'm thinking. My doc usually has me on Allegra for allergies, but since my eye has been so irritated, I stopped taking the Allegra, hoping it would help. I don't know what to do at this point, but even my husband said that I should just call the doctor since it's been going on for too long now. Ack.—*Chris*

Elizabeth, no, I didn't go to my doctor YET. I couldn't get an appointment when it was good for me, and he's been busy, so I pushed it off. It's STILL bothering me, so I know I should go! I don't have a fever, so I don't think it's an infection. I don't know what to think anymore!—*Chris*

PART III
IMPLANTS, SHELLS AND PATCHES

9

Issues with Implants

When an eye is removed, the surgeons will typically place a small ball, about the size of a ping-pong ball, into the orbit and stitch the eye muscles around it. This ball takes the place of the eye in the orbit, and gives it mass. It is against the implant that the prosthesis (the plastic eye) will fit around, much like a bottle cap would fit over a ping-pong ball.

There are various types of implants that are available for the patient's choice. The solid plastic smooth implant is still the most commonly used. Other implants, however, are made of such materials as coral or perforated plastic, with the idea that the eye muscles will actually grow into them and allow the implants to move somewhat like the eye itself would move. These implants typically have a titanium peg that juts forward from the implant upon which the prosthesis rests.

The downside to these implants, as opposed to the smooth plastic ones, is that on rare occasions they can become infected and cause problems. However, for those who want the extra, more natural movement of their prosthesis, choosing these more advanced implants are often worth the risks.

LETTERS AND E-MAILS

Hi, it was so nice to discover this web site, I too have been able to adapt quite well to my one eye. I lost my left eye to a melanoma in the retina. The prosthesis I now have sounds similar to yours although my implant is a bit different, it's made of coral. Coral is a porous material which the 6 eye muscles were able to attach to. It has been really fascinating to have this artificial eye fit right in place and move as well as my natural eye did people are completely amazed to learn that it's a prosthesis I also was free of any kind of infection, I took it easy after the surgery, got lots of rest, ate well and ensured that my immune system was in good shape, maybe that helped.—*Geraldine*

Dear Jay, I lost my left eye to retinoblastoma in 1952 when I was 3. My parents were told that the implant was a gold sphere. The prosthesis I received was the shell-type, no post to enhance movement. For the next fifty years of my life I had new eyes made for me by my old ocularists (now out of business). They always made me the shell-type eye, always explaining that it was the only eye that my implant would accommodate. Well, four years ago, I went to another ocularist, who took one look into the orbit and said "This [shell] is the wrong kind of eye for that implant." I said, like, "WHAT?" and he said "Sure, look for yourself." So I looked in the mirror and not only could I see the outline of the implant behind the scar tissue, (which I had never really looked for before), but also that it clearly was NOT a sphere but a cube-shaped device, with a post intended for a totally different kind of eye, which he then proceeded to make for me. I am wearing this new type of eye quite comfortably now and am told that the movement has improved immensely.

Now, obviously, the above raises many questions. The one that really freaked me out, though, comes from the fact that this new ocularist said that the type of implant I have wasn't invented till the early 60s. And of course I distinctly recall having the operation done in the early 50s, with no memories of any subsequent operation. I have scoured the web trying to confirm exactly when this type of implant was first used, have found zip. Any info you might have to help convince me that I am not in fact losing my mind? Great site. Fine work you are doing. Many thanks.—*John*

I am having my blind eye (since 09-1973) removed and fitted with hydroxyapatite ball. Then after 6 weeks meeting with an ocularist. I just want to talk to someone who had the surgery, is approximately 40 years old, whom I can just ask general questions. My surgeon has not-as of yet-replied to this request. Thanks,—*Michael*

I'm a 17 year old girl from India. I had my right eye removed 6 years ago (i.e., when I was 11).and in place of the removed one, the doctors fixed a glass eye, which was already made. Now this glass eye doesn't match with the size of my eye socket. Since then I've had this glass eye and haven't changed it even once.

I was really glad and happy to know that there were better alternatives for me like the bio eye from your website. I couldn't speak to anyone about this, and now after reading your website, it is like an answer to my prayer. Now what I wanted to know was if there were any hospitals in India where I could get the BIO EYE. I am desperately in need of it, and I would be really thankful to you if you could email me the hospitals in India where I could get the bio eye, and also the cost of it. Thanking you,—*Swathi*

My name is Jim and I live in Nashville, Tennessee. I have worn an artificial eye since I was 18 (I am now 52) I have tried all types from the coral implant with the sleeve and the peg to vaulted ones. I have an allergy problem of some sort whether it be from the material that the eye is made of or what I am not sure. I seem to have to clean my eye off constantly. We have removed the sleeve and the peg from the implant and have since gone back to the regular vaulted type. My ocularist is the only person that has ever made me completely satisfied with the looks of my eye. She passed away last spring and I am lost without her help. I have had an eye made by the gentleman that bought her business, and have not been completely satisfied with the fit or the color match. (he is by the way a super nice fellow, just not as good as my former ocularist was). I am a General Manager for an auto collision center, therefore I do have a good eye for color matches (only one though. lol). Anyway, I am having some more eye surgery in a couple of weeks and will have to get another eye, and was looking for an "expert" with color & fit issues.—*Jim*

Jay, I just went through your web-site, losteye.com. Thank you for taking the time to put this together. I am currently contemplating this type of surgery next month. Although the Dr. explains it in his terms, your explanation of the postoperative "what to expect", was what I was looking to find out about. I didn't find anything in your writing about evisceration (contents of an eye removed). This is what they are proposing for me. Here is a web site that you may want to add for information about the Bio-Eye Orbital Implant, http://www.ioi.com. Have you had anybody write in about this type of procedure yet or not that I could email to? One other thing, thanks for using the larger font to make your site easier to read. Regards,—*Wilbur*

Hi Jay, I was wondering if you've heard anything about people having adverse or allergic reactions to their eye implants (the ones made out of coral), or to their prosthesis. My husband had an enucleation of his right eye on 4/2/02 following the discovery of a tumor. He is 61, plays volleyball, and had been in good health up to this point. About 2 weeks ago he started having symptoms of sensitivity and pain in his upper chest area (muscles and skin), shoulders, and upper back. The area under his arm pits is especially painful, and sometimes he has shooting pains in his chest muscles. Recent blood work shows that he is cancer free, infection-free; there are no tumors or cysts in his skin; his doctor is stumped, and Jerry is quite frustrated. This has been a debilitating experience—worse than the recovery from eye surgery. Since there does not seem to be a medical reason for his pain, I'm wondering if he is having an allergic reaction to the eye implant, the way women have had reactions to breast implants. Thank you.—*Renee*

I had a morpor implant put in on Nov 4 2002 and I have had all sorts or problems getting my new eye to fit in fact I got another new one made 3 weeks ago now as the man I go to said it was not right and he gives a warranty. The follow week I got a extreme sharp pain in the outside corner of my right eye socket. it burns and stung and felt like a sharp knife was being stuck in there. I went up and took a bath soon after that as I was hurting and when I leaned over to splash water on my face I felt a pop behind my socket in the base. It felt like I had been hit right on my eye with a rubber band. The pain got worse and I went to doctor the next day and he said he thought it was a cyst that broke. That this type of implant tends to cause cysts and if you get one you will (or could) get another one. As they tend to fill up again and then break. I am now having a lot of sinus drainage and I wandered if this was from the inflammation draining out as that fluid had to go somewhere. They told me to not be alarmed if this happened again and blood drained down my face out of tear ducts. I said I would be alarmed.

Has anyone had this happen and does it make sense does it sound like I am having a reaction to the morpor? Thank you for listening and I would appreciate any help I am in a small town and I am sort of an "odd duck" for the doctor I have to remind them that a plastic eye can not see. when they say "oh do the best you can" so I do not get too much help here.—*Bea*

I have a coral implant. My WBC(white blood count) is unusually high-ranges from 12,800 to 17,800. This has been this way(noticed) since 01/2004. My doctor doesn't think its a problem. Had all my liver scans and abdomen CT-no metasizes. Could the WBC be high and this is my normal because my body is constantly fighting the "foreign bodies"-both the coral implant and the prosthesis? I have an older brother that was diagnosed with leukemia and I was tested to see if I had it or if I could be a stem cell donor for him. This is when I noticed the blood work being out of whack.—*Ron*

MESSAGES

Hi, I have been missing my left eye for about one and a half years now. I have an acrylic eye which eye can remove for washing etc. I also recently got a spare one from my oculist. I now like to ask a question whether an implant is worth of the money, I know it is very expensive. Does it move properly or are there any other benefits? My current eye does not move and it bothers me some times. My oculist also told me that there is a possibility with a traditional prosthesis wearer that the socket changes its form over time and then you cannot wear any eye at all and left with an eye patch. Any opinions or experience? Regards,—*JPH*

I would recommend an implant in principle JPH but you would need to get your surgeon to tell you exactly what the implant would achieve. You should find that it gives more bulk in the orbit so that you can have a smaller, lighter prosthesis. If you carry on without an implant, as I did for a few years after having one rejected, you will need increasingly bigger prosthesis and it is hard for the top lid not to droop. But find out as much as you can first. Best of luck!—*Chil*

Thank Chil, Is the operation for implant similar to that of enucleation or harder/more inconvenient? And how long is the recovery time? Enucleation in my case was to get rid of pain and as such of great relief. But I am not very keen to go through hospital and associated recovery episodes again. And how long it is expected to look normal again?—*JPH*

Hi JPH, I would say that the operation for an implant is harder to get over than the enucleation. Having said that, when I had a secondary implant I took two weeks off work but only needed to take one. If by looking "normal", you mean have a prosthesis fitted which moves, I would say that you can't necessarily expect to look normal in that your eyes will look different from each other, but there are lots of people out there with natural eyes that don't match. The socket has to heal before a prosthesis can be molded and I would expect this to be about 6 weeks. It may be that surgeons in different parts of the world will differ in their practice. You'd have to be sure to ask all the questions in advance.

I was told that an empty socket was not an option because eventually you would get problems like in growing eyelashes. But they give you a small clear plastic conformer which allows the eye to close over it. I don't envy you having to make decisions. There's loads of different knowledge and experience on this board, though and I hope we'll collectively help. All the best,—*Chil*

◆   ◆   ◆

I am 20 years old was born blind in the right eye. But the docs realized it only when I was 3, when I went for a regular checkup. As I grew older, the bad eye was beginning to shrink in size and was watering all the time. so much that it was affecting the good eye and that's when (when I was 13)the docs removed the bad eye. Since then I've had a prosthetic eye. My 1st prosthesis was very bad. The color didn't match not even the size. Now I have a prosthesis which looks OK. But there is no movement whatsoever and the eyeball looks upwards which makes it really odd. My ocularist says it is because my lower eye lid was drooping because it could not bear the weight of the prosthesis for so many years.

I was wondering if having the implant with the peg would do me any good. Whether there will be good movement in the eye. I've had a tough time at school because of the eye and I don't mind going through the process of having an implant and am willing to take the risk of any infection. Since I'm in India, I'll have to travel to the states for this. Could anyone please tell me how much the whole procedure costs and how long it'll take for me to have the implant and the peg (I'll have to plan the duration of my stay there). I have a sister living in California (Santa Clara), so I'll be grateful if anyone could refer to me any good docs in that area.

I've found this site extremely helpful. And the people here are so comforting and encouraging. I'm so glad I found it.—*Swathi*

Nobody can say if the procedure would work for you except for an eye doctor. I first had a plastic implant which they say my body rejected and I had it replaced with a much better one about 3 years ago. The healing time is a matter of weeks but they wouldn't drill the peg hole for at least 6 months and sometimes, as with me, they won't do it at all. It just depends on you and the way your body deals with it.—*Marmalade*

◆ ◆ ◆

I've had a coral implant 2 1/2 years now. From the start I felt the implant was the wrong size (18 mm). To me it didn't provide enough volume. My false eye appears as thou it's sunken into the socket. My upper eyelid also withdrew back into the space between my eyebrow and my prosthesis. As a remedy the eyelid muscle was weakened thru surgery and what was called a sled was implanted under and behind the coral implant also thru surgery. All this and my eye's appearance is such that it still appears sunken; so much so that in photos I appear as if I have a black-eye. To me the remedy would be a bigger implant (20 or 22 mm's). I know tissues have grown into my coral implant in the 2 1/2 years so I wonder how difficult it would be to remove the sled and implant and go bigger with another implant. You may wonder why I don't ask my Doc this but my surgeries were done in a charity hospital by Drs. doing there residencies and if I'm going to go thru this I want a much more experienced Doc to do it. Any Dr. referrals would be a big help if in fact this is feasible. Thanks in advance,—*Dre*

Hi Dre, I think it could be replaced. I am having a surgery in a week when the doctors will put for the first time the coral or MedPor implant. At the moment I've got an implant but it is much smaller. But I have to say that the doctors will find out during the operation whether it is possible, so fingers crossed. Take care.—*Anna*

Hi Drexler, this is my first post on this board and the reason I'm responding to yours is that I had a very similar problem after my coral implant. It was sunken into the socket, my eyelid was kind of drooping and I felt awful about how I looked. I was referred to a great plastic surgeon. I love this lady for what she did for me. She put in a floor implant, which was made from the same coral material as the implant. That brought the implant forward enough to correct the sunken look. She also fixed both of my eyelids so that they matched. The results were incredible. No one knows I have a prosthesis unless I tell them. Perhaps what you need is a good plastic surgeon to correct what you have, rather than a new, or larger, implant. I hope I've given you some information to go on, but please feel free to ask me any other questions. And good luck to you.—*Nancy*

◆ ◆ ◆

Hello. I'm new here. I lost my eye due to a faulty juicer (of all things) while working at a corporate health food store here in Memphis. This incident occurred 4 1/2 years ago. I had a craniotomy to ensure that my brain was fine and to insert a titanium plate into my skull to help rebuild it. My eye was enucleated shortly thereafter.

I originally had a hydroxyapatite (spelling?) implant. I eventually had it pegged. An exposure occurred and I had a graft (from the roof of my mouth) to try and correct it. This didn't work and the implant became infected. ETC. Needless to say, I've had numerous surgeries (just had my 11th) including a dermal fat graph, an acrylic orb insertion, and now another hydroxy orb insertion. This last surgery was done on August 17th. Yesterday I noticed ANOTHER exposure and today it seems to have grown already.

I'm going to try and get in touch with my doctor first thing this morning, but. I'm scared to death. I don't want another surgery! Does anyone have experiences like these? What kind of suggestions might anyone have? I took the conformer out because it seemed to be rubbing on the exposed parts, making them worse. Any advice/encouragement/personal stories would be greatly appreciated! Thank you.—*Lacey*

Dear Lacey: I still have my eye, but no vision due to choroidal melanoma, which was found in a routine eye exam. I'm looking at enucleation due to the rapid deterioration of my eye from radiation treatment. I am sorry for what happened to you. It seems like it was a fluke accident? The surgeries don't seem to be working? Have you sought a second or a third opinion? It is your right to seek enough opinions to make you feel comfortable.

Also, insurance doesn't always cover it. Mine has, but they will pay for the eye removal, but only 50% for a prosthesis. This website is so supportive and actually

I'm kind of a lurker here. I'm sure you'll hear from many more that will give you great advice. I just wanted to post and to give you support. I am so sorry you need to be here, but this is a great group to get information, support and to meet people with the same circumstances that you have. Don't ever feel alone. This group is here for you. All my best to you and wish I could say and do more for you, Hugs—*Sherri*

Alan is going to have his eye enucleated within the next three months, and obviously will have an implant after that. Being ignorant on this topic, I guess I always made the assumption that implants and the "after-market" eyes were pretty much maintenance free, aside from occasional cleaning and check ups. From some of the things I have read here though, I am starting to get worried that he is going to have life long problems. Are the problems I am reading about the exception, or is a dry/itchy/weeping eye, or constant pain/irritation going to be a part of life for him?—*John*

◆ ◆ ◆

I had choroidal melanoma two years ago and had my eye removed. My eye looks a little set back compared to my real eye. Also the fat or skin on the eyelid that I have on my real eye, disappeared over my prosthetic after the enucleation. It looks kind of hollow on the eyelid below my brow. I just want both my eyelids to look the same.

My last doctor kept telling me he wanted to wait for a gel implant to be approved by the FDA to put in the eyelid to fill it out. We've moved, and my new dr. says I need an implant under the actual coral implant to bring the eye forward and that will fill in my eyelid. But, she won't do it until I'm 5 years out from the enucleation! She said something about not wanting to disturb the socket. Sorry this is so long. Has anyone else had this problem and has your doctor fixed it before the 5 year mark? Thanks so much!—*mak*

Hi Mak, I had exactly the same problem after my enucleation for choroidal melanoma 12 years ago. Fortunately, I had an excellent ophthalmic plastic surgeon that fixed it for me. Five months after my enucleation, the plastic surgeon gave me a floor implant, which sounds like what your new doctor suggested. The implant fixed the sunken look that I had. I then had both eyelids done, because they were uneven, too. Now, both eyes and lids look alike. This was my experience. I don't know if your doctor feels there is some other underlying reason for waiting so long, besides disturbing the socket, but I think I would get a second opinion. Best wishes,—*Nancy*

I know there are different sizes to the implants. It's important that the doctor used the correct size for your socket. I know my doctor was concerned about it. He or one of his team had to travel to another state to pickup the correct size. My doctor used a MedPor. This was to keep the correct size behind the prosthesis, and to keep the socket from looking shrunken. Hope this helps. Regards,—*Michael*

◆ ◆ ◆

Hi Everyone, I have a question and I would REALLY appreciate it if someone would respond with a suggestion or some past experience. For those of you who have had your eye enucleated in the past and then rejected the implant, what were some symptoms that you were having to signal you that something was wrong with the implanted eye? I really haven't been feeling well lately and I have been having numerous tests done but they can't seem to find the source. I have developed a pixilated vision in my left (healthy) eye and I thought maybe this was a sympathetic situation to the implanted one signaling that something was wrong with the implant. My parents suggested that I take the prosthesis out last night to see if my symptoms change because I also have been having intense headaches all week but nothing changed. Ever since I put the eye back in it just hasn't felt the same. I don't know if I am jumping to conclusions and I don't want to alarm my ocular surgeon just yet. If someone who has experienced this or a failed implant could write back I would really appreciate it and maybe it would give me some form of relief. I truly appreciate it and love you guys! Hope everyone else has a good day Love,—*Jodi*

Jodi, I rejected MANY implants after my initial enucleation. I didn't feel symptoms with my healthy eye. I only felt intense pressure in my socket and then my body physically rejected the implant, right out of my socket. It was like a horror movie. If you're feeling pressure or pain in that socket, please, call your doctor as soon as possible! Good luck!—*Chris*

◆ ◆ ◆

Hello Guys, I had a surgery—coral implant—2 weeks ago and I have noticed that it doesn't move so well and that my eye-lid is not opening. Is it a typical/normal situation after a surgery, after 2 weeks? I am afraid that my eye-lid will be closed and that the coral implant won't be moving. Please reply.—*Anna*

From my experience, the eyelid was swollen and unable to open for almost a month, and very uncomfortable when I got my prosthesis fitted for it. It will take a while for the attached muscles to function normally because of the simple fact that they were cut and attached to something else. Not long, maybe a few months for full movement, but don't worry about it since it will all work out in the end.—*Tyler*

I'm hanging in through a crazy summer of implant rebuilding. One surgery didn't work out, so there were two. Now I'm waiting for the new eye, wearing a conformer that wants to move out and get its own apartment. Sigh. Does anyone have a MedPor implant? How long before it stopped getting shooting pains from growing in? Love,—*Alicia*

Hi Guys, I have posted that message a while ago. Now, it has been six weeks after my surgery and my eye lid is still half open. Is it normal? Is it OK? Is it supposed to be like that? Before my coral implant surgery my eye-lid looked normal now I am afraid that it will not come back to my old/normal looking shape. Please let me know if you had a similar experience! Thanks.—*Anna*

Hi Anna. I don't know what a coral implant is but I am sure that the movement will come back to you. I have no implant in my eye because of r/therapy treatment and even my artificial eye has a little movement. my problem is the other way to you my lid does not close properly as r/t killed off the good muscles as well as the cancerous cells but at least I am still here to moan about it hope this is of help to you. Love,—*Anne*

Hi Anne, thank you for your reply. I've visited my doctor yesterday and he said that my movement is very good and that in 2 weeks I can have my new prosthesis. He said that with the prosthesis my eye lid should open. We will see. I will keep you updated just in case someone else will have the same questions and doubts about eye lid. Anne, actually before my surgery my eye lid did not close properly and sometimes guys thought I was blinking and tried to flirt with them. Take care.—*Anna*

Hello Guys, just to let you know that I had my new prosthesis for 3 weeks. Only 3 weeks because I had another eyelid surgery. I am so happy because my top eyelid is open now and it looks OK. And I have another prosthesis which looks fine now.—*Anna*

Hi! I had coral implant surgery about 5.5 weeks ago, and I am going to the ocularist next week. I have a conformer in now, and I wear a little gauze patch and a patch from http://www.glamourpatches.net that fits over my glasses when I go to work. When they removed the silicon ball I got when I was five, it was encased in scar tissue and all the muscles were tucked behind it. No one knows if they were ever attached or if they just slipped off. At my follow-up appt, the implant had some movement, so I was pleased. I mean, the fact that those muscles were any good at all after nearly 30 years is a minor miracle. I don't know if there is anything to this I plan to ask the ocularist next week—but the lid seems to sit more normally depending on what position I sleep in! If I sleep on my back, I wake up and it looks like everything is further back than if I sleep on my side. So I've been sleeping on my side. It would make sense, since the coral implants are just like the others until they are vascularized, and I doubt my muscles are strong enough to hold the eye forward all night while lying on my back.—*Vivacemist*

Vivacemist, I'm SOOOO curious right now that I can't wait to hear your answer. I, too, had a silicone implant (30 years ago). I rejected the silicone ball, and my surgeon tried a groundbreaking new procedure-using silicone beads instead. I've had NO (zero) movement, due to muscle loss and it being a gunshot wound (BB gun). What I'm curious about, is, after 30 years of having the implant that I have, and having NO movement, is there even a remote possibility of the coral implant giving me some movement? Do you know?

As far as the prosthesis looking like it's deeper set sometimes, I agree with you. In my case, it depends on how I sleep or lie down, and it also depends on it I have a headache (it's deeper set when my head hurts for some reason). Anyway, your posts were very interesting to me, and I'm curious to hear more. Thanks!—*Chris*

◆   ◆   ◆

I have a question after my 1 month check-up yesterday from enucleation. I thought I was doing great, feeling good and back at work for a couple weeks but the Doc said that my body was rejecting my implant (pushing it out of the socket) and I have to have another surgery next week to replace it. Is this common? Should I expect the same type of recovery as the first time? The first time was due to trauma from a hunting accident. My Doc is sending me to a different surgeon a couple hours away because he feels he's better qualified. Thoughts or suggestions? Thanks!—*Chale*

Hi Chale, glad to hear you're feeling good after the operation. There is certainly a difference in outcome according to the skill of the surgeon. Your doctor should also involve you in the discussion about the material used for the implant. I believe the specialty is called oculoplastic and it's certainly worth a few hours drive to get the right specialist. Hope it goes well the second time around. Keep well.—*Chil*

Chil, thanks for the reply. The new doctor is indeed an oculoplastic surgeon so I'm looking forward to what the outcome will be.—*Chale*

Hi, I just read your post and I was wondering if you experienced discomfort or symptoms that made you go to your doctor and discover that you were rejecting the implant? I had my eye enucleated in May and as of 2 weeks ago I haven't been feeling right. I have this weird pixelated vision in my good eye and massive headaches and fatigue all the time. I haven't been able to see my doctor yet because he is away, but I wanted to know about your experience. Please let me know. And good luck with everything. Love,—*Jodi*

◆ ◆ ◆

Hi everyone, another question from the rookie. I have another 18 days (but who's counting?) before I get my prosthetic and have a new conformer issue I am hoping someone can help with.

Not to be graphic but I have been very ill with a nasty flu and cold this week (vomiting with a conformer in is extremely painful!) and now behind the conformer I can see what looks like yellow mucus (sorry). It is visible in the area where I have the air bubble. There's a fair amount of it in there and I wasn't sure if I should maybe take out the conformer and wash it off or go see my doc? I'm a bit uneasy about removing the conformer but I don't know that having mucus (or whatever it is) under there for the next 18 days is healthy either. I certainly don't need an infection that will postpone my new eye. I have had more pain this week than in the last while but I figured that was due to the pressure from being ill. Am I being over cautious? This stuff really needs to come with a guidebook! Any advice/experiences would be appreciated. Thank you!—*Sterretjie*

This is not an uncommon problem and I think most of us in here suffer with it at some time or another. With me it is always worse when I am unwell or the weather is very cold. My advise is to take the conformer out and give it a wash but take notice which way it is in and put it back the same way. The day after I got my very first conformer put in I rubbed my eye and it came out so I panicked a little but managed to get it back in. Since I've had my last op 3 weeks ago I can't get this conformer out very easily which must mean the op has been a success. MY old eye used to pop out very easily. I'm sure others will be here soon to offer more advice and support,—*Anne*

Being sick is gross. I hope you're feeling better. What usually happens to me is that any gooey stuff will leak out from under the conformer/prosthetic and manifest as the crusty eye syndrome in the morning which can be alleviated by a warm wet washcloth.

To encourage the stuff to come out without taking out your conformer if you don't want to take it out, use a warm washcloth that is almost dripping wet. You can roll up a bath towel and drape it around your neck to absorb the dripping water. Sit in a comfy chair, or prop up on pillows on your bed and lean back and tip your chin up. Hold the cloth to your eye, and while blinking, slowly squeeze that water over your conformer. This helps me to gently irrigate without causing more irritation by taking out my eye. And it can super-hydrate the skin around your eye, making it ready to slap on some nice rich eye cream to lessen the appearance of stress and crepe-y skin, so be sure to hydrate the other eye and send those crow's feet packing! Not that any of us here have any wrinkles. especially not me. Uh-uh, nope, not me. Love,—*Alicia*

◆   ◆   ◆

Hi Guys, I am really drawing at straws and so I thought I would try here with my fellow LostEye friends to see if anyone can offer some help or advice. I had my eye removed in May 2004. Everything went great, until October when I started to have this weird vision in my good eye. Its like everything that I see, especially solid colors will be made up of tiny dots. So if I look at a white wall, my eye is seeing white and grey dots mixed together. As time progressed, I started to get headaches, muscle and joint pains, extreme fatigue, weight gain, and a clicking and whooshing sound in my head. I have been to so many doctors and no one can figure out what is wrong with me. My surgeon, who I adore, assures me that it is not the implant. However, here I am in May and while I do have my other symptoms, nothing has been a constant expect for the vision. Once it came in October, it never left. Something in my gut tells me that all of my ailments stem from my implant. It all started 5 months after surgery, the time that it takes for everything to totally heal. I know that the surgery was a success, but I wonder if its possible to be having a foreign body reaction or a toxic reaction in my body to the implant? I know that this all sounds weird and everything, but I just don't feel well and I want to get better. I only have one eye and so as you all know, the fact that my healthy eye is not seeing correctly is very scary for me. If anyone can offer any suggestions or has heard of this before, PLEASE get back to me. I hope that all of you are well. Love Always,—*Jodi*

Hi Jodi, first of all, I'm really sorry to hear your going through such a rough time. I really don't know much about implants and their toxicity. But although the risk may be very small, I'd never rule anything out. I had a quick trawl through Google just now, and although I didn't find much about eye implants giving rise to toxic reactions, the plight of women with reactions to their silicone breast implants popped up constantly during the search. So who knows?

Even if you do go through all the medical examinations, i.e. thorough blood work etc, and they find nothing. Would you want to resort to have the implant taken out to see whether it is causing the problems? I'm sorry I don't have much info mate, I really hope you get sorted, do let us know, Take Care,—*Elizabeth*

Elizabeth, just being able to vent on here and the fact that you responded means a lot to me. Thank you so much for taking the time to read an respond and then check Google. I had actually spoken with a doctor about the breast implants and how women get toxic reactions to them and so I had known about that. Perhaps that's why we felt that the same could be happening to me from my eye. I don't think that I would have the implant removed unless I knew 100% that it was the implant that was causing this. I'm just going to keep on looking I guess. Thank you again so much for taking the time to write to me. Love,—*Jodi*

Hi Jodi, I wish I had some info for you but I don't. I'm so sorry for everything you are going through, please take care and keep in touch. Have you ever seen a Naturopath? Mine has diagnosed some odd things for me and really made a huge difference in a lot of areas. Just a thought, sometimes going off the beaten track helps. All the best,—*Starr*

Thank you for that suggestion about the retinal However, I have been to a retinal specialist and both he and my ophthalmologist assure me that my retina and my good eye are all fine. I went to see a neurologist recently who is thinking that some of my ailments could be caused by scar tissue forming around my implant and putting pressure on it. This would cause my headaches, pulsating noise that I hear in my head and possibly be affecting the vision in my left eye. I will be meeting with a neuro-ophthalmologist in July and probably having a specialized MRI performed that could present some evidence to back up this possible solution. Thanks to everyone who has responded and put in their two-cents.—*Jodi*

That does sound plausible. When I was pregnant, I had some headaches and increased phantom pain, both centered around my implant. I was told by my retinologist that it was likely due to swelling leading to increased pressure on the implant. I never did have any other symptoms but I certainly had some pain, and that is the only time I have ever had pain like that since my eye was removed. I'd forgotten all about it until I read your post (one tends to forget all the pains and discomforts concerning pregnancy and childbirth. the human race would die out otherwise).

I can see where scar tissue could have a similar effect, though I'm surprised that there would be that *much* of it. Good luck with tracking down the cause of this, keep us updated on how you're doing!—*Kelli*

Speaking of pixilation, and strange happenings. I get that quite a bit also in my good eye. I also get comet flashing going across sometimes. When I close both my eyes, I get strange distortion on my enucleated side. Like watching a T.V. with static. It scared me a few times, because I know I am blind on that side. At this point, I see it as my brain working overtime, trying to create a picture in my bad side to match the working side. If this makes any sense to any of you. My good eye has been checked 5 times since the enucleation. All the doctors say it is psychological. The brain is a very complex organ. The doctors really haven't skimmed the surface on it. If they knew more, then they would be able to transplant a donor eye. They just don't know enough about attaching the bundle of nerves back to the optic nerve. So much for modern witch doctors.—*Michael*

◆ ◆ ◆

About the peg, the latest I heard from Moorfields is that they have gone out of favor because they can cause a gap at the corner. I know lots of people on this site have had good experiences with the peg. This is not to prejudge the outcome of your next appointment but it's obviously best to consider all the options. Keep your spirits up.—*Chil*

About the peg, it isn't even considered until the socket has healed and the implant is settled. Then you can decide with the ophthalmologist if it's necessary or desirable and if you're a good candidate for it. So you have tons of thinking time and don't have to worry about it just now.—*Marmalade*

10

Scleral Shells

Many people lose the sight in their eye, but not the eye itself. Sometimes the eye retains its original size and appearance, but too often the eye will start to shrink or move about erratically and become strange or distracting for others to look at. Sadly, some are born with an eye in this condition. In these circumstances, an alternative to removal of the eye is to get what is known as a "scleral shell" which is sort of like a cap that fits over the eye and gives the appearance of a healthy eye.

MESSAGES

Hi, I just came across your site and have a few questions and comments. My story is that five years ago at the age of 19 I was driving at night and hit off-set head-on by a pickup truck, punching the hood of the car through the windshield into the shape of a spear, and into my left eye only short of death. Amazingly my miraculous surgeon had recently been to a medical conference and, unlike many surgeons at that time, he decided to repair what was left (not very much) instead of removing the entire thing (there was a common thought that sympathetic opthalma is a greater risk if the eye is left on a serious eye-trauma patient—it turns out that the risk of getting sympathetic opthalma is no greater than the risk of dying under general anesthetics, so it would have been pointless to have it removed. But this is one issue it could be helpful for you to raise.

Soon after the accident I started going to see some specialists, one of whom was a 'top' guy for Lion Eye. He looked at me with shock and proceeded to tell me horror stories, and insisted that I must have my eye removed immediately (by now I was recovering from the trauma, with practically no eye, but enough to wear a scleral shell). I was devastated at the idea of more surgery so soon after the accident. The next specialist I saw confirmed my surgeon and said he is amazed at how many doctors, in post-trauma situations, think they must remove the entire eye, when recent studies show otherwise. The Lion guy was trying to convince me to schedule the surgery before I even got out of his office. For a 19 year old I think it is good that I was able to keep what could be saved, as somehow I didn't experience a complete feeling of loss, though I am completely sightless in that eye.

In addition, the scleral shell I am fitted with goes unnoticed by 99% of all people I meet. It was comforting to read your description of the surgery though, because it remains a possibility that one day I may have to have the rest of the eye removed and have it posted (at this point I have little more than the socket, but it is enough to allow the shell to track almost perfectly). Anyways, I think your site is great, and I wish there had been something like that after my accident (though the book you recommended was the first thing I read back then).—*Gabriel*

I just read through your letters which you have posted, and as my earlier letter was not in a form which would be suited I'll write another one and forward it soon should you wish to post it. I would like to pass a message on if I could—that gentleman with the son who has a scleral shell asked what he could do, as it was painful and the son doesn't wear it. For starters he should get a new ocularist. A good ocularist should be on top of those things, have given the proper information, etc. It is true, with less traumatic trauma (like a BB) a scleral shell is not always feasibly as there are a lot of nerves that remain highly active in the eye—I was fortunate to have enough trauma that my damaged eye provides more shape for my shell to grip (texture and scar can almost be good in this case) and to have enough nerves damaged that it doesn't hurt. However, even for me I don't relish having adjustments made, but more importantly, I had my second shell made a year ago, and just like the first, it hurt like a mother for the first month as I got used to it. He should check with his ocularist (or get a new one, though usually that means a new shell, as most 'artists' that I've heard of won't work on shells they didn't make, for obvious professional standard reasons). There is still a good chance that if he really tries wearing it as much as possible that he will get used to it. (I'm amazed that evidently he was never fitted with a "practice" shell, clear plastic worn for the first month to get an idea of how good a fit to go for (the less pain the better the fit, more pain, slightly worse fit, but better than nothing). anyways, I just figured that scleral shells may be a bit different from the complete prosthetic so thought I'd share the advice.—*Gabriel*

◆   ◆   ◆

Hello. I am brand new to this forum, and am hoping I can find support and answers here. On Friday I has my first appointment concerning obtaining a scleral shell. At this appointment the ocularist used alginate to make a mold of my eye. The alginate made my eye VERY red and sore. It has never looked that bad before. The ocularist told me it might take a few days to feel better. My question for all of you is, if you have had this procedure, did it cause eye irritation, and how long did it last? Did you find anything to help it feel better? (I tried allergy eye drops, and found that they were NOT a good idea.) It is now Sunday night, and my eye is still very red and irritated. I don't know if this is normal, or if I'm having some sort of allergic reaction to the alginate. Any feedback would be greatly appreciated. Thank you!—*Renee*

Thanks, Mindy, for your reply. My eye felt a lot better beginning around the 5th morning after the fitting, and hasn't bothered me again. I felt no irritation at all during the actual fitting. I hope this doesn't mean I'll have a big problem with the shell itself, but I think you may be right, it may have been an actual allergic reaction to the alginate mixture. How did you do with the actual eye, even though you had irritation during the fitting? Was it difficult to get used to wearing? Was yours a prosthetic eye, or a scleral shell? Thanks again!—*Renee*

I think I have the shell. It is the one that fits over the base they attach during removal of the bad eye. I have really had no problems. At night mine does get a little matter, but the only time the eye ever irritates me is when an eyelash or something gets stuck behind it. They are very easy to remove and put back. So I can fix the problem quick! Good Luck!—*Mindy*

◆ ◆ ◆

Decided to have the Scleral Shell put in my eye. Most of the time keep the eye shut to block out light and irratants. Hope I am doing the right thing since the eye is holding pressure and not having any pain. Tired of walking around with dark glasses. Are there many people on this board that have one? How long do they last?—*Sueanne*

Hi Sueanne, what is the condition you have which causes your eye problems? What kind of shell will you get? Mine is a hand painted one that can be taken out whenever, sometimes called an Occlusive Contact Lens, but my other Eye Dr calls it a shell so that's what I call it too (its shorter! lol.) I was born with Optic Nerve Hyperplasia, and developed diplopia (double vision) about 4-5 years ago. I had prisms and the good old pirates patch to control the diplopia until I was eventually given the shell. My shell, although great for blocking out light and stopping the double, etc., has caused a few problems. I have to use artificial tears all the time because my eye dries out so quickly, which is a real pain in the hoop and if I can find any tears quickly enough it is really sore! I also have an area around my iris which looks like the beginning of an ulcer because it is constantly red and when I put the shell in it rubs on this area. If there is another course of surgical action that can solve my problems I will be opting for that because I am finding the shell hard work.

Cosmetically, the shell is great. I had its colour mastered digitally, comparing it to the images taken of my other eye. The only time I find it noticeable is in a dimly lit room, or on a very sunny day, when pupil sizes will be different. Although most people would know that something is there, they will not be sure what, and eye movement is nearly 100%. However, with all that said, I am still really trying to persevere with it, because it gets rid of the debilitating diplopia. As for how long they last, I am planning on asking that myself at my next visit. So really, it depends on yourself as to weather you have any problems with it and how you manage those problems. Hope that helps a bit,—*Elizabeth*

Hi, I am the office manager for an ocularist. A corneoscleral shell eye, in our clinic, is custom fabricated on sight. We don't use stock eyes of any sort. If the eye is not a "stock eye", they will take an impression of the socket with a material that sets up with the consistency of an egg white. This doesn't hurt, but may feel cool and a little weird at first. Once this is set, your ocularist will remove the impression and begin to create a mold of this material. We use dental stone for this impression. In our clinic, the whole process takes 2 days. The first day consists of the impression (and takes 4-4 1/2 hours) and creating the molds and creating the eye itself out of acrylic plastic. The second day takes about 6 hours. The second day is what we call the paint day. The ocularist will paint the artificial eye to match your live eye. There are some ocularists that will make an I in one day, and often within 4 hours. However, it has been my observation, that these eyes tend to be made from stock eyes. Many people dislike the results because this type of fabrication doesn't fit well, resulting in eyes that cause the eye to look unreal.

I suggest that you inquire of your ocularist if they use stock eyes or fabricate them from scratch. Sometimes the lower or upper eyelid can cause an eye to not fit well and requires surgery to correct. Your ocularist should show you how to remove and insert your artificial eye. Instructions on the proper care for your artificial eye. This eye should be polished once a year, however, some people require their eye to be polished twice a year. Your corneoscleral shell should last about 10 years, requiring a revision in 5 years. This, of course, depends on your age, illness, weight loss or gain, and/or the build up of protein.

As to the other persons post here regarding dry, irritated eye socket. Have you ever heard of Sil-ophtho (sill-off-tho) Oil? The works better than artificial tears, however, there are other oil drops like Lacrilube too. Inquire with your pharmacy, ocularist or eye doctor on how to obtain a bottle. It should be available over the counter, and doesn't require a prescription from a doctor.—*Teddy*

Want to thank you for the information you provided. The doctor was happy the way I handled everything. Guess knowing what to expect really helps. I have a detached retina. After four operations no luck. Hoping this shell will work for me without any problems. The eye has shrunk so it will need some building up. Will keep you posted on the results.—*Sueanne*

◆ ◆ ◆

Hi Dave, I had surgery on my iris many years ago to open the pupil up and create a more central opening (I have a little bit of sight). It really was a functional change and was not really intended as a cosmetic improvement. Ask your eye doctor if this is appropriate for you. I'm amazed how often doctors do not tell you about cosmetic options unless you ask. Please research any Surgeon you consider.

I'm checking out a scleral shells for myself because my eye lid is starting to droop in addition to having a misshaped iris and scar. If your eye pupil isn't too bad, consider commercial color lenses in both eyes. They helped soften the differences between my eyes. Some lenses are pretty opaque and might improve your appearance enough to make you feel better. I hope this will help you get the ball rolling! Best wishes,—*Amy*

◆ ◆ ◆

Hey All, I have been having lid irritation for the last several years. I use Tobradex ointment often. I read on the web that old "shells" can cause lid irritations & that made sense. My old scleral shell is over 20 years old. Surprisingly, this ocularist said old age wasn't an issue with shells (again, I read otherwise on the web). So I just had a new shell made last week—but I can't wear it. It's too large I think & there is a wobble every time I blink. I think it is too think & too large for my socket. It is very different in shape from the old one which did fit comfortably.

I figure the up-and-down wobble has got to be dragging against my eyeball and causing some of the discomfort. My ocularist said it wasn't very noticeable & let me leave for home with the "bounce". I was so tired & sore—I just wanted to come home. He said the eye would settle in & I believed him. After an hour—the eye began to feel really tight. By the time I got home—I was miserable. Took it out & it was so large that it hurt extracting it. I waited a few days & reinserted it again—even though I didn't want to. I wore it overnight to try to get it to "settle in". Still misery.

Did I just get a bad ocularist? He's 3 hours away & I'm not going back. He used a Sharpie to mark on the wax model & I didn't think about it until I got home—but I bet he used that same marker on all his clients. If so, I just got exposed to body fluids from everyone who was there before me. Has anyone had this kind of problem?—*EJ*

Hi EJ, when you said that it hurt extracting your shell, was it like you had to "peel" it off your eye? I had a shell and had EXACTLY the same symptoms as you, which my ocularist called "Clamping". I was in AGONY. I went through artificial tears like they were smarties, and it basically wasn't fun! It will not get any better on its own, so my plan would be go see an ocularist ASAP. It could be that your eye is just taking a while to get used to a new shell after all these years, but still, it sounded so like what I had I thought I would share. I hope you get sorted. Take Care,—*Elizabeth*

Thanks Elizabeth. Actually, it was swollen lids that caused the pain during removal—in conjunction with the new prosthesis being larger and having little tabs (for lack of a better description). It looks monstrous in diameter with the little protrusions flaring out. It almost looks like it has corners. It just doesn't look eye friendly (I know that much).

I am having all kinds of problems with lid irritation. Does anyone out there have chronic lid irritation? When the shell is out, I'm fine. When it's in, after a few hours the swelling and itchiness resumes. I'm speaking of the old shell as well as the new one too. The lid problem is what prompted me to get the new shell. I figure it had to do with the 24 year old shell (but this particular ocularist said age didn't affect the shell). My optometrist has prescribed Tobradex ointment & Lotemax (a steroid). They help clear up discomfort as long as I don't wear the shell. I wish I knew what to do other than just leave the eye out. I am about to the point of just wearing a patch. Keeping the eye shut all day is so fatiguing and uncomfortable.—*EJ*

◆ ◆ ◆

Hi All, Does everyone get a good fit for their new shells the first visit to their ocularist or do they have to go back several times for either additional grinding down or for an entirely new eye? Does anyone have a great ocularist in the South east who could get the right fit on one visit? Maybe mine is just hard to make because it has to be so thin. I don't know—but I really need some wisdom. Many thanks. Any help/advise would be appreciated.—*EJ*

Hi EJ, I had a scleral shell made recently here in Philadelphia. My first "finished" shell had my eye looking off to the left! My second "finished" shell has me looking slightly down! I go back tomorrow to have this fixed. I think he's going to create a new mold and build up the existing shell. We'll see, I won't be shocked if he starts over. I can tell by the look on my Ocularlist's face that he is sorry he told me he could fit me. He is not really sure why we're having all the troubles but he did say these thin shells are the most difficult to fit. He is committed to getting this the best it can be and I'm grateful for all the effort. I would be more upset if he was less a perfectionist. I've spent over 14 hours in his office (so far) but it's worth it. The shell is beautifully painted and really does look natural. I'm also very lucky that the shell is comfortable. It's really strange having a normal looking eye after 30 years. Best of luck to you. I hope you end up with a beautiful and comfortable shell. ~*Amy*

◆ ◆ ◆

Hi All! I lost my left eye about 37 years ago as a 5 year old. Not many problems all in all. I've wore a scleral shell up until a short time ago. I have had discomfort so stopped wearing it. I am seeing the blind eye daily now and noticed that its movement is very odd at times. I wore a new stronger prescription glasses & couldn't believe it when I looked in the mirror today! Both eyes were tracking the same! I mean WOW! The left one normally looks off to the left since the muscle stopped working right 30 years ago. Get this: I took my glasses off to look up close & the eye floated back to its usual blind gaze off to the left. I put the glasses back on and boom! The eye shifted back to almost perfect alignment. I went through this process for 10 minutes. No wonder my shell isn't feeling right. My blind eye is getting a stronger signal from my brain somehow when I focus wearing these glasses.

Anyone! Please tell me what is up with this? Is this good or bad? Has anyone ever experimented to see if you get some realignment if you focus at different focal lengths? This is really bizarre. My blind eye feels a little bit achy today—but not bad. It actually feels pretty good. I'd love to hear from any of you regarding this. Thanks in advance,—*Kate*

♦ ♦ ♦

I know that some of you read my story. I had a bad experience with my first eye and haven't been able to wear it since around 2003. Finally, with my new insurance, I was able to get a brand new scleral shell. It was made in April over a two day period (they didn't have to go through the whole process with me since I already had an eye) and then I went for a follow up in June to make sure everything was okay. They did a fabulous job! I couldn't be happier!—*Christine*

Hey Christine, I am so glad about your new shell success. How has it been for you? Hope it's great. I am still having lid irritations. I thought this was due to the old shell I was wearing (over 20 years). I have a beautiful new one but I'm still experiencing some eyelid burning. How about you?—*EJ*

It's been wonderful! So much better than my first one—it's so perfectly that I don't even know it's there anymore. My first one was a stock eye and the iris was painted directly on to the eye making it look very "2D" and not like a real eye. Even the iris was bigger than my real one. The only problem is that my eye gets 'goopy' when my allergies act up. But other than that, I've been very pleased with it. I just need to take it out after I've had it in for 8 hours working on a computer all day.—*Christine*

♦ ♦ ♦

Hey everyone, I went to see my specialist yesterday as I had been feeling my prosthetic shell wasn't looking as great as it did 16 years ago when I first got it (got it when I was 7). He admitted that my eye has shrunk somewhat and I have been booked in to have a mould taken of my eye. SUPER DUPER YAY, should take 4-6 appointments and I will have a brand new eye, one that is of better coloring and that opens a bit wider. I'm all excited.

Does anyone else here have the prosthetic shell? I know the movement isn't fantastic but I've accepted it now and I like the way I look. Laters—*Cindy*

♦ ♦ ♦

Hello everybody, I just discovered this website and I really like it! I was born with a left eye that is smaller and is blind…When I was 17, I got my first scleral shell and it made me really happy. After some years, the color started changing.

Not that funny as it almost turned yellow, spooky, you know. Luckily, my boyfriend thought it made me even more special.

A few months ago I visited a specialist to make me a new one. Now I have that new shell (only for three days), but every time I take a look in the mirror I'd like to run away. I don't really like it, although the color is great and I m sure the specialist tried to do his work really good. What I wanted to know are there some people here that had the same experience? And how long did it take to get used to that new look? Many kind regards,—*Isabelle*

I recognize the feeling of being almost frightened by the first sight of a new prosthesis. Mine is the whole thing rather than a scleral shell so there is more difference in terms of shape. I think it's because we build our hopes us so that we are almost expecting to be disappointed. I also think that our view is distorted. It's like an anorexic looking in the mirror and seeing herself as fat. Your boyfriend sounds like he has the right idea. Listen to him and not your inner voice.—*Chil*

◆ ◆ ◆

I only wish that I had found this forum earlier, when I was having real trouble accepting that a) I couldn't join the ambulance service, b) I was unable to drive (for however long it took to sort things out) and c) that the operation hadn't fixed the problem. I still had double vision and It didn't seem that I was going to get anything done. Having a forum like this would have been great in helping to thrash out some of the problems. It was only after I accepted things in my head, and stopped getting angry, that the ball started rolling and I got this shell.

I go back to see my surgeon soon, and the next step in treatment, if the shell doesn't work or I can't handle it, etc., is to put a permanent lens into my eye. I am not quite sure how that works or what it entails (I know its more surgery, but I don't know weather it's like a cataract procedure or what). I know surgeons are quite reluctant to do surgery if the situation is ok at the minute. But I am not quite sure of the long term status of one of these shells, you know, can you wear it until you are 70?

I would like a long term solution to the double vision problem, and although the shell is great at the moment, it is a bit of a nuisance, e.g., taking it out and disinfecting it/cleaning it every night, the artificial tears all the time by day, and the problems with it sticking or going up above my eye lid/round the side of my eye when its windy or when I am watching television, etc. The only problem with the "permanent" solution is, if (heaven forbid) I loose sight in my good eye, I would be totally blind, whereas if I still had my eye, I would have at least a little light perception.

I know most of you already have a full prosthesis and so you've already sorted out this scenario for yourselves, so any help would be great!—*Elizabeth*

This scleral shell covers my pupil and iris completely when I wear it, so no light passes through (unless its shifts itself via the wind or something!) and so I don't get double vision. Essentially these leaves me monocular, as I was before my muscle snapped and my eye moved off its suppression, causing my brain to show me a picture it had been blocking off for 14 years. So I am not really worried about the monocular bit, I have sort of already overcome that!

I don't know if its a full enucleation the surgeon was talking about, he just said it would be to "put a lens *into* my eye" and that was what made me think of it being like a cataract operation, only instead of replacing a cloudy lens with a clear one, taking the natural corneal lens and making it opaque, so that no light would get in.

That kind of operation sounds a bit weird and so I don't know which one would be better or worse, the lens in my eye or enucleation. Its not even the cosmetic side of things that worries me (with this scleral shell people ask me all the time, "Have you got a glass eye?" because of the lack of pupil reaction and the fact that the color is a bit off) Its just the fact of leaving myself *totally* blind if anything happened to my good eye. Maybe this is a pretty irrational fear?—*Elizabeth*

◆   ◆   ◆

Hi Amy, you mentioned about scleral shells, I have to say, that Scleral Shells and Occlusive Contact Lenses are not all they are cracked up to be, mine hurt a lot, and artificial tears did little to ease the discomfort. It used to clamp on to my eyeball (Aoooooow!) and when its windy or anything it had the tendency to fall out (sometimes mine just fell out when it wanted to, windy or not!) or slide to the side of your eyeball, making it in my opinion WAAAAY more trouble than its worth. Also it does look like you have prosthetic eye to the onlooker, so if its cosmetics v. that offered by a full prosthesis your going for this is something to think about.

My eye never looked funny naturally but I needed it occluded because of double vision, this was acquired by putting a black intraocular lens inside it, to "turn it off", however I have to take Pilocarpine to make the pupil small so that no light gets in around the lens, making me have a "Wonky" eye to the onlooker. However, I am much happier now than I was with the shells/contact lenses. The Ocularist never told me at the start how much of a nuisance they were.

The only time Id say not to go for an evisceration/enucleation would be if you have any sight (however small) remaining in that eye, because that's always a back up if (Heaven Forbid) something happens to your good eye. Just a few points to keep in mind.—*Elizabeth*

◆　　◆　　◆

Hello & Welcome! I am so very sorry you are having this problem. First of all, please find a good ophthalmologist if you can. You didn't mention your country or city of origin, but if you'll let us know, perhaps someone here can recommend a good doctor in your vicinity. Many of us just hate to go to the doctor, but your doctor should be your starting point.

Often headaches are caused by the complications of a blind or partially blinded eye. A good ophthalmologist can evaluate your situation. For example, you need to find out if there is increased pressure in your problem eye. And since you have only one eye, it is imperative that you see an eye doctor yearly at minimum to preserve the good remaining vision you have. A yearly doctor's exam can prevent much suffering & even blindness.

Children with a "lazy eye" are often treated by covering the stronger eye, but you are apt to harm yourself by trying this. Please make an appointment with a doctor just as soon as possible. Do let us know how you're doing. We care.

I've been blind in my left eye since age 5. I wear a scleral shell or dark glasses to cover the scar & the "drift". I know how you feel about it and I want to encourage you. The fact that your eye has drifted more may mean that your brain is trying harder to reconcile its two vision inputs (even if one is very weak). Wearing a scleral shell may be an alternative for you. Perhaps patching the bad eye might alleviate the headaches. Your doctor can help you sort this out. Again, let us know how you do. Best wishes,—*Elizabeth*

◆　　◆　　◆

Hi, Jay, I just discovered your Lost Eye website and found it very informative. My daughter was a crime victim in 2001 in which she suffered a severe injury resulting in a detached retina and trauma to her left eye. After 4 operations, the doctors were unable to reattach the retina and, as a result of the trauma, her eye was disfigured. They did not recommend removing the eye but, rather, fitting her with a scleral shell. You are so right, her ocularist is not only a true artist but an angel. I was absolutely amazed at the results.

Like you and many others in their letters, she hasn't missed a step in her life. I am so proud of her determination and commitment to carrying on without dwelling on the past and in self-pity. I really don't know if I could be as positive if it happened to me.

Thank you for your time. I will recommend your site to my daughter.—*Susan*

11

Patches and Eye Coverings

Most people who lose an eye will never wear a patch. After I had my surgery, I wore a simple patch around the house for a couple of days, and then opted for dark wrap-around shades instead. However, some people prefer a patch, and may even wear it over their prosthesis. Other people, for whatever reason, cannot use a prosthesis and thus use a patch to keep dust, etc., out of the orbit.

As you will read below, finding a good patch is not as easy as it would seem. While there are a lot of cheapie medical patches and pirate costume patches, it is sometimes difficult to find a good patch that is also comfortable, looks good, and fits well.

LETTERS AND E-MAILS

First of all, your first few pages were very helpful. One of the most fearful things to me was thinking that I was walking around with a hole in my head for 6—8 weeks. When I read about the gel, it was a bit bothersome (actually very), but I guess I will get over my squeamishness because cause ya gotta do what ya gotta do.

My surgery is this Thursday. I don't want to deal with the plastic insert and would prefer a patch. As I was loosing my vision I would periodically use a drugstore "pirate" patch which I am not only used to, but it's easy to get a clean and fresh one immediately. I noticed they were not mentioned by you, and wonder if they are a problem. Sincerely,—*Judith*

Thanks Jay. I read your account on the web site. It sounds like you are a go-getter and have done well since the surgery. I do like your idea of having them write above each eye which is which. I plan to take my daughter with me when I purchase glasses. She likes to give fashion advice. I suspect she'd be appalled if she saw me in wrap-around sun glasses, but there will be no choice if I go for enucleation. My protective measures will just have to be upped a notch or three. Thanks again.—*Judith*

I have lived with only one eye since I was 5, and therefore have no recollection of what it is like to see with two eyes, and therefore nothing to compare against or feel bad about. To me, I have no problem perceiving depth, and I never have.

My problem is, since all the muscle was removed, I am left with an empty eye socket that regular eye patches—designed to be worn over an eye—will not cover this. Although I have a decent artificial eye, I would rather wear an eye patch for sports (because the loss of a patch is more weatherable to the loss of the artificial eye which takes ages to produce). Do you know of any sites that cover the sale of non-cupped eye patches for sport or regular wear?—*Anon*

Thanks for a great site. I have only read a few pages but will certainly read the rest soon. A couple of the things I read really hit home. The part about not needing a support group if you've already had your eye out except for how you think people perceive you is the biggy for me. I had my eye out in 1994 and most days it's not a big deal.

I'm having surgery in a couple of weeks to reposition and have a skin graft done on my hydroxyapatite implant. I can deal with it, but it's the thought of having to leave my eye out for 4-6 weeks while it heals. I got fitted for a contact for my "good" eye so I can wear sunglasses instead of a patch. Dumb idea?? I would love your opinion. Thanks and keep up the good work!—*Joan*

Hi Found your site while searching for information regarding eye patches. Have a friend that lost an eye in a bull riding injury about 3-4 years ago. My concern is he does not ever wear either his prosthetic eye or an eye patch—finds them both uncomfortable. He has recently started back riding bulls and I believe he really needs to wear a patch because of all the dirt and dust and germs. How would you suggest I approach this matter with him or should I just leave it alone? He is only 25 and a really nice looking fellow and he doesn't do himself any justice by not wearing either—think I will just tell him like it is and add the fact that all those young cowgirls would just think an eyepatch was kinda sexy. Thanks for any suggestions.—*Concerned*

My husband just had his left eye removed on Friday (8/5/05) he is home now and resting. I am worried that he will become more depressed when I have to go back to work tomorrow. His own parents didn't even come for the surgery and it really did a number on his emotions. I was hoping someone could let me know what I have waiting for me in the next few weeks and also where can I find an eye patch. I have looked all over and have come up empty handed. Please help with any info you can. Thanks,—*CK*

A very good friend of mine, whom I haven't seen in almost 2 years, lost his vision in his left eye. I am planning to visit him this summer and was wondering if you could tell me what I should expect. From what I've read and heard from my friend, the loss of sight in his one eye doesn't cause him any problems. That's great! Amazing! But, should I expect him to look any different? Do people who lose sight in one eye usually wear a patch? I don't feel that I can ask my friend my question without making him feel uncomfortable. Thanks for helping me out! Best of luck!—*Amanda*

Hello! After years of pain, I am finally having my eye removed on June 11th. I am only 31, and would like to know if you know of any websites with fashionable eye patches for the first month. Or are there any that just stick on and dont wrap around? Thank you,—*Mindy*

I have an eye condition that I periodically need to wear an eyepatch sometimes for several days at a time. I have been looking and cannot find a good source for colored or attractive eyepatches, I know I have seen other people with red ones etc. Any good resources would be appreciated. Thanks—*CJ*

My brother was in a vehicle accident which has left him blind in the left eye. He feels more comfortable wearing a patch over the eye. The only thing that I can find for him are the cheap inexpensive ones you can pick up at any local pharmacy. Do you know where I can find a black leather eye patch, something that is more durable than the ones we have been using? If so, please respond. Thank you.—*Kathy*

Hi, I have recently lost my right eye, upper lid and lower lid to cancer. I am looking for eye patches since it will not be possible for me to use anything else. So far I have had not been able to locate patches, for under my glasses that are solid color. I have tried on line and in my area . Also tried the ones that are on your site. But those sites don't respond. Can you help! Do you have any suggestions? Thank You,—*Gail*

Thank you for your website. My uncle just lost an eye due to cancer. He is extremely depressed and trying to adjust to his depth perception. He also has an uncomfortable black patch that he wears. Do you know of any sources that sell comfortable eye patches besides a black pirate looking patch?? I have searched the web and have not had any luck. Sincerely,—*Darlene*

MESSAGES

I'm a 55 year old professional woman who went through much the same experience as "Frances" on page 1 of the messages. My doctor recommended I wait 3 months from date of surgery to get the prosthesis fitted over my implant, and I too have the clear plastic shield in the meantime. Instead of an uncomfortable and oh-so-obvious eye patch, before I had the surgery, I had eyeglasses made in a nice trendy frame but with shaded tinting, like back in the 70's. The tint creates a shadow that hides the bad eye. I also opted for regular instead of non-glare glass. The reflection serves as a mask also. As my eye opened, showing just a blank (sort of like Night of the Living Dead), I put a very small piece of regular frosted scotch tape on the inside of the glass right where you could see my open eye. With the tinting and the reflection and the tape, unless you're really looking into my eyes, it now just looks like my glasses need cleaning. Not one person who knows nothing about my surgery has asked what's wrong with my eye. It was well worth the extra investment to feel normal.—*Janet*

◆ ◆ ◆

My wife has another three weeks or so until she gets to the ocularist. in the meantime, here is what she is doing. She is finding static cling vinyl "stickers" (the stuff they make the reusable holiday window decorations out of) for her glasses lens. We sent some images to a guy in Ohio to have them made, but they didn't turn out as well as we had hoped, so we have purchased some sheets of clear vinyl at the local hobby lobby and some stickers from there and Wal-Mart. She had a heart for valentines day, an American flag, her companies logo, a smiley face, and today she has a butterfly. We have several other things and they work great! My favorite is a great big eyeball but some of her coworkers thought that was a bit much, oh well! Anyway, she thought it would put people at ease and lets her make the best of a bad situation.—*JB*

◆ ◆ ◆

Hello again. I'm trying to work out in my mind why I prefer to wear a gauze and tape covering rather than a black patch, a fancy patch or one of those Band-Aid colored teardrop shaped things. To me, IN MY CASE ONLY, the black patch says, "This is permanent." The white patch says, "Temporary." Fancy patches, like the sweet little beaded fabric ones my mom sent me, saved all these years, lovingly made by Great Grandma say, "Big Old Nerd." The beige bandage says, "Gotcha!" (This is what they say to me about myself.)

I couldn't explain this to my husband very well. We stopped at a drugstore on the way to meet buddy Rachel for lunch, and I got some Tylenol and some of those beige patches. I put one on in the car—it felt pretty good—held the conformer in, feeling secure. Rachel was already at the restaurant, so when I walked in, I looked for her. John didn't say anything about it then, but he told me a couple of days ago that he watched the people watching me. They looked, saw that something was different, then when they looked closer, they were weirded out by what they saw. I noticed none of it, but John said he understood why I preferred the white patch after that. The visual cues we use, at a very basic primate level to identify each other as members of our species happen so fast we don't know we're doing it. Upright bi-ped, two legs, two arms, a head, two eyes. whoops! The camouflage of the beige is startling, as if there is no eye at all. Instead, there's a healed-over space. I'd rather give a visual clue that says "healing owie."

I have no idea if that makes any sense. I think that whatever makes us feel the most comfortable is what we should do. I'd be more inclined to try an "around the head elastic" patch if I wasn't so completely sure that I'd accidentally strangle in the elastic within three minutes. I can't even wear a headband or a scarf without endangering myself and others. Love,—*Alicia*

Alicia, I don't know why I never tried the patch before, during my MANY years of surgeries and recovery. I had the gauze and tape method, which brought about MANY problems for me. My eye "sweated" underneath the gauze and I was allergic to many of the tapes, which left my skin raw. Thank goodness I haven't had to go through that since my last operation 12 years ago. The beige patch sounds like the way to go! Sounds great. Good luck with everything!—*Chris*

Hi Alicia, I was worried about you. You usually post more often. Am glad you are recuperating. I think I so know what you are talking about. The white eye pad with tape does say that you will be okay in a few days, and no one notices as much. Once, when I was in the mall wearing the dreaded black eye patch (which I only wore for two days), this STUPID woman came up and just started rambling about what a poor thing I was to have a lazy eye and how she used to have one too. I just let it ride, but later wished I would have said something like "Lazy? This one's dead sweetie".—*Roadrunner*

Hi Alicia, I agree with you about black and white patches. It is very actual for me at the moment as I am wearing an eye-patch for at least 4 weeks. I do prefer white. Today I tried a beige one—did not feel comfy, for me it looks like telling everyone: "I do not have eye". White is like "I just got a surgery and will remove it soon". I've got a black one but I do not like it. I think I will stick to the white gauze and a tape. The problem is that my skin is very sensitive and the tape doesn't help. But so far this is the best for me as well. Do you have any problems with your skin around eye—especially a nose? Cheers,—*Anna*

Hi, Anna, I've been using cloth tape and 4 x 4 gauze pads folded in half and secured with tape. I cut about an inch or so off the length of the folded pad, trimming the inside in a < shape to fit along the inner corner, and) shape for the outer. I put the tape on the front so it overhangs the edges. Then I trim the extra tape away, leaving about 1/4 inch all around to press onto my skin. So, it's kind of like a big oval band-aid. When I used the "gentle adhesive" beige patches, I tore off a little skin under my eye, no matter how careful I was! If that adhesive was gentle, I'd hate to see what their "extra-strength" is like!

My new best friend has been a warm washcloth. It loosens up tape for removal, and helps get any sticky stuff from the tape off. It also just feels great over the conformer. The swelling has gone down considerably since the cortisone shots last Wednesday. I'm four weeks healed now, and I feel more free to rub the inner corner—what relief. I think it's a "thing" in my family, because I've seen my mom and recently my sister derive great enjoyment from rubbing their eyes. I remember thinking the night before the first surgery that I'd miss it. Must be a tension reliever or something. Does anyone scuba-dive? It's something I've always wanted to do but have been afraid of the eye being an issue, what with the pressure and all. any insights? Big hugs to all,—*Alicia*

◆ ◆ ◆

Hi, I'm a 23 yr. old married female from VA. USA. I am a mom, and a college student. I was born w/a rare disease in my left eye called "Posterior Lenticonus". I am clinically blind in that eye, and mainly have only peripheral vision in that eye. But looking at me, you can't tell anything is wrong. I have about 20/20 in the right eye with glasses or contacts. My left eye strained my right over the years, causing me to wear glasses for the right. I'm just looking for new friends, and anyone else who may have this disease. Feel free to email me if you have this disease or any other eye condition.

I also want to start making homemade fashionable eye patches for people who are sighted in only one eye, and wear an eye patch. Does anyone out there know whether or not it makes a difference how eye patches are made? Can they effect one's eye if made incorrectly, or are they mainly just material that cover the eye? Thanks!—*Betsy*

◆ ◆ ◆

Though I may have been able to keep my natural eye following radiation treatment for malignant melanoma, my vision is very limited, if it can even be called vision. Moving around left me in a state of frustration trying to interpret what I saw. I discovered patching the bad eye made me feel more comfortable, so I set on a search for a eye patch. My lucky day was when I found http://www.perfecteyepatch.com on the web. The patch is a cover which attaches on one end to the earpiece of the glasses and the other end slips over the nose piece. Comfortable. Doesn't slip around. Won't mess up the hair with an elastic band. Washable. Doesn't look just awful. Comes in an assortment of colors or prints for children. I wanted to pass along my discovery for those who are struggling with patches.—*BeJay*

◆ ◆ ◆

I've had a glass eye for quite some time now (since the age of 4, although I lost it to cancer when I was only 5 months old) and have always had problems with the socket. My current false eye has been causing me increasing amounts of trouble over the last couple of years; and not just comfort issues. Since the age of about 17 I've had an increasing paranoia over the fact my prosthesis has close to zero mobility, so I've decided that rather than putting up with a weeping socket and people staring It would be better if I got a patch instead.

I was wondering if any of you know how I where I could get a quality eye patch. I'm currently in the process of moving and don't have contact with my ocularist (sp). I currently living in the North East of England, and would prefer not having to travel too far to get one. Thanks,—*Dancing*

I'm in Thornaby just outside Stockton, I recently started studying anthropology at university there. I've looked at the sites this page (I found the link about three minutes after I posted) but none of them really have what I'm looking for, and it's also a bit dodgy I clicked on the 'adult' link thinking it meant adult-size patches. I tried searching the web, but I just keep finding pages about pirates (who are way better than ninjas) and how 'badass' patches are, I think one of the topics on this forum has a link to one of them.

I spend a lot of time hanging around gothic clubs so bright colors and patterns are pretty much out of the question. I was hoping to find somewhere nearby where I could get custom patches, my left (false) eye is slightly sunken so I'd like to get something that would sit comfortably. But thanks anyway,—*Dancing*

◆ ◆ ◆

Hi, I'm new and would like to say hello to everyone. I am 46 years old. Can any one help me with locating an eye patch? I have searched every where online and so far have been unsuccessful finding a quality leather eye patch. I purchased a really nice leather eye patch two years ago from Patchworks, Inc. but that site disappeared online. Any help would be appreciated.—*Rusty*

Welcome Rusty, can't help you on the leather patch but I made one out of a sleeping mask. Altered it pretty good!—*Tommy*

Hello Tommy, good idea! Unfortunately I am now spoiled by wearing a beautiful, stylish black leather patch. I am dreading going back to something less comfortable. The guy who made this patch disappeared from online and I have no way of contacting him. His patches were everything I ever wanted in an eye patch. I'll keep exploring and make do if need be.—*Rusty*

◆ ◆ ◆

Have just found out that my operation will be in January. As the weather will be quite cold at that time I have been looking for a site which sells eye patches and have found one in the UK this is it www.reliabletechniques.fsnet.co.uk I know some people have been asking for a site so I hope this helps—*Anne*

◆ ◆ ◆

My husband lost his left eye four years ago due to a fungal spore that somehow got trapped in his sinus cavity and destroyed his optic nerve. The infection grew into his skull causing fluid from his brain to leak into his spinal column. To remove the infection they had to take his eye which was already destroyed by the infection. We were told there would never be a way of using a prosthetic eye. He has used eye patches since the surgery, but it has been very difficult to find them. Please send me web addresses or some info if you know of any. Thanks,—*Shannon*

Hi Shannon, if he wears glasses, here's a suggestion. My wife lost her right eye to cancer in February and didn't get the prosthetic until April. In the meantime, we went to hobby lobby and bought some clear static cling vinyl (can get 8 1/2 by 11 sheets), cut it to the size/shape of her lense and then attached stickers to it. Smiley faces, stars, shamrocks for St. Patty's day, angels, peace signs, teddy bears, etc. anything to have some fun with the situation. Also had some static cling patches made by simply emailing images to a company that works with the static cling vinyl. If you are interested I can look up the company and get that info to you! Hope this helps,—*JB*

Thanks Shannon, I'm still searching. I wish I could find something decent to wear for a few months behind my glasses. Why can't someone make a decent patch?!—*Christine*

When my son had his surgery, we got two patches from Patch Pal. She was very friendly and the patches were easily trimmed to fit his small glasses but would have fit adult glasses as well (I tried it out on mine). My son also enjoyed choosing his own "design" and we could always offer that he could wear the "stars" or the "train" which helped with his desire to wear it before getting his prosthetic.—*Bethy*

◆ ◆ ◆

Hello everyone. I lost my left eye in January of this year, and I just found this site a few days ago. I was snow tubing with group of friends and we lost control and ran into each other. The air stem on my friend's tube punctured my left eye. After 3 days in the hospital the doctors decided that the damage was to severe to save my eye, so on the fourth day after the accident my eye was enucleated. I was released from the hospital the day after, and the pain was more than I was told to expect, but nothing I couldn't deal with. I'm slowly getting used to the monocular vision, but I'm having more trouble dealing with my appearance. I didn't have any insurance coverage at the time of the accident, so I won't be able to get a prosthetic anytime in the near future. So as it stands now I'm stuck wearing an eye patch indefinitely. I managed to find a patch that is not overly big, and somewhat attractive as far as eye patches go I guess, but I would really like find something that is more comfortable and feels more natural to wear. Any info anyone could give me would be greatly appreciated.—*Matt*

Hi Matt, you seem to be pretty positive after your enucleation and that's great, but don't be afraid to air your fears or worries here, everyone is willing to give their advice and tips. As for the eye patches, there have been a few threads all about where to get suitable patches, so have a wee look through the archives.

RE: The insurance issue, It never ceased to amaze me about the US system, if you accident had of happened here in the UK you'd have your eye by now! I'm sorry that you have to wait until you get funds sorted out, it seems quite unfair!—*Elizabeth*

Hi Matt, welcome to this forum. It is a great place to exchange experiences with people who have been there. Like Elizabeth, I am also still amazed by the US health system. I am from Holland and here you would have had your eye too. I cannot imagine being left without an implant. It is so unfair. I do not wear eye patches, but like Elizabeth said lots of people here do and they have mentioned several websites you can visit for great eye patches. Good luck,—*Willeke*

Hi Matt: I just wanted to say hi and that this is a very supportive group. Your attitude sounds great for this being so recent. What about glasses? I have glasses that are clear with one lens shaded out. I also wear sunglasses when the sun is out. I prefer that as I look pretty normal then. I had enucleation back in November that didn't heal correctly, so I understand about appearance. I bought a really nice chocolate suede patch with a braided trim. It's very professional looking and comfy. the website address is: http://www.lenfante.com. I did take a long time to get (6 weeks) it was worth it. Another site to try: http://www.eyepatchheaven.com. Those are cheaper, but some were a little to cutesy for me. Hope this helps,—*Sherri*

◆ ◆ ◆

I suffered a stroke-like episode during the early morning while sleeping. I am told it was more than a t.i.a., because there was permanent damage (the right retina was killed). It's been over 3 years of tough adjustment. There is a tiny "window" through which I can actually see and if I turn my head, I can even read this writing, but this is a very small window. Because my muscles are controlling the eye progressively less, this is causing more of a distraction. I have corrected 20/20 vision in my left eye, but "see" or am aware of some things through my right eye that would normally be outside the field of vision. I drive and read better if I close the eye.

Therefore, I am considering a patch. A black patch sounds kind of ominous, and I am thinking of very dark blue if I find one, which would match the color of the good eye. I guess a soft cloth patch would be best. Can anyone tell me where I could get one or advise me on this problem. Also, I am totally confused by this site's layout. Thanks,—*Duane*

Hey Duane, check out Lenfante.com, I love the patch I got from there, I got camel color for the front with a black inner lining so it would not reflect light into my eye that I patch because of the distorted vision from eye cancer surgery. I really love the patch I got and am planning to get more. They are $25 dollars each. If you need some that are inexpensive Wal-Mart pharmacy has one for about two bucks, I get tired of wearing the ones from Wal-Mart because you can feel them too much and they reflect light, that's just me though. Best wishes!—*Barry*

◆   ◆   ◆

Hi folks, Thank you in advance to all those who are able to lend a helping hand. My grandfather had brain surgery to remove a tumor that had been growing for nearly 15 years without anyone being aware of it. The surgery was successful but it left certain side effects that are irreversible and permanent. His face has partial paralysis, which, amongst other things, causes his right eye not to close, not even to blink. He has problems keeping it moist and something as simple as a ceiling fan is an irritant to his eye.

He is still able to see out of it without any problems but has been relegated to using a pirate's patch which has completely eliminated irritants to his eye, such as the moisture and wind. However, I want to find him a clear eye patch if possible so that he can have the use of both of his eyes. If anyone is aware of where I can purchase a clear eye patch I would be grateful for a hint or tip. Thanks again to all who respond.—*Sasha*

I have a few ideas that are outside of the box so please check with your grandfather's doctor to see if they are okay. You might try www.lenfante.com. If you click on contact us sort of near the top right of the page you can send an email telling her your needs and she may be able to custom make something. I left my phone number with a request to talk via phone and she called me within two or three days. I am very happy with the patch I received and it was $25 dollars.

I'm not sure about this next suggestion, but you might think about safety goggles, you might find inexpensive ones in the garden areas of Wal-Mart or Kmart, but if I remember correctly I have seen some with a very nice quality of lens in the special section of Wal-Mart where they fit you for prescription lenses, they are usually located in the front of the store. I believe I remember seeing very nice quality safety goggles located right by all of the frames you can chose for prescription lenses and I think they were around $12 dollars. If you go this route I would get the best lenses possible so your grandfather will have the best quality goggles to look through. I would ask his doctor if looking through this lense will adversely affect his vision.

I have also seen ocluders that cover one eye but all the ones I have seen have a frosted lense so that would not work, but you might find one that has a clear lense if you search Google. The ocluders I have are made like an eye patch but have a frosted like plastic lense, they are very uncomfortable to wear. It might be ideal if you can find safety goggles that only cover one eye, I'm not sure if they exist though.

Out of everything I have mentioned the safety goggles are the only thing that sounds like a good possibility, and I would ask your grandfathers eye doctors what they think about that. I would also be asking them as many questions as possible about keeping your grandfathers eyes moist. I wish you the best, it is very nice that your grandfather has you there to help,—*Barry*

◆ ◆ ◆

I thought of one other thing. I am 4/200 in one eye after cancer surgery, but before my vision got that bad my doctors advised me that patching that eye could cause problems over a long period of time. I'm not saying that anything that you have done so far has caused any problems. I just hope you will find a solution so your grandfather will not have to patch the eye for a long time, and I applaud your efforts in seeking a solution. Your grandfather's eye doctors may not agree with what my doctors said about patching an eye that has vision, and also every persons medical condition can be somewhat unique, so I hope you will work with his doctors regarding the solution that will be best overall.

I just remembered that I think I also saw safety glasses along with the safety goggles. The safety glasses wrap around far enough that they might block any wind or breezes, and they will be more comfortable than goggles, you might want to alternate between the two.—*Barry*

I think the safety goggles are a good idea. Also, the lady at lenfante.com is super for making customizations so definitely give her a try. Also, I remember seeing a "Patrick Moore Style" monocle which had a tight piece of elastic round it, so it fitted like a patch but was just as effective as a monocle (and didn't require the effort of holding it in with your cheek muscles). I also read of a Bells Palsy Sufferer who used the clear lid of a yoghurt put and made a patch out of it so she could drive for short distances. I hope you find a solution, because using artificial tears is neither practical nor fun.—*Elizabeth*

Yeah, the best people to talk to would be the doctors he's seeing, and those in the Orthoptics Department, as they have all manner of patches/prisms/lenses. Talking to the manufacturers (e.g. 3M) would also be helpful. It is definitely possible to get clear adhesive dressings, and so maybe they could be workable? Again, talking to the hospital and the manufacturers would be an idea.—*Elizabeth*

◆ ◆ ◆

I'm 42 and I've just partially lost vision in my right eye to wet macular degeneration—right over the macula, which I understand is not uncommon. My doctor like a very sharp guy, but very busy and his staff has not been very useful outside the direct problem I'm having.

I'm looking for a few things: 1) A good optometrist on the westside of Los Angeles—I've just moved here. 2) A good eye patch—I can't drive or read with my right eye open any longer—I've got 3 cheap eye patches at this point and I don't like any of them. I'd be happy to pay for a few really good comfortable ones. 3) Probably most important—I want to get good protective eye gear to wear while playing basketball. I play every weekend and I'm afraid of eye injury, now that I'm down to one functioning eye—been jabbed in the eye too many times over the years while playing. Is there a recommended "best" protective prescription goggle out there anyone's used? A lot of questions, I know. I'm glad I found this website.—*Sam*

I live on the west side, too. because As far as eye patches, I only use them "between eyes" like I am now and I use the opticlude patch that has the little girl on the box. There are some links in the archives here—do a search for eye patches. They have all kinds of protective stuff too.—*Alicia*

Thank you so much! That's all really useful to me. I've got P.P.O., I can go wherever I like. I'm pretty much stuck with eye patches—on the good side, I still have some useful vision in the bad eye—on the bad side, I can't drive or read with that eye open. So I'm going to need patches for a good while—I hope. It should have occurred to me to search the site for that.—*Sam*

I think you will really like it, I got the one with the adjustable band, I may try the braided cord later. Since I have partial distorted vision in that eye I asked her to put black on the backside so it would not reflect light, and I have camel color on the front side that people see because it sort of blends in with my skin. They are very comfortable, I have to adjust mine occasionally to keep it in the right spot but it is well worth it. I hope you like it a lot!—*Prism*

I have partial distorted vision that I block too, I use a patch but I also do something else that you might like from time to time. Before you try this please check with your doctor to see if it's okay. First I have someone at an eyeglass store remove one lens out of a pair of sunglasses or other glasses, the lens I have removed is the lens on the side of my eye that was not affected by the cancer. I remove the lens from that side so the lens cannot be broken and get in my good eye. Wal-Mart always does this for free.

Then I take electrical tape and put two strips on the backside of the remaining lens so it will block vision in the eye with very distorted vision. I drive much better with a patch and a patch also works better outside for me, but the eyeglasses with the electrical tape to block the image on one side works for me inside when I'm just sitting around.

It might not work for you but I thought I'd let you know just in case. Because my vision is so distorted it helps me to change things up from time to time and letting some light in seems to cut down on pain that I have some time when I use my eyes to focus for extended periods. I really think you should ask your doc to be sure it will be okay for you. I think you mentioned he is only interested in certain aspects of your condition, and I have run into the same thing with my docs, you may be able to get him to answer you via phone or letter if he is hard to get in touch with.

I think you asked about safety glasses for basketball, have you thought about one of the masks like the pros wear when they have injuries, that might be best and the safest if you can find one at a sporting goods store, if you can't find one that way maybe it's possible to contact one of the pro teams and ask their trainer. If you think goggles would be the best, Wal-Mart has both goggles and safety glasses I believe. Since you haven't been wearing a patch long I want you to know that pirates costumes were the most popular Halloween costume in the US last year, it's good to be in style.—*Barry*

Barry, this is too funny! I was just dropping by to brag about my new invention, and you've described it! Mine is a pair of clip-on sunglasses with the right lens knocked out, and the left is covered by a sticker that I colored black with a Sharpie pen and trimmed to size. Since I wear glasses, it's uncomfortable to wear a patch, but it's hard to read and work at the computer with my distorted vision. I had a fit of frustration last night while working on a take-home exam and this is what I came up with. My boss says I look "very Matrix." I was planning on getting this patented and retiring early, but looks like you beat me to it. Want to go into business together? You handle the U.S., I'll handle Eastern Europe? The ever so lovely and stylish,—*Ya'ara*

Hey Ya'ara, thanks for the fun way that you described how we have the same idea about making our own glasses, great minds think alike I'll let you have the patent rights and if you get rich I'll be your blind in one eye chauffer I wanted to mention that a patch from lenfante.com may also work very well under your reading glasses, they don't stick out as far as the store bought patches and they are very comfortable. I love mine so much I told the lady who makes them that she is an angel. I am happy to know that we are both in style together, setting fashion trends on two continents.—*Barry*

Hi Barry, we really are on the same wavelength. I just ordered from L'Enfante myself today, after reading all the good things Prism says about them. Do you have a flat patch or a cone-shaped patch? I went for flat because of my glasses, and am worried that it will irritate my eye when I blink. I wanted to ask L'Enfante to embroider it with the words ASK ME ABOUT MY LASIK but then I thought, "I'm the only person in the world who will find that amusing."—*Ya'ara*

Hey Ya'ara, I have a cone shaped one. It doesn't stick out nearly as much as the store bought patches. It also has a lot of give because it is made of ultra suede, but at the same time it has enough stability to maintain the cone shape. If you want to change the order I bet you could email them and she will change it for you. I think she usually has a two week delay in filling orders. We will be in style together,—*Barry*

◆ ◆ ◆

This is a very minor complaint in the Grand Scheme of Things, but I can't find patch for my left eye. L'Enfante sent me a very pretty one—but to keep my glasses from going askew when I wear it, I have to move it so far over that it doesn't function as a patch. At the moment I'm making do by covering the left lens of my glasses, which looks oh so professional and attractive. My eye doc here says yes, an intraocular occlusive lens would work, too bad we don't have them in Romania. Grr! I am pinning my hopes on something called the Mins lens, which I stumbled over at http://www.eyeassociates.com/mins lens.htm I'm trying to talk their docs into making me a pair if I send them my official prescription. Hugs to all,—*Ya'ara*

◆ ◆ ◆

Hi, I lost my left eye in '96 & due to the nature of enucleation, cannot fit a prosthesis. So I've worn custom made leather eye patches ever since which are generally OK, you sort of get use to them. However, has anyone heard of the following or will it always be just a dream of mine. Mirror-type glasses that don't allow people to see in but you can see out clearly, including at nighttime. Clear night vision is critical as sunglasses are no good in the dark for people like us. Leave that to the rock stars.

If such glasses were possible, then I could do away with the patch which has two main drawbacks: 1. People (especially kids) tend to stare and either become noticeably uneasy or bombard you with pirate queries/jokes. Or, 2. Patches tend to sweat and become uncomfortable in a working environment, especially in summer & warmer climates. Anyway, any info or advice will be much appreciated and thanks for the site, it's great! Regards,—*Julian*

I think that if you wear mirrors it looks as curious as a patch or frosted lens on the lost eye side. I have a pair of glasses with frosted lens, I wore them before I got my prosthetic eye. And still wear occasionally, if I feel like not wearing my prosthetic eye. And a patch is one alternative. But I think I would not wear mirror lenses, you must have them on both sides and it sure looks curious, especially during hours of darkness. Regards,—*JPH*

Thanks JPH for your view. You're probably right if one lens is different from the other, e.g. frosted as in your case. That's why I was suggesting both lens be the same, i.e. mirror finish. Providing I can see clearly out of my good eye I wouldn't give a hoot if some people think it strange to be wearing mirrors at night. It'd be no stranger than a patch & at least provides an alternative. So the search continues. .if anyone else out there knows of any glasses like this? Cheers,—*Julian*

Hey Julian, if you find the glasses that you like you can cover the back of them with electrical tape and that way no one can see in. You might also try lenfante.com If you email the lady that does the patches she will even custom make them for you, including the exact size that you need the patch to be. I would be sure to get the a patch that is cone shaped so you will not feel your eyelash touch when you blink. No eye patch is perfect but the one I have from L'Enfante is about as close to perfect as I have found. It is the coolest patch in the heat and is washable too. I hope it works great for you.—*Barry*

PART IV
CAUSES

12

Choroidal Melanoma

Many people lose their eyes or eyesight in one eye to various cancers and diseases. As related earlier, I lost my left eye to choroidal melanoma in 2000 after going in for a routine eye examination to renew my contact lenses prescription. Within a month after being diagnosed, and after many tests and meetings with various physicians to explore alternative treatments, my eye was removed (enucleated). Eight weeks later I got my new prosthesis.

When cancer is found in the eye, it creates many concerns for the victim who has to worry not only about the cancer spreading (metastasizing) from the eye through the body, but also in determining how to treat it. In the past, enucleation was the only option for eye cancer. Now, treatments involving radiation, lasers and photon beams have been developed which can destroy the cancer but leave the eye intact.

Sadly, these treatments still usually result in the vision in the eye being totally and permanently destroyed. They are also not foolproof in the sense that it is impossible for the physician to determine whether all the cancer was eliminated. In my own case, my tumor was too close to my optic nerve to attempt these alternative treatments. This was very fortunate for me insofar as a later biopsy revealed an additional growth of cancer on the optic nerve itself which would not have been treated and possibly would have spread throughout my body. This is by way of saying that the safest way to deal with eye cancer is usually enucleation, but this is a tough choice for victims. There is also the stress of having to make what amounts to an immediate decision so that the cancer is treated one way or another before it spreads.

The purpose of this chapter is not to catalogue or describe the various types of eye cancer, but rather to demonstrate how victims of eye cancer deal with the fact. There is fortunately a good deal of information available on the internet about eye cancer, with perhaps the best resource being that of Dr. Paul Finger's Eye Cancer Network at http://www.eyecancer.com which was the first resource that I found after being diagnosed and for which I was very grateful. Dr. Finger corresponded with me during my time of stress and decision, and helped to recommend the very good surgeon that ultimately provided my treatment.

Letters and E-Mails

Hi, I'm contacting you hoping you might know of an organization that could help. I am a case manager with a patient who has lost one eye to cancer and has tumor near optic nerve for his remaining eye. Radiation therapy is scheduled to begin next week on this tumor. Treatments will be 5 days per week for 6-7 weeks. The treatment center is approximately a 2-1/2 to 3 hour drive from patients home. The clinic has recommended patient stay in the area of the hospital during the weeks of treatment. The problem is the cost of doing this. Many cancer organizations have funds available for just such situations, i.e. one time $750 for transportation costs for treatment, or partial assistance for temporary housing such as my patient needs. I have been unable to find any organization with funds available for eye cancer patients. Are you aware of any help? Thanks so much!

◆ ◆ ◆

Here's a message I got from a contact that might help:
For starters feel free to have them call the National Cancer Information Center in Austin at 800.227.2345 and make sure they ask for a Cancer Information Specialist. You have to be there a year and pass several certification exams to be a tiered CIS. Off the top of my head here are your answers. Please understand I am not at work with my computer on and the ACS databases at my fingertips so I'm flying by the seat of my pants. But I've done this for 15 months and know this stuff by heart.

For FREE lodging he can try http://www.nahhh.org and they will provide a list of lodges/hotels/motels across the nation that offer a free/reduced cost place to stay. For transportation he can try http://www.airlifeline.org and he'll probably be able to find private pilots who can fly him there and back for free. Commercial airlines like Southwest, American etc fly greater distances, but private pilots or company pilots usually fly short distances.

The ACS also has a program called "ROAD TO RECOVERY" where volunteers will drive patients to and from appointments. However, with the distance involved it is unlikely. So his best chance to request MILEAGE REIMBURSEMENT and we can cut him a check to cover gas if he sends us his receipts. It's not a solution, but with gas prices like they are (thanks to EYES =P) it will help some. For $$$$ assistance he can try *http://www.cancercare.org* or call them at 1

800 813 HOPE and they can give him tons of financial referrals. Hope this helps amigo. God bless you.—*Anon*

I have started a support group for people with choroidal melanoma. would you be willing to add the website to your support groups worldwide section? I would greatly appreciate it. http://health.groups.yahoo.com/group/ChoroidalMelanoma/?yguid= 186561376

I was diagnosed with choroidal melanoma in November 2004 and had my plaque treatment in February 2005. I still have a lot of questions, and am hoping that with a chat board more people can find support, answers to questions, and maybe a little bit of fun while we fight this horrible disease.—*Dana*

Our oldest son, Chris was diagnosed with amelanotic choroidal melanoma at age 30. He elected to have the radiation plaque surgery. All was well and the tumor continued to shrink, and as recently as last December his oncologist in Philadelphia announced that Chris was doing "remarkably well" and could now cut back his quarterly testing to every 6 months.

This February, Chris became aware of a marked & rapid deterioration in what was left of his vision in the left eye. His wife, an Optometrist by profession, his dad and I all attributed the sudden & rapid changes to what his first surgeon had advised. At approx. 2 yrs., the remainder of his vision would begin to fade, but stated that it would be gradual. It was not. Approx. 2 mos. passed and Chris went to Houston for a check-up about 2 mos. ahead of schedule. The news was our worst fear; the tumor had grown and was nearly twice the size from the initial diagnosis.

Chris had the enucleation on his left eye on May 9th. The first good news was that the tumor was still encapsulated within the orbit. Second best news is today, on his second follow-up w/one of my eye surgeons said Chris is doing very well, and in approx. 10 days or so, he will be ready for measurements for his permanent prosthetic. The absolute best news though is that the pathology narrative indicates a very low ratio of malignancy.1 out of 40 cells. Praise God!

You may or may not have already heard from my son, Chris, but I personally wanted to let you know that your website is a Godsend, and he's been in contact with another gentlemen very close to his age, also diagnosed with choroidal melanoma. I hope my note finds you doing well, and that God will continue to bless you with continued good health and a happy, full life! Sincere Regards,—*Dorothy*

Thank you so much for your website. I'm a 54 year old female that was diagnosed with melanoma in my left eye in 2000. It was a whirlwind of tests, second opinions and before I could turn around good I was in the hospital 2 weeks later to have my eye removed. Like all of you, I was very afraid of having the wrong eye removed. My doctor assured me that he intended to go all his career without doing that. He went thru all the steps that they would go thru. It was a tremendous help. Even though they had marked my eye to be removed with a dot, he came in and asked me which eye, he looked to make sure and then he took a big huge black marker and drew around my eye. That alone was reassuring.

The difference for me has been that he wanted to wait for 8 weeks to make sure my eye had healed to get my prosthesis. My eye has a clear plastic shield where the prosthesis will fit. I've worn an eye shield over the outside of my eye while I have been waiting. Things were ok until this past week when it just became too prolonged. I replaced the shield with an eye patch. It is much better. I'll be getting my prosthesis on Feb. 9. That will be one proud day for me-like Christmas, birthday and all the holidays wrapped into one.

Thanks so much to Jay for providing this website. I now know what to expect and am looking forward to it without any fear of the unknown. It is really good to know all of you have gone thru this before me. It gives me hope and lets me know there is a lot of life left to live. Thanks!—*Frances*

I have just read your website and am really impressed. I am 47 years old and was diagnosed on Jan 26th with melanoma of my right eye and the cancer was on my optic nerve too. I had my eye removed in London. I agree with everything you say. I was terrified and my worst time was pre-op. Once it was over I was fine and what you say about depression and how everything is the same is so true. The only difference here is that we are fitted with a temporary eye for a few weeks which is not made for us and I found that the worst thing. Once I got my 'own' eye I was fine and I have super trendy tinted specs. I have pre-carbonated glass in them they are completely shatterproof.—*Anon*

Read your web-page with interest. In the summer of 1993 a routine eye test revealed an abnormality behind the pupil of my left eye and like you I was sent post-haste to my local hospital. After a second opinion and many tests, malignant melanoma was diagnosed. Six weeks after the initial diagnosis my left eye was removed. I wondered how I would cope. To my Knowledge I had never met anyone with one eye-apart from the lady the hospital asked to call on me just before I went in for the operation. Her diagnosis had been different from mine, but her artificial eye looked fine. She also had no qualms about removing it for inspection

In the early days worry about the cancer far outweighed the problems that resulted from losing an eye. Though I recognize the need for speedy action in cases like mine, I do believe the mind needs time to adjust. I don't suppose I have fully accepted how I look, although most people say they cannot tell the difference between my real and artificial eye. I shall know I have fully accepted it when I can leave home without my tinted glasses.

Because there was no one to talk to about my fears and how I felt seven years ago when it was happening to me, I set up a local group (with the help of the local blind association) called ONE VISION. We offer support information assistance and understanding to people with monocular vision. The word spread and soon calls were coming in thick and fast from all over the UK Our work continues and at present discussions are being held to decide if we should become a registered charity

I must say I really laughed when I read the bit about you writing on your forehead before the operation. You seem to have a really good positive attitude, that really helps. I was very negative at the time and without the daily support of husband and family I would have found it difficult to cope. I hope your web-site goes from strength to strength and I hope to set up something similar here in the UK. Best wishes!—*Wendy*

Jay, I have to thank you for all the information on your website. A week before Christmas, I was diagnosed with a tumor. It was so big I had to have my right eye removed immediately. At 25, this has been quite an experience. The great thing about your website is that every fear and phobia you mentioned, I have had. Next month, I fly to Utah for a prosthetic, and the fact that I know what to expect is priceless.—*Anon*

I also was diagnosed with the same condition (only big tumor) two years ago and am very happy to see this website. The loss of an eye is better than the alternative. I have found it does pose unique challenges in activities where depth perception is an issue. I refuse to accept that I can't do something I did before, although my lack of acuity has had an effect on my performance for things like tennis where something comes toward you. When I was enucleated my physician gave me Frank Brady's book which helped to prepare me for some things. I believe something good can come from even the worst situations and greatly appreciate being alive today, now and for as long as I am blessed to be in this world. Great Site!—*Anon*

I had my eye removed in 1999 due to melanoma. At that time, I did not think I would live to see the millennium. I just went to get glasses (I am 40 years old) and thought I couldn't see well. The next thing I knew, they were removing my eye and telling me my chances of survival were poor. Being a single parent with an 8 year old, I was devastated.

Now two years later I guess my prognosis is still poor. After about six months of very serious depression, I made a decision to "live" for as long as I am blessed to be here. Most of the time, my life is very normal now. Every day though, I really don't have an eye and always have a Cat scan "shake" in my refrigerator. I found the letters very comforting. It's nice to know I'm not the only one out there!—*Anon*

Jay, this is a wonderful site and resource for someone going through the experience of losing and eye. Like you, I am a very active 35 year-old man that had never heard of "eye cancer" before. I was actually riding my bicycle about a month ago, which I put a few thousand miles a year on, and noticed some floating vision in my right eye. The next day I noticed it more while I was riding again and contacted an Ophthalmologist the next day. He saw me a day later and saw the melanoma right away. He said I was lucky to have caught it because I had actually torn my retina, which was actually what brought me in to see him. The tumor was totally unrelated to my symptoms but wouldn't have been found otherwise.

Its been a month since my enucleation and my life has started to go back to normal. I have been back to work for over two weeks (the first week from home) and have been riding my bike at least every other day for an hour or two. I tried riding my mountain bike on some relatively easy, wooded trails and had some difficulty with rocks and roots. That will take some getting used to again but I am confident I will be able to do it. I am looking forward to doing some racing again this summer and fall.

In the last six weeks I have had a couple of those "why me?" days. I already wear corrective lenses (used to wear contact lenses) so I had routine eye exams annually and just had one four months before my diagnosis. I wondered that if it had been picked up then would I have lost my eye? I didn't dwell on it long because it wasn't going to make the cancer go away or bring my eye back.

Your section on visiting the Ocularist will be helpful because I do that in a couple of weeks. I have been a little anxious about it and your experience puts it in a good perspective. I am actually really excited about it because I want to get back on with things. Your site is a great reference for people who have gone through this ordeal or are about to. I will be sure to recommend it to my doctor when I see her again in a couple of weeks. Sincerely,—*David*

Dear Jay, I too lost my eye to Choroidal Melanoma. I had enucleation surgery one week ago today in Miami, Florida. My surgery went extremely well (so they tell me). I wanted to thank you for providing this website because I have been pretty in the dark about this. One of my options for treatment was to go to Boston and have proton-beam radiation. However, I am only 28 years old and I have a three year old daughter. I also found out three days after my diagnosis that I am expecting again. Needless to say this has been a difficult couple of weeks. I also felt that my best chance to beat this was to have the eye removed. I have been so worried about the cancer spreading to other parts of my body. So far my tests have all come back fine, but I know that is no guarantee for the future. Do you have any information of the incidence of spreading and survival rates? I would really appreciate any (good news) you could send me. Thank you!—*Amy*

Jay, I corresponded with you a few months ago. Like you, I am a very active 35 year-old professional that had no symptoms and bam, I'm losing my right eye because I have a 12.8mm choroidal melanoma. A couple of months after my enucleation (which I have adjusted to just fine) I followed up with an oncologist my surgeon recommended here in the Philadelphia area. He had me go through a series to tests and CT and MRI scans (which all took a few weeks) and I found out that it has metastasized to my liver. In a big way too, about 40%. I started an immunoembolization treatment process last Friday. I tell you all of this because my chest x-rays and blood work is still all normal. If I continued to rely on those I still would not be diagnosed and I would probably only have months left. I don't know what your follow up has been or the people you speak to through this site, but I think everyone who finds out they have choroidal melanoma should start immediately having semiannual CT and MRI scans of their liver. Just some suggestions.—*David*

Jay, I wanted to let you know your web site has been very helpful. I am going in for surgery on the 16th of Oct. for removal of my left eye due to Choroidal Melanoma. I have spent much time on your site and have been very much encouraged by yours and other's comments. I am a pilot and will have a lot of work in front of me to return to flying status. I have been in touch with the FAA and was also encouraged to find that all other major airlines have pilots with one eye. I opted for removal because the cancer is very close to the optic nerve and radiation would destroy my vision within a few months. So the best chance for stopping the cancer is to get rid of the eye. All this probably sounds very familiar to you, but it has been a real learning curve for my wife and me in the last 3 weeks. Thanks once again for your work and site, it was and is greatly appreciated. I will keep you posted on my progress.—*Tom*

◆ ◆ ◆

Hi Jay, Thanks once again for your web site. It was a great relief to find the Letters From Friends section and read that I am not the only person in the world faced with a decision of losing my eye or my life. Here is a tally of the last few weeks since I was diagnosed with Choroidal Melanoma in my left eye, and some of my thoughts and fears. Please feel free to post them on the web sight if you wish, either in whole or in part.

In 2001, I went to my ophthalmologist because a few weeks earlier my FAA doctor told me at my age (53) and 33 years of commercial flying; I would probably need some distance correction for my next aviation medical exam in another six months. I thought he was probably correct in his evaluation and I had noticed some blurring in my lower left eye in the last few weeks. I thought some dirt or something I had gotten in my eye and caused some minor discomfort for a few days, may have even scratched my lens and caused some surface scare, which was now giving me some blurred vision. A little change of prescription on my glasses, a little suave for my eye, and my wife and I were off to lunch.

Soon my eyes were dilated and the normal vision test were completed and the nurse was about to cheerfully leave the testing room, I placed her hand to the lower left area of my left field of vision and informed her I if she would wiggle her fingers, I would not be able to see them move inside a space the size of an orange. After a few quick hand tests she said, "Oh, I'll go get the Doctor". This was the first red flag of what was shaping up to be a very bad day. Shortly the doctor was looking in my eyes with a very strong light and glasses, and informed my wife and I of a mass inside my eye. He said he could make an appointment with a laser specialist, and within two hours we were sitting in an examination room with a laser surgeon when he informed my wife and I of a Choroidal Melanoma in my left eye that was to big for him to operate on. My wife and I just looked at one another as I informed the doctor that I was an airline pilot. As we were leaving the office the doctor said he could get me an appointment first thing in the morning with a man who was a specialist in this type of CANCER. Thinking about total blindness and death due to an inoperable cancer as the only end was beyond belief. It was a very sad day, and a very long night.

The next day, my wife and I made our way through the early morning traffic to meet an eye cancer specialist. From this point the news for the next few days would slowly get better, or at least there would be some options other than dying from cancer. The first piece of good news we got was that this type of cancer was hereditary and was something formed just after conception and I had about a one in six to eight million chance of getting it, and this type of cancer will either show up in one or the other eye, or the pancreas, and most often during childhood. If it does not display itself during childhood, it will show-up after SO or so due to a lowered immune system because of the aging process. Also the chance for it to show up in the other eye is one in fifty to sixty million (statistically not measurable). After a few painless test that included a visual inspection, an ultrasound on the affected eye, a computer 3D image of the tumor, a fluorescein angiogram (dye injected through your arm that goes to your eyes and is then photographed with a very high powered flash camera), the doctor was able to determine the size and approximate location. Later that day we once again met with the doctor and he was able to give us a general idea of the treatment. But first there were a few more questions that needed to be answered. The cancer was very close to the optic nerve so an MRI was set for the next day (an MRI of this type can show resolution down to 2mm) to see if the cancer had begun to grow down into the optic nerve canal. Another big question was if the cancer had spread from my eye to any other parts of my body. This question was answered at least for now with a blood test, EKG, and two chests X-rays. After a few days of processing and anxious waiting, we returned to the doctor and got some long awaited results and news.

That same day we got some good news. Our doctor and the doctor who is the MRI specialist were both waiting outside the MRI room and after some time the images were ready for reading, and the results showed the cancer was still 2mm from the edge of the optic nerve and did not appear to have traveled into the optic channel. This was good news.

A few days later, we met once again with the doctor and got a much more detailed explanation on treatment options. The choroidal melanoma cancer was classified as a medium to small size (about the size of a pea) and had been growing for about a year. The blood test showed no spreading of cancer was active in my body, chest x-rays were clear, and EKG was good. Since the cancer was confined to the inside of the eye but very close to the optic nerve, and had not spread to other parts of my body, the choice of treatments was easier to define.

1) One type of treatment is called radiation brachytherapy (pronounced brake therapy) and is actually a small device that looks like a small coke bottle cap about the size of a wooden pencil eraser and has some very small radioactive pellets glued to the inside and a thin gold shield attached to the other side to contain and direct the radiation, this helps to prevent damage to surrounding tissue. This shield or bottle cap is sewn on the outside of the eye and left there for about 3 days, and then removed. In a perfect procedure this would normally give about a 90% success and the tumor might even shrink some over a few months, but vision loss will occur . In the cases where the cancer is very close to the optic nerve, the radiation shield has to be notched so it can be placed partially around the optic nerve. The problem with doing this is that the effectiveness of the radiation is not yet known, so there are no statistics on long-term success and sur-

vival. Additionally, due to the close proximity of the shield to the optic nerve, there was almost a 100% chance to lose all my vision in my left eye within a few months of the procedure and a 20% chance of eventually losing my eye within 5 years. Not really a place you want to be if you have cancer.

2) Another type of treatment is called enucleation. This is the medical way of saying eye removal. As unpleasant as this sounds it is a fairly simple operation, usually done under a general anesthetic, and has been one of the preferred methods for many years. During this procedure after the eye is removed, a pre-sized orbital implant (a porous ball that acts like your bone) is inserted in the socket and the muscles are stitched to it, and then a large contact lens is placed over it to act as a protection from the elements for the first few weeks and allow the doctor to view the wound and observe your recovery. This procedure has a 90% success rate for long-term survival, but loss of an eye is a scary thing, especially if you are an airline pilot.

The doctor said a decision did not have to be made that day or even during the next week or so, since this is a relatively slow growing cancer at this stage. My wife and I were thankful that a hasty decision did not have to be made. So for the next few days we had many discussions about the pros and cons of the two options, and also spent some time discussing a few other traditional and non-traditional treatments. My doctor was very helpful with all the technical aspects of the procedures and all the stats, he also discussed the case with his partner who participated in some of the long-term studies of this type of cancer, but he said the decision was totally up to the family. This seemed strange at first, but now I can understand his view. We spent much time talking to friends and explaining all the options, and much time in prayer. After a week or so we finally reached a decision. Since my vision in the left eye would be lost, and the chance of occurrence in the other eye is highly unlikely, and the cancer appears to be isolated to and in the eye, why not remove the eye? So on about the 8th of October we set the surgery for the 16th. At first the doctor said it would be a day surgery operation, since I was in good health and not too old, however after some thought about the operation and given our distance from the hospital, he was quick to comply with my wishes to stay in over night. This decision made the week of waiting a little easier.

The morning of my enucleation, the drive to the hospital was a quiet one, but it was 5 A.M. and we had already been up for an hour. Check in at 6:00 A.M., completed check in by 7:00, change clothes and lie down on the rollaway bed at 7:15. After a few questions from the nurse and having a small red dot placed on my forehead over my left eye, an I.V. was inserted in my right arm and only produced mild discomfort. After a brief visit from the doctor it was off to the operating room. Medicine into the I.V. and out likes a light.

Next thing I remember I was in recovery, very little pain, mostly just some pressure on my eye. About 30 minutes later I was wheeled off to my room and into a hospital bed. I must say that the decision to stay overnight in the hospital was one that brought my wife and I a lot of piece of mind, even though it was not required. That day I was given some pain killer type pills, but I was still only experiencing a mild headache with an occasional higher level of pain, but very easy manage. Later that evening I received a 1/2 dose of morphine, which really knocked me out for the rest of the night.

The next day, I was out of the hospital and on my way home with almost no discomfort. My wife and I were met at the house by my mother, sister, daughter, and friends, all were wearing eye patches. We had a good laugh and the rest of the day I spent walking around the homestead and talking to family and visitors. No real pain, an occasional pain pill did the job. That night before going to bed it was time to remove the patch and clean the area. It was a little of a shock to see the place where my eye had been for the first time. The affected area was dark red and gave the appearance of Arnold in the movie "The Terminator". After a few minutes I got over it. The good news there was no pain, just a numb feeling in my eye socket. Took a pain pill and slept all night.

Within three days, I drove around the local neighborhood. It was a little scary but I had practiced it before my eye removal. I would suggest you do that before you become monocular vision, it will that some of the apprehension away. By the way there is no requirement in the state of Texas to be re-licensed to drive.

A follow up office visit to the doctor and all looked fine. The pathology report will be back in 3 weeks or so. A long time to wait, but the doctor feels good about the operation and seems to have reason to feel good about the pathology report. After all we caught the cancer early and had a good description of its size and structure. The earlier the better for cancer. Have not had any pain at all for 3 or 4 days.

Two weeks later I got the pathology report back and all looks good. No evidence of cancer in the optic nerve. It was a very good day. No pain in the eye, now it is just a matter of getting fitted for my prosthesis in another three weeks.

Within a month of my surgery, I got fitted for my prosthesis. It is absolutely amazing, the prosthesis looks so real it is hard to tell which one is false, movement is very good, but of course not as good as my real eye. The level of self-confidence is much higher now that I can see the finished product. The fit is a little tight for now, but the fitting and finishing with take several visits. Overall I am quite happy and the whole procedure was painless.—*Tom*

◆   ◆   ◆

Hi Jay—Thank you for your words of support. I have been doing some meditations and positive thinking exercises and I feel better. I also contacted the Cancer Clinic and have arranged for some counseling. My is malignant melanoma and was contained in the eye. I don't know if that is the same as choroidal melanoma. I am also trying to take better care of myself i.e. better diet and exercise.

Does it hurt to have the new eye fitted? Does it take a while to get use to it? When I first arrived home I managed to trip a few times but I learned to take things a little slower. I simply couldn't see things on the lower right side but other than that I haven't had too much trouble with depth perception. Pouring things from a jug into a glass can sometimes be an experience. I have decided to move in with a roommate for awhile as I find I do not like being alone. Thank you for you support. I feel this happened to me as a wakeup call and I hope that I can help others in the future who go through this. I have been told by others that their life changed after this and they all said for the better so I find that very encouraging. Take Care,—*Vicki*

My name is Joe and I'm a 35 year old male. I was diagnosed with choroidal melanoma (medium sized) last week and I'm simply overwhelmed with the work to be done researching how to go about getting better. I have a medium sized tumor in my left eye and I can't decide if I'm going to go for the radiation treatment or not.

I was hoping to hear about your experience and to see if you've tried any naturopathic therapies or any other alternatives. When I was diagnosed in the hospital, the only choices offered to me were radiation (in the form of a plaque) or removal of the eye. I am hoping to hear from other who have successfully tried conventional therapy and other things—holistic, naturopathic, ayurvedic, etc. Much thanks in advance.—*Joe*

Jay, thirteen years ago, I was diagnosed with choroidal melanoma. I opted for the radiation treatment. The radiation did it's job and did little to destroy what vision the tumor had left me. The residual vision can, in certain light conditions, cause severe double vision, requiring that I immediately close the "bad" eye. At other times, I hardly notice the problem. I have a depth perception loss, but perhaps my work is more demanding of that feature of sight. I'm an electronics engineering specialist and work with surface mount, very tiny parts. While doing chores around the yard the loss is not apparent. I have decided to look for a totally light occlusive patch and found your site. Any help would be greatly appreciated.—*Ray*

I was told in 2001 that I had and ocular tumor. It started out as a routine check up, they noticed what they thought was just a retinal tear. Which was bad enough. They immediately sent me to a specialist. He in turn sent me to to a retinal specialist. I was diagnosed with choroidal tumor. Cancer. A tumor measuring 8.9. This all within hours. The only signs were circling bright light. Then 2 weeks ago I felt like my eyes were strained. I had a few headaches, but my job can be stressful.

This doctor was very straight to the point, no emotions as he said what he found. My husband and my emotions did a temporary shut down. Then to be told I needed to get the "Hot Spots" checked immediately was total shock. I was set up for a second opinion with one of his collages on the following week on the 23rd. We met this extremely gentle and caring doctor who eased into what was to come. I was lucky to have him examining me that day. I was let know in a caring way that the only chance of keeping this from spreading was the removal of my left eye. I've just turned 41, have a loving husband, 2 beautiful daughters ages 22 and 10, and one angel of a granddaughter who is 4. I also chose to just take it. So as of tonight at 10:00 I go to the eye surgeon tomorrow the 24th, and it's planned for surgery to be the following day.

Of course I'm nervous, but knowing life is still out there after the eye. Thank you for this site. My mind is so much more at ease and my fear not so intense. My husband found this site one night is our search for information. Again my thanks.—*Tammy*

◆   ◆   ◆

I wrote to you about a week ago. I had just found out I had choroidal melanoma. The surgery was done on in 2001. I went home the same day. Also like one of the others who have written in had blood work done and chest x-rays done. Both came back negative. But thanks to one of the people who wrote in about having CT scan done, my husband ask my surgeon about having a PET scan. She felt it was a great idea as blood test do not show up as quickly. I had it done on the 31st and sure enough it showed 2 small spots on my liver. I go for the CT scan on the 5th. I just hope it was caught in time for maybe just some radiation or something on that line that will zap it before it goes to far. So anyone out there that has been for blood test, get the other done. Thanks for your site.—*Tammy*

◆   ◆   ◆

I have written twice before, but I wanted to put an update on the scans I had done. A week after my left eye was removed, I had a PET scan done. It showed 2 small spots on my liver.

A CT scan was ordered a week later which, luckily and by the grace of God, it showed nothing. I couldn't understand why the PET scan showed something but the CT showed nothing. At the time we were told I just assumed the 2 spots were cancer. But when I ask my surgeons assistant, which she is an excellent and caring person, as is my surgeon, reminded me that they never said cancer only that there was something that shown. I was so relieved. I go back in 6 months for another CT scan. I go next week to see if I've healed enough for the "fake" eye.

I want to thank you for setting up this site. If it wasn't for this site we wouldn't have known to ask for a PET scan. And if those spots had of shown up on the CT scan, at least there could have been something done early. Which can mean the difference between life and death. Blood test do not always show up early enough. So no one should go by blood test alone. You can take it a step further. You must take it further.—*Tammy*

Hi Jay, I've just been told I have eye cancer in my left eye and are waiting for an app. down in a hospital to have the radiation treatment. Hopefully the tumor won't be too large. They have measured it at 11 so isn't very small. I had never heard of this cancer before last week and find it quite a scary thing, especially when it involves your eyes. Is the radiation very painful and what is it like to have only one good eye. I love the outdoors and have a small farmlet with donkeys on it. I was wondering if you could tell me about your experience and might help me put my mind rest a little. My eye at the moment has blurry vision, is hot for a while and have constant headaches. I'm getting real tired and trying to lay down at least once a day to rest my eyes a little. Look forward to hearing from you.—*Glenice from New Zealand*

Hi Jay, well here I am nearly a week after they operated and took out my eye. I must say I have had a few bad days with how I am feeling in myself but guess that will get better as time goes on. To make matters worst I have a hip replacement and had to have all my teeth out a year ago because of my health so am feeling like a broken down bit of machinery at the moment. This has been the hardest thing to get my head around I have to admit. My question at the moment is—when I am looking at things or trying to read what I can see thru my good eye is a haze (like on a hot summers day when you can see the heat in the air) I can only read 1-2 pages of large print before the words start to swim—is this normal to start with? My other eye has been quite sore over the last few days but guess I can't expect much else. We have an appointment with the specialist tomorrow so will ask him about this but feel you can't get a better answer than asking someone who has been thru it. They took some tissues from behind the eye socket last week so will know the results of those tomorrow and will ask about the scans. They said last week that the chances of it traveling from the eye socket are slim but when they tell you that the eye cancer is rare then slim doesn't really come into it and will feel more assured when I hear a clear result tomorrow.

By the way here is a little about myself—I am 48 years of age, live with my husband on a farmlet with donkeys and numerous other animals, have three teenage children and we have just sold our house (two weeks prior to finding this out) and are moving on the 22nd Feb. up North. It is 6-7 hours drive and as I am not allowed to drive for three months will be a passenger on that day instead of a driver. How long ago did you have your operation and how are you getting on? Looking forward to hearing from you. Kind Regards,—*Glenice*

◆ ◆ ◆

Hi Jay, I enjoyed your web site. I am losing my left eye next Tuesday to cancer. I have a good out look on life and do not worry about the things I can not control but your web site is an inspiration to all people that are in this boat. I know I will adjust and I have always said "Don't take life too serious because none of us are coming out of it alive" Each day is a gift to be enjoyed. Thank you for the site and your efforts to help others deal with losing an eye. God Bless you,—*John*

I would like to ask you some questions about the loss of your eye. My wife recently underwent surgery for removal and reconstruction of the eye and orbit due to a choroidal melanoma. A biopsy of the bone tissue removed indicated some migration of the cancer cells and the doctors recommended bio-chemotherapy as the adjuvant treatment. She has just completed her 3rd cycle of treatment with one remaining. Would you mind telling me about your situation and what adjuvant treatment, if any, was recommended? Thank you,—*Stephen*

Thank you so much for your site. I will have my eye removed due to cancer in the next week . I have been going over all of this in my mind every second of the day. Your site is wonderful and has put to rest some of my fears. Thank you again so much,—*Noreen.*

Dear Jay, I want to thank you for your site. Your positive attitude is a true inspiration. My name is also Jay and I am 33 years old. I was a bit surprised your site did not discuss "suspicious" nevus at all. I believe choroidal melanoma is a choroidal nevus before turning malignant. I have a "suspicious" choroidal nevus that shows high risk for turning into choroidal melanoma. It was discovered while I was in college 10 years ago when I noticed my vision in my left eye wasn't as good as the vision in my right eye. My retinal specialist examines it every 4 to 6 months and so far it does not appear to be malignant but my doctor believes it is only a matter of time before it turns into a choroidal melanoma. My nevus is so close to my macula that radiation treatment will probably ruin my useful vision in that eye.

I read at the University of Iowa website that 30 to 50% of people with choroidal melanoma die within 5 years even when the primary melanoma is treated! There seems to be a high incidence of it spreading to the liver or other organs even when the melanoma is caught early and treated. Thus, I am wondering if there may be value in removing my eye before it turns malignant. Especially since they think it will turn malignant and since a sizeable portion of choroidal melanoma patients metastasize even when the eye is removed. It seems in many cases by the time it is melanoma, it is too late even when the eye is removed right away. My thought is that if my eye is removed before it turns malignant, the cancer will not spread. It seems that in many cases by the time doctors realize it is melanoma, it may have already begun the spreading process.—*Anon*

I am having my right eye removed due to a large melanoma on June 13, 2005. I want to thank Jay for this site and use it as my main resource center. I have read both the books on Hope and a Singular View and found them very helpful. I would recommend them to all my family and friends so they can understand what I am going through. I have 6 more days to D-Day and am scared to death and at the same time I know that I will make it thru this journey thanks to everyone's support and help.

I am off for the surgery and then come home. Thanks for allowing me to write and offer my support to everyone else going thru an eye removal. Everyday is precious and rewarding. All for now!—*Lynn*

Hi, I am a 25 year old that was diagnosed w/melanoma on my optic nerve of my left eye. Two days ago I had it removed. I am a college student and mother of 4. I have to say the next few months are looking pretty scary. However, I am sure I will prevail. Your website is very encouraging. Keep it up!—*JCrawford*

It has been about six months since my right eye was removed with a melanoma, the surgeon said I have 20/20 vision in my left eye with glasses, I am a young 75 year old racing motorcycle mechanic, I am finding it very hard to come to terms with the lose, I only drive my car down a back road to take my wife to the rail station, is my worries of losing my good eye normal, and how long do you think it will take to adjust, I am normally a very positive thinker, and I try to be a perfectionist in what I do, I am beginning to think a bit negative or maybe worried, thank you for reading my email. Regards—*Edd in South Australia*

Three weeks ago my right eye was removed due to a cancerous tumor 20 cm in size attached to the optic nerve and the eye. I returned to work, marketing and sales, wearing a pirate patch yesterday. I travel 90 miles round trip besides visiting clients every day. In the past I have driven as much as 350 miles per day. But the 90 miles per day is exhausting me. By 3:00 in the afternoon I try to be home just so I can rest. My doctor tells me it may take six months to a year to return to my old self. Can you tell me if you have experienced being exhausted such as I have mentioned and if so how long did it take you to get over it? Is there anything you suggest for me to try? I eat healthy and did exercise frequently until the removal. My blood pressure is 120/80 and am in good health. At 56 years old I do not want to start a new career. Any words of wisdom would be greatly appreciated. Gratefully,—*Ric*

I was just told that I need to have my left eye removed due to a tumor. I can't say the past few days have been the best, but with the help of friends, others who have had an eye removed and your site, I feel more at ease with the whole thing. I read most of the letters from others and can't help but be encouraged. I would like to know if you know of any golfers who have had an eye removed. I would love to talk to them either by phone or email if possible. I'm wondering if I can get my game back to where I left off in the fall. Thanks again for your help.—*Guy*

Hi Jay, I just read one of the letters from one of your friends. I saw that one person had the blood work done and chest x-rays as well and the cancer still showed up in the liver. Well my level of fear has gone up 100 times. I guess I just need to talk to someone. I have arranged for a CT Scan for tomorrow. They are very positive that it is only in my eye, but were happy to any tests I wanted to put my mind at ease.—*Guy*

Guy: The cancer scared the hell out of me—much more so that the loss of one eye. I was just glad to get the cancer out of my system. When they do an autopsy of your eye they ought to be able to tell whether the cancer has possibly spread or not down your optic nerve. If it has spread, then obviously you are going to be much more aggressive in looking for it. If they do, THEN I would do the CT scan. If they conclude that it didn't spread, then you can take a deep breath of relief. If you are at a good medical facility, let them ultrasound your liver and look for cancer. The advantage to the ultrasound is that you don't get an unnecessary dose of radiation. Then, I would wait one year after the surgery and then get the full body scan and have them look at your liver. Unfortunately, I been right in your shoes but I lived through it alright. Call me if you need to.—*Jay*

Jay: Had my operation on Thursday. Everything went very well. Very little pain so far. Trying to get used to focusing with one eye. Thanks for everything. Could not have gotten through this without your website and the pep talk.—*Guy*

My son, who is 38, had his right eye enucleated just 5 weeks ago due to a malignant melanoma. His blood tests & liver scan prior to his operation were all clear. He is now recovering and has recently had a shell fitted into his eye socket. However, it was exactly 3 weeks from being diagnosed to him having his operation, and I think the seriousness of what has happened is now beginning to take its toll. He appears fine when he has visitors, but his wife tells me it is a different story when they are alone. It sounds as if he is sinking into a depression and his wife and young family are trying their best to lift his spirits. Counseling has been offered to him but he says he is ok and does not need it. Is it usual for depression to set in post op, and how can we help him if he won't help himself?—*Catherine*

Hello, My name is Christine. I am 43 years old. At the end of August at once I had a hazy sight on my right eye. I thought it was something of a cold I had and did not worry too much. The following day I had the same hazy sight. I went to a oculist and she told me to go to the clinic at once. The retina of my right eye was damaged. After several examinations at the clinic the doctors told me I had a melanoma in my eye (cancer) and my eye had to be removed. I thought I was dreaming, this was a nightmare.

Today it is 3 weeks after my eye was removed and I live in fear although the cancer has not metastasized. I also have a fear of loosing my other eye. I am also afraid of having a eye prosthesis. Here in Belgium there is not much known about those things. Through my search I found this site, which I find very interesting. If anyone can help me or give me some information or experience in anyway, I thank you in advance. Or if there are people who also live in Belgium, any information you can give is welcome. Next Wednesday I have my first appointment for my eye prosthesis. Until now I did not look at my wound, I find it very scary. I also sometimes feel very dizzy, is this normal? Thanks for all the help.—*Christine*

Wow! I finally found a place to learn more and hopefully interact with others like myself! I had a large choroidal melanoma and had an enucleation in March of 2000. I have a prosthetic and joke about it all the time. The truth is I would feel better about myself and maybe even a bit more secure to talk to others—learn of long term prognosis and recurrence. I just found out I have another tumor this time it is behind my uterus. I am almost at my 5 year mark so I am more than a little scared. I am also thrilled to have found your website. Thanks for being here!—*Susan*

Hi there: I saw your name and email address on the Eye Cancer web page. My name is Lisa. I was diagnosed with choroidal melanoma in my right eye back in June, and have had brachytherapy and laser treatment since then. I've only talked with one person that's actually had choroidal cancer, so just trying to see how people with the same type of cancer have been faring. Looking forward to hearing from you.—*Lisa*

Thank you for this site. Most encouraging. I had Googled surgery enucleation recovery time [without quotes] because I want to know how long it will be post-surgery before I'll able to engage in my regular activities, like teaching and TaeKwonDo. I have yet to see the oncologist and have a final diagnosis and recommendations for treatment, but from what the ophthalmologist and optometrist were discussing, it sounds as if the tumor is growing and is close to the optic nerve, so, like Jay, I'm probably not going to mess around with radiation, but get straight to the point and go for enucleation.—*Judith*

Going to have enucleation instead. It seems the way to go to avoid the cancer going to the liver and other places. I am sure glad I ran across this web site. Wish me luck.—*Gene*

Hi I am back from my appointment with my ocular oncologist. Unfortunately the news is not good. The cancer has spread inside the eye. There is no cure for eye cancer. The only option is surgery to remove the eye and part of my face. This is drastic and extensive. I will consider other solution such as clinic trials before. I will keep you posted on my decision, Thank you once again for your support.—*Andre*

I have CM and am so excited to have found your website. I have been struggling with losing my eye and having this cancer for the past 9 months and need to be able to talk to others who really understand. Please help me. Thank you.—*Lisa*

Jay, I got your name from the eye cancer website and thought that I would send you an email because I am scared to death. Just diagnosed with this melanoma by the doctors this week. And I am to have a CT scan of my brain and liver as well as a chest x-ray. I am just turning 58 and am very active and do not look forward to losing my eye. Could you send me your suggestions as to how to handle the stress and how you had your melanoma removed. Thanks so much.—*Lynn*

Could you please help me find information I had my eye removed from choroidal melanoma 2 years ago. I would like to find other people in my situation I appreciate you.—*Nicole*

◆ ◆ ◆

Jay, add me to your list. June, 2002 right eye, Choroidal Melanoma 14mm spindle, A cell type and it was all contained in the eye. Now I am cancer free. I'm 35 years old. From initial diagnosis it was six days later I was at the hospital. I have a temp prosthetic in now and recovering great. I was in process of applying for Term Life Ins. when this happened. Now I've been denied coverage. I'll probably have to wait five years to reapply. Adjusting to one eye has been interesting. I find I have to sit strategically in restaurants so I can see the wait staff approaching. I try to sit where my right side is against the wall. Otherwise, I get startled if I don't notice them standing there. I am more irritable than before and I am trying to cope with that. My left eye was my weak eye and it is still getting stronger. Sometimes I close my right eye so I can focus more with the left which seems to help! Anyway, I appreciate your web site. Thanks.—*Michael*

Jay: Where to begin. My name is Gary. All my life (I'm 39) I have been proud of my baby blue eyes that God has given to me, they are the same shade of blue as my recently deceased mother, whom I loved dearly. Today I am told by doctors that to remove the cancer in my right eye, it needs to be removed and 6 weeks of radiation is to follow. Needless to say I have had brighter days. Jay how did you handle the news when they told you that your eye needs to be removed? Was yours due to cancer? If so, how are you today? How long ago was your operation? Did it take long to adjust to having just one eye? Sorry for all the questions, but that's all I have are questions. How's your other eye handle the strain put on it?—*Gary*

◆ ◆ ◆

I have just been diagnosed with Choroidal melanoma and will be treated with proton beam radiotherapy next week…I was wondering if any of you have had the same treatment and/or same physician and what advice you might offer.

What were your experiences during and after treatment? How long ago were you treated? Were you able to keep your eye or has it been removed? I am also interested in follow up after the treatments. My cancer has not metastasized, but I am wondering if I need more follow up than my eye specialist has recommended. What yearly appointments have your doctors recommended? (i.e. liver scans, lung x-rays?) Thanks for any help you may be able to give me.—*BW*

Dear Jay: I have just read your website and am really impressed. I am 47 years old and was diagnosed on Jan 26th with melanoma of my right eye and the cancer was on my optic nerve too. I had my eye removed on 8.3.00 in London. I agree with everything you say. I was terrified and my worst time was pre-op. Once it was over I was fine and what you say about depression and how everything is the same is so true. The only difference here is that we are fitted with a temporary eye for a few weeks which is not made for us and I found that the worst thing. Once I got my 'own' eye I was fine and I have super trendy tinted specs. I have pre-carbonated glass in them they are completely shatterproof. I am on my daughters computer now and I have to go, I will be in touch again and tell you more about things here. I believe you may have had an e-mail from Wendy from North of England, I chat to her on the phone from time to time. Yours with admiration,—*Lynne*

Jay: I'm a 51 year old civil engineer. I was diagnosed with choroidal melanoma last week. The tumor is on the retina by the optic nerve. I saw a eye specialist and the only treatment option I was given is removal of the eye. I'm scheduled for the removal surgery on August 24th. My daughter found your web site and I've read it with great interest. I find it very informative. You've included information that I haven't heard from my doctor. I want to thank you for putting this information on the web. It gives me a very good idea what I can expect over the next few months. I'm greatly encouraged by the information you have provided. Thanks again and I'll be watching your web site and let you know how I'm doing as I work my way through this.—*Larry*

At the age of 23 in 1998 I was told I had a ciliary body melanoma, I was treated with proton beam therapy and all seemed well, I moved on and went back to work, I continued with my check ups until this very day, however in October of 2004 I was devastated to learn that the cancer had spread to my left orbit. My very worst nightmare had come true the very thing that I feared for six years had happened. After a biopsy my worst fear confirmed in January 2005 I was admitted to a hospital to have a enucleation of the left eye and contents, followed by 27 Radiation treatments. I found my life experience pretty hard to take, but a life changing one, and I feel lucky in a sense that I am still here.—*Natalie*

MESSAGES

Hi, I really like the positiveness of this site. I was diagnosed in, 2002 with choroidal melanoma. I had proton beam radiation and surgery in September and October. I'm legally blind in my treated eye. I had a few weeks of depth perception problems, but now everything is pretty much like before. I do a lot of computer work and read a lot. It hasn't affected my artwork at all. Thanks for all the great information here. My 6-month check-up is next week and I'm looking forward to it being over. I still have to go every three months for tests. Thanks again!—*Sherri*

Hi Everyone! When I first was diagnosed with this melanoma, I was in such denial. I mean, I am 31 years old vibrant and healthy. I also was pregnant with my son. I just couldn't believe it. And then I had 5 specialists tell me the only option to save my life would be to have a enucleation! I don't know actually what was going on in my mind: scared, terrified and not understanding. This couldn't be happening to me. Why ME? So it took some time to get used to, and I did. You always as a human being I have learned can handle what life deals you because God doesn't give you more than you can handle. And that is so true. I have had my surgery and am home and hold my son and look at my husband and other children and Now Go on with my life. Any one struggling and upset please feel free to write me and talk about it I promise you will feel much better. Don't take life for granted as it is a gift worth treasuring every second! Thanks,—*Nicole*

◆ ◆ ◆

I've been blessed with compassionate doctors, good friends and co-workers, and a loving family. My personal timeline. On one day, I had an eye appointment. The next day, I was diagnosed with ocular melanoma on my optic nerve. I was tested for cancer elsewhere in my body. None found. Referred to a surgeon after multiple opinions. Became a member of LostEYE.com. Great/smart move. A month later, I had my eye removed successfully and started my quarterly follow-up with a cancer center. A month after that I got my prosthesis.

What am I saying? Everything went according to plan. I didn't need any additional treatments. I live in Pittsburgh, PA and have found the best of the best. The surgeon, along with his staff, was so compassionate. He explained everything and yes, I did have him mark the eye to be removed. I was in & out of the hospital in 7 hours. No problems. My ocularist made my prosthesis just 2 days ago. It feels great with just a little discharge and everyone is so surprised by its natural appearance and that it moves. He did say initially that my lower lid was small. He compensated for that and completed the prosthesis in a total of 6 hours. Yes, I am blessed to have such good care right in my hometown. I have read how many of you have had to drive or fly great distances to get care.—*Rich*

My timeline eye appointment August 7th; eye removed from melanoma on August 25th; prosthesis on October 15th. The difference is that my lower lid is "too loose" needs a tuck soon, I wish my prosthesis was tighter, I'm so concerned it's going to fall out mid-conversation with someone, I have to be so careful but this is the beginning. I feel so lucky actually, and grateful, after the horrible not-knowing and you know what I mean by that 14 tests in 4 days, ruling out cancer in all the organs, and then waiting for the results. The anticipation of those reports were worse than the surgery without a doubt. Take care. Everything is put into perspective isn't it, and this is a small bend in life!—*Loralsar*

◆ ◆ ◆

Hi! I lost my vision in my right eye due to treatment of a large choroidal melanoma. This is recent, so some days I'm very positive and others aren't so well. I now have glaucoma in my good eye. I have young children and I'm an artist. Everything I love to do is with my eyes and I'm a very visual person. I found out recently that my cancer is a more aggressive version (Epitheliod sp?) not the spindle variety. My goal is to see my young children grow up and finish high school. I've had wonderful medical care in the form of treatment, but no compassion what so ever. I am now in the process of finding a more compassionate doctor.

On the trivial side, I lost all my eyelashes on the treated eye and being a woman it has made me feel shy. I'm pushing forward and trying really hard to be optimistic, but I've had my days. This week a lump showed up on my spine and I have x-rays next week. It appeared almost over night, so I really feel it is due to a back injury I had years ago. I wonder and just keep telling myself that this will be o.k. too. My vision loss hasn't effected my work and for the most part, life is totally normal. More emotional, but normal. I've learned to cherish everyday and even to embrace the yucky stuff we all have to go through. Thanks for letting me vent. I truly needed to tonight. Hugs,—*Sherri*

◆ ◆ ◆

Today marks the 12th anniversary of the day I got the diagnosis of choroidal melanoma in my right eye. I had the enucleation four days later. I'll never forget that day in the doctor's office when they told me what I had, and that the best course of action was to remove my eye. It was quite a journey, that first year after the surgery. Thank goodness I had the best ocular oncologists, ocular plastic surgeon and ocularist. These folks saved my life. When I start feeling a little sorry for myself, I always try to remind myself of how lucky I really am. I post on the CM board at eyecancer.com, and in the past week, two or three people there have found out that their cancer has spread. I get my check-ups every six months, and say a little prayer of thanks when they come back clean.

This board has been a tremendous help to me. I have never met anyone, personally, who has experienced what I have, so when I found LostEye, I felt like there was a community I finally belonged to. Everyone here has been so supportive and caring. I can't thank you all enough for having the courage to share your experiences and the strength to offer your support. Best wishes to all of you,—*Nancy*

◆ ◆ ◆

Hello, my name is Christine. I am 43 years old and live in Belgium. At the end of August at once I had a hazy sight on my right eye. I thought it was something of a cold I had and did not worry too much. The following day I had the same hazy sight. I went to a oculist and she told me to go to the clinic at once. The retina of my right eye was damaged. After several examinations at the clinic the doctors told me I had a melanoma in my eye (cancer) and my eye had to be removed. I thought I was dreaming; this was a nightmare.

Today it is 4 weeks my eye was removed and I live in fear although there were no metastasis. Also, I have a fear of losing my other eye. Last week I went for my prosthesis and it is very strange that a strange object is in your eye at once. Sometimes the water runs out of my eye, is this normal? Here in Belgium there is not much known about those things. Through my search I found this site, which I find very interesting. If anyone can help me or give me some information or experience in anyway, you're very welcome. Or if there are people who also live in Belgium, any information you can give is welcome. I also sometimes feel very dizzy, is this normal? Thanks for all the help.—*Christine*

Dear Chrissie, Welcome to the board, even under these unfortunate circumstances. I'm sure you will find some comfort here. I also lost my right eye to choroidal melanoma 12 years ago. At that time, working with my other doctors, was a doctor from Belgium, who was really my primary doctor throughout my ordeal. This was a few years ago, so I don't know if he is still there. If you are looking for a doctor that knows about CM, I would highly recommend him. He studied with two of the leading experts in the field and I thought he was great. Good luck to you and keep us posted on how you're doing.—*Nancy*

Hi Chrissie. I am very sorry to hear of you're loss. I also sorry to say that most of us fear the loss and injury of our other good eye. Hopefully this will diminish in time. I too am in the early stages of my loss. You will start to get used to the prosthesis. It takes a bit to get used to something foreign being in you're eye that is not you're real eye. You will need to use rewetting, and lubricating drops for the loss of water in the eye. You can use any rewetting drops that would be used for contact lenses. My loss was pretty traumatic. I injured it, and the next day it was taken from me. The reason they rushed you to have it done because it could lead to sympathetic ophthalmia. In you're case it was the cancer. Regards,—*Michael*

Hi Chrissie, I am Willeke and I am 32 years old. I lost my eye little over a year ago due to CM (Choroidal Melanoma) and I got my prosthetic eye 5 weeks after surgery. I never had a temporary eye and maybe that causes the irritation you have on the operated "eye". Mine doesn't and never did bother me in any way. I clean it about every two weeks with some soap. Every two to three months I put it in salt warm (not hot) water and that cleans it really nicely. Polish it up with a clean dry cloth and it shines just like your real eye. Maybe you should check with you ocularist about the irritation or contact your eye doctor. Good luck. Let me know if you have questions.—*Willeke (from Holland)*

◆ ◆ ◆

Hey all: Quick question. I was told after losing my eye to CM that I need to get annual chest X-rays, routine blood work (tracer cells, RBC and WBC, etc.), and abdominal CT. This is (I suppose) to make sure there is no metastasis Is anyone else doing this? I'm being followed by both my primary dr. and my oncologist. Had a couple of scares in seven years(skin cancer-another story), but I thank God that I'm still here. I get the feeling sometimes by my primary dr. that I'm too concerned with my health. It's a "feeling" like—you only lost your eye, get over it. Nothing was actually said-just my gut feeling. BTW, I've changed my primary doctor. Anyone else get this feeling?—*Ron*

◆ ◆ ◆

Thank you for your website. I lost my left eye, to ocular melanoma, July of 1999. I was cancer free until July of last year. Get those 6 months check-ups! I have 19 melanoma tumors in my lungs. This is uncommon as it usually comes back in your liver first. I have been in a clinical trial at Mayo-for 5 month. A GM-CSF study. I am not responding to this treatment, so I am on chemo now-Temodar. If anyone else has experienced this type of cancer-please write me. I have never talked to anyone with this type of cancer. Thanks for any help. God Bless,—*Sue*

Hi, I'm sorry for your recurrence! I was just diagnosed with choroidal melanoma, had the eye removed, they said if it returns it usually goes to the liver etc. They told me there was no treatment, but you are getting chemo? How is it going?—*Mary*

Dear Sue: The first place you should go to is the occu-mel list. A wonderful supportive group that is up on all the treatments. It's a list-serve. Type it in Google to find the spot to get on or go to eyecancer.com and there is a link on the homepage there. I have choroidal melanoma also. A very large tumor and had proton Beam radiation. I fought for scans, as I am young and have children at home. I think my doctors thought I was crazy to ask for this test or that. There is hope! Others that are going through what you are on the occu-mel list and get you up to date on all the new treatments. I wish you the very best and please don't give-up hope. There are still procedures that are possible.—*Sherri*

◆ ◆ ◆

I was just diagnosed with a melanoma of my right eye after a regular eye exam a few weeks ago. I am having a Cat scan of my brain and liver as well as a chest x-ray to make sure that the rest of me is clear of cancer. And I am scared to death. I am an owner of 3 fitness facilities for women in CA and will be selling 2 of them ASAP. We were in the process of selling them before this diagnosis. And I am recovering from spinal fusion of last year. I anticipate going back to my doctor at Stanford to discuss treatment of the large melanoma and am terrified of losing my eye. I have found this forum to be most helpful as well as emails from Jay. I will keep you all posted and am asking for support and good thoughts for me in the next few months. I know that it is like to work towards a goal being an athlete and motivator to our 1300 members, but every little bit helps. Thanks for your support and thoughts,—*Lynn*

Lynn, first off, welcome to LostEye, its just a pity you are having such a rough time! Have you tried the www.eyecancer.com support group? they have good info on all the forms of eye cancer, though we have many eye cancer sufferers on here too. Feel free to post ANY of your questions or worries on here, we are all more than happy to help. Do keep us informed of how you get on, and I really hope that your CT/MRI and CXR all come back clear, do let us know. Take Care,—*Elizabeth*

I am going to the oncologist to rule out cancer in the liver after my results of the liver CT scan. My eye oncologist says that I need to have a liver panel done and complete physical. The brain CT scan and chest X-ray were clear thank goodness. :lol: I am still struggling with all the stress involved in not knowing if the growth is a true melanoma and to have a biopsy done on it before it is removed. Too many ifs and maybes, and the light is too dim at the end of the tunnel. And my male partner is having a tough time dealing too. Any books out there to read on how to handle with stress with myself, my businesses and my partner (no we are not married either)! Thanks,—*Lynn*

◆　　◆　　◆

Thanks to those who generated this site. I am a male age 46 from Hamilton, New Zealand. I have had my right eye removed two weeks ago. The process, while daunting at first, has been helped immensely by this site. I was diagnosed with a melanoma sitting right in the centre of my eye. Any other therapy was not an option as I would have been blinded and the percentages of being around in five years lessened.

Now two weeks down the track I am feeling very confident with my life ahead with one eye. I have not had the big tick saying that the cancer had not spread yet, but all my tests and scans have come back negative so far. I obviously have not had my new eye fitted yet, but am interested to know what the process is in getting this fitted etc. To any reading this and are about to or are contemplating eye removal as an option to a particular problem, all I can say is, so far for me its not as scary as I thought. I can see a lot more with my good eye than I thought I would be able to. I can drive a motor vehicle. I can still walk, talk and laugh. Its not the end of the world for me or you. To all the other group members "Shine On" and enjoy each new day as a gift.—*Seaspray*

◆ ◆ ◆

Hi, I just went to the specialist this past Thursday, I was being seen for a Choroidal nevus which was located right near my center of vision in my left eye. My vision has continued to deteriorate. I can still see, but everything is very blurry. I still have peripheral vision. Now, after two years of being the same size, it has grown 3/4 of a mm in width and thickness. They are saying it's a melanoma now and the eye will have to be removed. My doctor had his associate come in and take a look at it and they both agreed. They didn't offer any other options. I think that the news shocked my husband more so than I. I had just kind of figured that this is how it would end up, that the eye would have to be removed, I just thought that it wouldn't be for a few more years or so. I have to meet with the ophthalmic plastic surgeon who my dr. referred me to on July 13th. My doctor suggests that I get the procedure done this summer. Any great words of advice or wisdom to share on how to cope? Is there anyone out there who lives in AZ? My husband thinks that it would be good if we could meet with someone who has had the procedure done.—*Renee*

Well, that's pretty much what happened to me except that (1) I didn't have any warning, and (2) I wanted the cancer out of my body as quickly as possible before it metastasized. The problem with the tumor being close to the optic nerve is that the plaque treatment isn't an option, meaning that enucleation is it. While certainly dramatic, enucleation certainly isn't the end of life and most of us who have had the procedure have gone on to happy and productive lives.

My suggestion is that you do seek a second opinion, if only for your later peace of mind in wondering whether anything else could have been done. Personally, I think that once the decision has been made to enucleate, that you should do it as early as possible so that recovery comes sooner. Ask many of the people here and they will say that one of the best days of their lives was when they got fitted with their prosthesis and felt 99% of normal. Also, the longer you wait, the worse the stress and worry will be. Good luck!—*Jay*

◆ ◆ ◆

Hi folks. I was surfing the web and found this site. Had my eye removed do to cancer in 1998. Still have medical checkups every 6 months. A positive attitude is very important as is the support of family and friends. I wish that I would have known about this site back in 1998.—*Dale*

Hi there, I had my eye removed for the same reason in October 1988 and I'm still going strong. Almost 17 years now. woohoo!—*Marmalade*

Hi, I had my eye removed due to cancer in November 2004. It was originally treated with proton beam radiation in 2002, so that was three years ago. It was great to hear from people that are doing so well years later. I'm on interferon therapy right now as I was deemed at high-risk for reoccurrence. I'm a very positive person, but this treatment has gotten my down at times. It was a much needed breath of fresh air to read your posts. Thanks so much and here's to many more years of NED for all of us. Hugs,—*Sherri*

◆ ◆ ◆

While searching for info on ocular melanoma and enucleation, I found this forum. What a relief! I found a group of positive people helping each other. Many of you have been without the use of one eye for a long time. This is all new to me. Five weeks ago I was diagnosed and told that I would lose an eye since my ocular melanoma was on my optic nerve. At the same time the Dr. said we needed to "make sure" that the cancer was no where else. At that time I thought I was going to die by years end.

I have had various tests and now know that the cancer is not any where else in my body. I also have had other opinions which confirm the need to remove my eye. Tomorrow (8/2 I will see an eye surgeon to set up the operation. I believe my family and I are prepared for what is to come, at least as best we can. Obviously I am nervous and unsure. I have gotten this far by reading the input from all of you. Thank you. I look forward, if that's the right word, to being a part of this group.—*Rich*

Hi Rich, I am sorry to hear about your diagnosis. I hope your surgery goes well. I am in the same boat as you, but had my surgery in Feb 03. I found that many things did not change, but maybe a little reevaluation as to what is significant. I hope all works out well for you.—*Roadrunner*

13

Other Cancers

Sadly, choroidal melanoma is not the only cancer that causes the loss of sight. Other forms of eye cancer will require treatments that will result in the loss of sight, and some particularly deadly types of cancers require removal of not just the eye but portions of the skin and bone around the socket. Yet, people cope with these tragedies as they do others.

Letters and E-Mails

I like your site. I am a 57 year old male. One week ago I lost my left eye to squamous cell cancer on and around the eye. The procedure was called a complete exenteration. The eye was removed, along with all associated tissue, including muscles and lids, right down to the bone. I am currently shopping for a eye patch. It will be months before the skin (and scar tissue) creeps in to cover the bone. Then, I can consider a prosthesis. Do you have any advise on patches? I can't get by with just dark glasses because my socket is open and must be protected from contamination.—*Anon*

In 10/03 a biopsy was performed and it came back with two undifferentiated squamous and adeno carcinoma of unknown origin. All of the tests came back negative other than the biopsy. While there has been some confusion and conflict among the various doctors(going to local county hospital-no insurance) about what type of cancer and an importance of the unknown origin. They all seem to agree that this a rare situation and that the eye needs to be removed as a tumor and then some radiation and hopefully the cancer will be gone but will monitor me frequently. One eye doctor said in fifteen years he has only seen three eye patients where the origin was unknown.

While not elated over removal of the eye I am resolved that this is in my best interest for the moment. No chemo is in the plans, no cancer has spread into other areas of the body, and I would rather loose one eye than my life and would rather be cure than go through long bouts of chemo (which I feel destroys the body, it's like poison, though some do well undergoing chemo). They want to put a prosthesis over the right eye that can be removed for future testing of cancer reappearance.

Anyway, just wanted to know of someone else's experience and things to be considered and to know about adjustments, etc. emotionally, its been up and down, however, without denial. I am okay about loosing the eye as opposed to having cancer throughout the body. Thanks for sharing with others.—*David*

This is a great website with lots of encouragement! I have a situation that is a little different and would like to see if you or any of the folks communicating with you might have some suggestions. I was diagnosed with what I am told is a rare form of cancer and had to have my eye and the contents of the eye orbit removed. I am currently going through radiation and chemo and I am seeking info as to what cosmetic options might me available. At the surgery in September of this year the doctor removed the contents of the orbit and then used the eyelid itself as the covering for the back of the socket. So far the only option I have been given is to go back with a magnetic type pf prosthesis. I am a 37 year old otherwise very healthy man and would much rather have a more permanent option for the long haul. Any help would be greatly appreciated.—*Mike*

Will have my right eye removed (along with bone and tissue) in 3 weeks at due to cancer of maxillary sinus (adnoid cystic carcinoma). Have been through radiation & many chemos since Jan.03 when diagnosed at home in TN. I'm so glad I found this website. Thanks.—*Linda*

I started the New Year with a bang. I went to eye doctor for glasses and ended up at the ophthalmologist. I have ciliary body and Iris melanoma. They want to take out my left eye. I am afraid. No one will tell me what to expect. How do they put in the new eye? Does it hurt all the time? How will my vision be with having only one eye?—*Karen*

◆ ◆ ◆

Hi, my name is Karen. I was diagnosed with Iris melanoma 1 month ago. The doctors want to take out my left eye. The tumor is of medium size and is also in the ciliary body of the eye. The pressure in the eye is high. I'm scared out of my mind. The doctors wont tell me the percentage of people that survive, without this cancer coming back in your liver . This cancer is so rare I can't find anyone that has had it. Any information you could give me would be of a great help to me Thank you.—*Karen*

◆ ◆ ◆

Jay, thank you so much for the email. You made me feel better about the whole situation. I was so depressed. I was already planning my funeral. Your story about how you've maintained a normal life is very helpful. I thought my future at best, would be that of a handicapped person I tried to put my letter on the bulletin board. I don't know if I did it right. I have never used a computer before in my life. I just started playing with my kid's computer last week. I'm 38 and computers were not invented in my day. My vision has been affected, sorry for errors in this letter. Thanks again,—*Karen*

I had a basal cell one on the lid of each eye. I had radiation, which went well, was ok for about 6 weeks, then my eyes were so dry I had such a severe sensitivity to light. Dark glasses don't help, I have tried every eye drop in the book, even Restasis, and I do not respond to anything. I had to stop driving outside of my complex, even recently not comfortable driving just a few blocks within it. Have to watch TV with dark glasses on, and my eyes are so dry they hurt all the time. Drops hardly relieve the pain at all. Did you have similar condition? Do you know someone else that did? Do you have any secrets that I don't know about? Your input would be appreciated!—*Bette*

Dear Jay: I am Subhankar from all town called Guwahati (Gua—hati) in the northeast part of India .I am 31 yrs age Male. Recently I have been under going treatment of alveolar soft tissue sarcoma of the right orbit (right eye cancer) . It is a rare form of eye cancer. I was told that the tumor I in a preliminary stage and the size was 25x16x17mm. In spite of a major Neurosurgery the tumor could not get removed, the Neurosurgeon had advise for complete removal of the right orbit (right eye). The Ophthalmic surgeon has denied it saying it would not help as the type of cancer is very nasty & dangerous . The metastases occurs in other part of the body along with the brain. My longevity depends on my physiology & age. And unfortunately my age group falls under the very danger category. But I am not losing hope . I was advised by some other doctor here at India that if some how the tumor get removed it might enhance my longevity by quite a long period. Therefore I could not but look out for any other option available in other part of the world .On searching the eye cancer site for a help I select your name . I though I will get a honest suggestion from a person who could feel the agony & the sufferings going through them, therefore I seek you advice if at all I seek some medical suggestion What will be the best Doctor or Institute in your country where I get suggestion . Would you kindly advise me on the same. I will be eagerly looking forward your valuable advise. God is great will definitely give strength to people like you and me. Have a good day. Thanks—*Subhankar from India*

After having a conjunctiva papilioma (lid/caruncle) removed from my right eye, the pathology report showed several fragments of tissue all showing papillomotous squamous cell carcinoma in-situ extending to all lateral portions of the fragments. I have been treated with mitomycin eye drops, but, have not been able to tolerate them because of a severe allergic reaction, so, am desperate to find an alternative. The doctors here do not seem to know of an alternative. Any assistance would be appreciated Thank you.—*Norma*

Hello Jay: I am not sure how to start this letter but my name is James and I live in Florida USA. I found your web page wile trying to find info on Dept Perception. I have to agree with you about the myth. My problem is my job requires very precise up close work. Having only one eye is a real challenge. While reading your page on Removal Surgery & Recovery I knew very well what you were talking about. I was losing my sight in my right eye over a few months so I went to a local Eye Doctor to find out why. I am 48 and thought I had Cataracts. Because it was my right eye with the problem the doctor examined that eye first. It was not long before I know it was a little more than Cataracts. I was having trouble seeing because I had a uveal ciliochoroidal melanoma and it had retinal detachment. My tumor is large(20.5 x 19.5 x 7.7mm) I had the plaque radiotherapy on 01/21/03 about 3 weeks after finding the tumor. My sight was 20/200 almost 0 before the surgery and now it is 20/400 or in other words 0 . You were right I can not use my eye and still have the worry of reoccurrence and enucleation.—*Jim*

Hi Jay, I am writing to you from Edinburgh in Scotland. I am a 57 year old woman and I have been diagnosed with a tumor in my right eye I have been told that it is Conjunvical Melanosis. I started treatment 3 weeks ago chemotherapy drops, this all came from pigmentation which I have had for 7 years. I hope you will communicate with me and tell me your experiences, although I have had no pain taking drops now I am off first day my eye is running not badly but running any thoughts? I see the doctor next wed. and have a three week break of drops. Best wishes.—*Isobel Douglas*

Dear Jay, I guess I don't know where to begin. I am a 46 year old mother of 6, grandmother of 6. I lead a very healthy, active life. My youngest children are 11 and 9. I work full time as a teaching assistant in the local elementary school. I am never sick. I went to my eye doctor a week ago to have my glasses adjusted. Just a routine visit. No real complaints about my eyes. I didn't even wear glasses until my early forties. Then my arms just got too short! Anyway, this has been an incredible week. I went from a suspicious area on the retina of my right eye, to a diagnosis of a cancerous tumor on the retina. My doctor is recommending radiation treatment or removal of the eye. I live in Oregon and the closest place for the treatment, because of the size of the tumor, is in San Francisco. Needless to say this has all been very weird. I have no physical symptoms of any kind. I even see fine out of the affected eye with my glasses. I enjoy extremely good health. I eat good and exercise daily. My doctor expressed urgency about starting some kind of treatment .My family and I have discussed it and I have decided that my best bet would be to have the eye removed. I am OK with this. My family and friends are freaked out. I came upon your website totally by accident, but I must tell you that you have been a great source of information and inspiration to me. I have recommended that my family and friends all go to your site so that they can better understand what is going to happen and that I will be OK. I am going to have my eye removed in the next couple of days and then get on with my life. I am now confident that this won't change things much for me except that I have a new appreciation for life and getting the most out of every day. Thanks again,—*Connie*

◆ ◆ ◆

Jay—Thanks for answering my email in March. I just finished the proton beam therapy. In addition to the proton beam therapy my doctor also did some laser work as my tumor is next to the optic nerve as you indicated your was. My tumor measured is 13 X 8 X 3.5 and was called a spindle cell melanoma and has not metastasized. My doctor said he is going to try to save the eye, but due to the proximity to the optic nerve there are no guarantees. Therefore I would like to find out as much as I can so if the time comes I will be more prepared than I was last month when out of the blue I found I had melanoma. Some of the questions that I have from someone who has been there are as follows: 1. Did you have any treatments before they decided to remove the eye. 2. What were the deciding factors in removing the eye. Did they think that the proximity to the optic nerve would just destroy the eye or were they more worried about metastasis? 3. How long were you in the hospital when they removed the eye and how long before the put in the artificial eye? Any other concerns that you have had and found answers to I would be interested in. Thanks again for any help you may be able to offer.—*Connie*

My mom has just been told that she has eye cancer. I can't remember the name of the cancer. Apparently it eats away like a mole over time. She has had it about two years. Her lower eyelid is dropping down with it. She is booked in to have surgery one day and the next she is having skin grafts to build up what they have cut away. She is very scared and so am I.—*LS*

Hi Jay, I found out the other day I had several neoplasms in my right eye. I find out tomorrow what type of cancer it is. My biggest fear is that I may have cancer somewhere else in my body as well and it metastasized to my eye. I'll probably find out in a couple weeks. It's the waiting and not knowing that is hard. Because of the large size of the tumors I think enucleation is going to be my best option. I found you're web site very useful and informative—you answered a lot of my questions about the loss of an eye. Even though I am a health care professional myself this has been a very difficult time for me (I think I know too much about what is going to happen) I am the Director of an Eye Bank/Transplant Center—pretty ironic huh?! I've done enucleation surgery (on cadavers) myself. But I knew very little about living with monocular vision . I have been searching the web the last couple of days, trying to learn as much as I can. Your web site made me feel a lot better about the possibility of life with one eye, since I am hoping the only cancer I have is in my eye. [if not—I plan to fight it!] I'll let you know how things turn out and will share my one eye experience with you so that you can continue to help others as you helped me. Thanks again for the info.—*Bob*

Hello Jay. I lost my eye to cancer in January 1999. I have to tell you that I did not drive for a few months and when I visited your web page I didn't believe it. Of course I was being defensive. I am happy you did so well. I am doing much better now. You are the first person I have run into that is about my age. I am a 38 year old female, married with three children. I was pregnant with my third child when I was diagnosed with melanoma located on my eyelid. I had several cryotherapy treatments in both Atlanta and Boston at the Massachusetts eye and ear clinic. Unfortunately, the cancer spread to the conjunctiva and started penetrating the sclera. So it was decided to remove the eye. The only problem is that they also had to remove the muscle and surrounding tissues. I am left with a hole in my face the size of an egg which goes back several inches. I visited an ocularist in Alabama, who is a very nice elderly gentleman who crafted an artificial face piece that holds an artificial eye. The prosthetic is then attached to a pair of men's eyeglasses. This is a viable option, great for going to the grocery store, but not what I would call attractive. The face part is made from a very hard plastic and is not very comfortable. Frankly, there are all sorts of issues. I have had no luck trying to find other alternatives. Also, I would like to have contact with other patients like myself that may have information that would assist me.—*Gina*

I found your site to be most inspiring. I too work in the legal arena as a court reporter. (Okay, sometimes it is a zoo)! Although I have not had to have an eye removed, a nevus was detected on my iris about 6 years ago. Funny thing to me, I had had the spot since childhood and never gave it a second thought. Was only caught with a routine eye exam. I started seeing a specialist who followed me for growth and any change in appearance. Two weeks ago I go in for my routine yearly checkup. Doc says the spot has grown and needs to be removed. I underwent outpatient surgery and now awaiting results from pathology. The surgeon thinks it is a spindle type cell. That's the best kind, I understand, if you're going to have any, and having a melanoma on the iris is better than most, considering it stays contained within that area. I am a bit self conscious about how my iris looks now. If you think of the iris as a pie, 3/4 of pie is now black like the pupil. To me, very noticeable. After reading through the letters on this site, I see how fortunate I am and pray that the melanoma is benign, or at least hasn't spread. Thank you, Jay, for this site. Good luck to you (and remember, to speak slowly for the court reporters! ha).—*Debbie*

Hi everyone, my name is Tommy. I lost my r. eye along with all tissue, (eyelids, eyebrow) and part of the bridge of my nose to skin cancer in 1996 at age 34. I have what they call a "free flap" covering my eye socket. I drove heavy equipment for 5 more years until an abnormal heart condition forced me into early retirement.—*Tommy*

MESSAGES

Hi! I don't post here much, but could truly use some help. I'm looking for information or a forum for someone that has posted on another message forum I am on. He has had surgery on upper lid and under eye for the above mentioned cancer. He would greatly like to talk to someone that has gone through this.

As for me, I have both eyes but lost my vision in right eye to treatment of Proton Beam for Choroidal Melanoma. I have had complications due to the radiation treatment and even though the tumor is shrinking and my scans are clean, I will lose my eye eventually. I've already adjusted over the last two years to depth perception issues and I function quite well. O.K. a little coffee spillage here and there and I hate to parallel park, but I can deal with these annoyances.

Right now I'm in a wait and see mode. I'm on prednisone and pressure lowering drops. So far I have no pain. I knew from the beginning that I may lose the eye. I thought I was getting comfortable with the idea. I feel kind of panicky about it again. It's not out of vanity, because my eye looks really bad right now. I've learned a lot from you guys and know life will go on with one eye, probably pretty much like it is now, since I have no vision at all in treated eye. I think it's the surgery I'm concerned about and I've already had surgery for my eye. Just thought I would post that and see if anyone had any info. on the above cancer and if anyone had any suggestions for pre-surgery jitters.—*Sherri*

Dear Sherri: I don't know about the cancer you asked but I had a malignant melanoma in my eye had eye removed and then radiation therapy for the few cancer cells which had escaped the eyeball into my socket. I didn't have much time to worry about the operation as my eye was removed a week after seeing the specialist but I am sure you will be fine. The pain is not too bad the worst part is looking to the side but this eases after a couple of days. Let us know how you are getting on.—*Anne*

◆   ◆   ◆

I started the New Year with a bang. I went to eye doctor for glasses and ended up at the ophthalmologist. I have ciliary body and Iris melanoma. They want to take out my left eye. I am afraid. no one will tell me what to expect. How do they put in the new eye? Does it hurt all the time. How will my vision be with having only one eye?—*Karen*

I had an iris melanoma. I had had a freckle since I was a kid and never gave it a thought. I too went for new glasses and was sent to a retina specialist. He followed it for five years, and this year, in January, said it had grown and changed color and recommended surgery immediately. So within a month I was in surgery having the melanoma removed from my iris. I think it looks funny, but most people don't ask about it and those that do, think I have had a tear of some type. I will continue to follow up with the retina specialist and hopefully it won't spread. He believes that he got it all. I still have vision in the eye but it is blurry. I had to follow up with an oncologist, who sent me for a PET scan. I am happy to report that there was no other cancer found.—*Anon*

14

Disease

Disease is also a significant cause of the lost of sight in an eye. Sometimes the disease is such that it takes many years to take away sight, while other times the effect is unexpected and immediate, such as during a stroke.

When disease does take away sight, the issue then becomes whether to have the eye removed entirely or not. Often, an eye that has lost sight will slowly shrink and cause pain. Thus, many people will eventually choose to have their blind eye removed entirely.

LETTERS AND E-MAILS

Hello! At first, many thanks for your excellent website! Well, let me tell a bit about myself. I am a 19-year old female from Germany and I am about awaiting the removal of my left eye. It became necessary due to glaucoma and a corneal transplant surgery where have been several problems. During operation my eye started bleeding a lot and I lost more than half of eyeball volume. I have no medical knowledge, so I can't explain the exact reasons for that happening. Now living with a blind eye, a clouded cornea and a shrinking eye, the doctor asked me to let the eye be removed because it makes more problems (and sometimes pain) than it is helpful. And, of course, it is very unsightly, people always look at me because of this. So, after a period of thinking about it, I decided to let my doctor do the enucleation. Although the eye a damaged a lot, it was really a difficult decision I made. The operation is scheduled for the end of April.

Your website helped me a lot to get information and learning about other people's feelings. Additionally, I agree with you all, it is also my fear that they remove the wrong eye! But I know from the hospital (from my corneal transplant) that they ask you which eye should be operated to make sure that they mark the right eye and make no mistake. My second concern is about how I will look like after surgery. But after I read you site, I concluded that it might be not as bad as I had imagined. And the third thing is that I agree that nervousness before surgery is more present than after surgery. Well, there are several weeks left until then but I am starting about making thoughts about what I will go through. Again, thank you a lot for providing the information. I think you will hear from me when I underwent the surgery, I will tell about my experiences. Greetings!—*Sandy*

I was born with glaucoma. I had a lot of problems with my eye pressure when I was growing .Then at age 25 I had to make the biggest decision in my life. It was a hard one to make. I was told if I did not have my eye removed it would exploded because of the pressure in my eye was uncontrollable .I was very frightened by them words. I did not know what to expect or how I would feel. I'm now 41and I still have problems dealing with my artificial eye. I was wondering if there were any support group out there. Thank you,—*Brenda*

Jay: Found your website while surfing the internet—thanks for your good work! I lost eyesight in my left eye while undergoing a procedure to repair a vitreous detachment—without warning the sclera wall tore, flooding the eye with blood. Two surgeries (One of which was an emergency surgery) were unable to restore my vision. A subsequent journey to the hospital convinced to continue my life with my remaining eye.

I drove for the first time on Nov. 15—not too traumatic, but will require some additional practice to restore my confidence. Being left-handed and having a smallish nose have come in handy! Eleven years of experience (with many in-service sessions) as a Lutheran Nursing Chaplain and as Nursing Home Administrator certainly are taking on a greater meaning now. If you know of others who have had a similar experience to mine, please inform me. Thanks,—*Fred*

◆   ◆   ◆

I am a 33 year old male who has no vision in my left eye due to a surgery for retinal detachment in 1995. My first surgery was in 1985 which corrected the retinal detachment. I was also born with a lazy eye, so I never had clear vision in my left eye, matter of fact the only way I could see out of that eye was to close my right eye and even then vision was very poor. Since my last surgery I have had no vision in my left eye, I wear a very strong prescription in my right eye, now the center of my left eye has turned white. I would like any information you can send me on this condition, and steps I could take to apply for disability. Thank you.—*Lamar*

Your web site is quite interesting, and you are very brave. What you went through must have been so difficult. I'm at a loss as to what to do about my eye sight. About seven months ago, I had a Central Retinal Vein Occlusion in my left eye. It's left me with such poor vision in my left eye. I can't seem to bounce back. I can see out of both eyes, but my left only sees a hazy blur, with lots of black spots flying by. It makes me so sad.—*Theresa*

I lost the sight in my right eye at age 58(unfortunately, my stronger eye) due to a stroke-like episode or t.i.a. This is becoming much more common, and is sometimes called an eye attack. Unlike a t.i.a., it causes permanent damage. A piece of cholesterol or plaque will come loose (usually while sleeping and often with sleep apnea), travel up the carotid artery and destroy the retina.

My eye doctor believes that work is proceeding on a computer chip to replace the retina. I am wondering if anyone lost an eye the way I did, and whether anyone knows of a possible breakthrough in the manufacture of a computer chip. Thanks for your attention.—*Duane*

Hi, I lost my right eye a week ago! I woke up after a nights sleep and my vision was gone! I immediately called my eye doctor (surgeon) MD, who stated take two aspirin and get to the office while breathing into a paper bag to expand the veins. Also tried were five nitro pills per my family MD I have one pair of glasses for distance and am going crazy taking them off and on, now I will try bifocals! Any info would be appreciated! Thanks—*Don*

My husband, Hugh, lost his right eye during brain surgery to remove a mass on his pituitary gland. We had no clue that this was going to happen. This happened in February of 2004. We have had no one to turn to that this has happened to. He was a police detective and I am a teacher. He just turned 57 years old three days ago. He could not return to his former job because he can no longer carry a gun. He had to retire and is now on Social Security Disability. All these changes plus the loss of his pituitary gland functions have taken place in this last year.

Is there anyone out there who has gone through anything like this? I would like support for me and him even though it has been a year. We are just trying to make it through all these life-changing events together with JESUS to help us. We would welcome any support from anyone who has been here.—*Josie*

Hi, Jay, Thanks for your site. It's very empowering and I'm going to bookmark it. I'm one-eyed now but will likely have a vitrectomy to hopefully restore vision lost (Feb 28) to a severe vitreous hemorrhage. I haven't had surgery in 3 decades (I'm 42) so reading your surgery story was extremely helpful for me (and I agree, enucleation should be a banned word). I might touch base w/you in the future to see if you'd like to be interviewed if/when I score a magazine assignment about life after losing an eye. I admire your resilience.—*Marie*

Hi, Very happy to have found your website. I just found out yesterday that I have neovascular glaucoma in my right eye. My doctor gave me the requisite drops, etc.; but he did say that I may have to consider enucleation. (I lost sight in this eye after six unsuccessful retinal detachment surgeries twenty years ago in grad school). What freaks me out about this (besides feeling like a freak) is that in 2001 I lost sight in my good (left) eye and had two vitrectomies, retinal tear repair, and an inert gas bubble inserted into the eyeball where there had been the vitreous. Had to remain with my head in a downward position for 12 weeks. Thank God that I now can see well out of the left eye, although I always am afraid that I'll be blind. The diode laser treatment for the right (glaucomic) eye is dangerous because of the possibility that it would affect my good (just repaired!) eye, so my doctor said that enucleation is really the best alternative.

Do you know of any support groups in my area? I asked my doctor and he had no idea; also had no idea of therapists for people confronting blindness, or fear of. I have two daughters, one 17 and one 14 and I think they are having a hard time with the possibility. I am still relatively young (une femme d'un certain age) and relatively attractive, and if aging isn't enough, this is two standard deviations away from the norm! Thanks for doing the site; I look forward to reading every single word and every letter. Best,—*Larisa*

I have been diagnosed with CRVO in my right eye for the past two years. I am only hoping and praying that someone, somewhere will find a cure for this disease. Thank you for all your help.—*Carol*

I have not lost an eye, but have lost sight in my right eye due to temporal arthritis . Is there a difference here? I note numerous success after loss of an eye stories, but none from temporal arthritis victims who retain the eye but no longer have sight in the eye. Help!—*John*

Jay—Found your website while surfing the internet—thanks for your good work! I lost eyesight in my left eye while undergoing a procedure to repair a vitreous detachment—without warning the sclera wall tore, flooding the eye with blood. Two surgeries (0ne of which was an emergency surgery) were unable to restore my vision. A subsequent journey to the hospital in Chicago convinced me to continue my life with my remaining eye. I drove for the first time on Nov. 15—not too traumatic, but will require some additional practice to restore my confidence. Being left-handed and having a smallish nose have come in handy! Eleven years of experience (with many in-service sessions) as a Lutheran Nursing Chaplain and as Nursing Home Administrator certainly are taking on a greater meaning now. If you know of others who have had a similar experience to mine, please inform me. Thanks,—*Fred*

I am a 29 year old mother of 2 little angels and married to the most wonderful man in the world. I have proferative diabetic retinopathy and recently had a vitrectomy. After that everything went wrong. Two days later I got a staph infection, major inflammation, and now so much scar tissue on the retina that it detached and the sclera is covered as well. Needless to say that my eye has started to shrink all within a month. Now they just want me to go through the motions. I am very scared and full of panic because I don't know anything about this process. As a last resort, I am going to Miami right away to see a doctor. If anyone can provide me with any helpful information or advice it would be a blessing. Thanks,—*April*

MESSAGES

Wanted to share my story with you as it's a bit different than the others I've seen. Would love to hear from someone with a similar medical history. It was Friday afternoon. I had this weird sensation while mowing my lawn, and realized a gray darkness was moving in on my vision (kind of like a shade being drawn). Within 1 minute I had no vision in my right eye, had the phone in my hand, and was in the hospital ½ hour later. Something had restricted the blood flow to my retinal artery—a "retinal stroke", though the root cause was unknown at the time. The next morning I awoke and thought—it was a dream (nightmare?)! Then I realized that I still had no vision in the eye. I cried and felt sorry for myself for a few minutes. Then I got out of bed, showered, and went to the golf course. Less than 18 hours after losing the vision, I was on the golf course, playing in a charity tournament.

My thought was—I don't see with my eyes, I see with my heart. Well, 5 weeks and many tests later I found the culprit—my heart! As my cardiologist puts it, I was an "extremely healthy 35 year old woman". Except for one thing—I had a hole in my atria, and an atrial septal aneurysm—the artia of my heart didn't develop properly before birth. These defects lead to a blood clot, which traveled up my neck to my retinal artery. I never knew I had a problem prior to this. I am extremely lucky to be functioning—had the blood clot traveled to my brain instead of the retinal artery, I could be in a nursing home right now, learning to walk/talk/speak again.

In the last 12 months, I've had my heart repaired (one year ago today!), traveled extensively both in the States and overseas, have run for public office (and won!), and continued to maintain my very active lifestyle. I also golf regularly, jet ski, read, work, travel, and do everything I did before. Sure, driving is different with one eye—I live on Lake Ontario, where we got almost 200 inches of snow last year (and 4 wheel drive is a necessity!). But I've adapted. And I feel very, very lucky. This is just a hiccup in my life.

I realized I have a choice to make every day—I can wake up and feel sorry for myself, or I can be thankful for another morning. I'm happier now, in fact, than I ever was when I had 2 eyes. I've stopped waiting—for the perfect job, a husband/child, more money, etc. Instead I look at how much I do have, and how blessed I am. If it took losing an eye to learn how to live, I'd do again tomorrow. I have a second chance—some people never get that option. Anyway, thanks Jay and friends—this website has been a great resource. I'd love to hear from someone with medical history similar to mine.—*Jessie*

◆ ◆ ◆

Hi Christine, What was the name of the childhood cataract you had? I was born with a childhood cataract in my left eye called Posterior Lenticonus. I have never had it operated on, and I am 23 now. Sometimes I think about operating because I'm clinically blind in that eye, but worry about the risk. Thanks for your story also. Take care.—*tanunson628*

I'm 25 yrs and lost my eye due to an accident I had in the backyard when I was 10yrs. I myself have 'issues' about my eye and I too worry that people notice. I have since learned that accepting who you are and what the circumstances are help you more rather than trying to fight it. This doesn't mean that you have to like it but simply accept it. That said, I truly admire where you have come from and what you have been through, you are an inspiration to the rest of us. Thanks for your posting.—*Mike*

Hey Mike, that was great advice . I think we all have issues . and you are right you don't have to like it but you need to accept it. It's great to have someone else from England on the board!—*Cindy*

◆ ◆ ◆

I haven't been on the site for a while. I went to see the oculoplastic department in London and they casually tell me I've got raised pressure and an excavated disc which looks like glaucoma. They sent me a follow up appointment which happens to be 28th May when I will be on my way to Canada and I'm really worried about the delay. If I need to start taking drops to lower the pressure I want to start doing it now. They also said that the steroid drops my general practitioner prescribes me when the irritation in the prosthetic eye gets too bad will raise the pressure in the good eye. The visit to the oculoplastic dept was to sort out the irritation. Seems I need a mucus membrane graft to enlarge the anterior fornix but this seems like the least of my problems now.

Am quite apprehensive and wondering how long I can carry on driving. Nothing wrong with my eyesight yet. It's so scary to have something go wrong with your one remaining eye. The National Health Service seems so cumbersome. Does anyone have any experience of glaucoma?—*Mary*

Hi Mary, first of all, HUGE Hugs to you! It sounds like your having a really tough time at the moment! I would say hassle them for an earlier appointment, you really want to get on top of this and leaving it for another 6 weeks doesn't sound like a great plan to me! See if something can be swung with regards to that being the only eye you see out of anyway, and just let them know that you need the earliest appointment you can get.

Did they tell you what your IOP is? Steroids will cause IOP's to rise, but if it isn't a continuous treatment the problem shouldn't persist. (I was on oral steroids for a good while and after treatment stopped the IOP in my good eye came near back to normal). I take Pilocarpine (Pilogel 4%) in my bad eye, keeping the pressure down and keeping my pupil teeny. Its not a major inconvenience, though it does hurt ALOT on application, and lasting for about 10 minutes or so. (But really I think that's just me, and its not really supposed to do that! lol). Glaucoma is a manageable condition and if treatment is started promptly then vision loss can be kept at a minimum. Here are a few sites that may be of interest: The Glaucoma Research Foundation www.glaucoma.org Glaucoma UK www.iga.org.uk and, a really informative discussion group with resident Glaucoma Specialists who meet each week: http://www.wills-glaucoma.org/support.htm Its tough having something going on with your good eye and I really hope you get sorted soon. Do let us know how things go,—*Elizabeth*

Thanks so much for your support and sharing your expertise. I've got myself an appointment for this Friday by bypassing the NHS and going private. I'm against it ideologically but I can't take chances with my sight. Thank you for the links too. I found a brilliant one which I'll made the subject of a new thread because it's so cool. Best example of interactive use of the web I've ever seen.—*Mary*

I don't have any experience but was in the same situation. I was told that I was a "glaucoma suspect" and had to take a visual field test. The results were good and everything's okay. But it was definitely nerve wracking when we only have one good eye. I will make sure that I go get this checked and take the visual test often. Good luck to you.—*Andrew*

♦ ♦ ♦

I'm so excited that I found this message board. I wish I would have found you guys earlier. Before my surgery at least. A little about me, since I'm a newbie and all. I was born with 75% of my retina scarred for reason we have never figured out. At 19 I was diagnosed with neovascular glaucoma and retinal detachment. I went through a laser surgery to relieve the pressure, leaving my pupil permanently dilated. I think they call it a white pupil or something like that. Then last June I started having spontaneous bleeding in my eye. They couldn't get it to stop and I was nonresponsive to all the medications I was on so I decided to have it removed. I don't think it was a difficult decision. I think I was more troubled over the fact that I didn't feel any sentimental attachment to the eye. It was my right eye for Pete Sakes! And I was more than willing to part with it. But I digress. They did an evisceration (I think that's how you spell it) The pain subsided almost immediately, well within a day of the surgery. I was back to work a week later. I haven't had my prosthetic for even a month yet. I got it as a birthday present. well not really I got it two days before my 24th birthday. I "took it out" for some cheesecake and bowling. I'm so excited about having it. It shocks me that people don't really notice. But sometimes I can't help but feel self conscious of it. Like if somebody looks at me for too long I start thinking "They know, they know its not real" Any tips on dealing with that? I think that's the hardest thing I've had to deal with thus far. I'm so excited to have found you guys! This is awesome. I'm actually feeling giddy. I have pictures up on my homepage if you would like to take a look. I documented most of the progression of the eye with milestones after the surgery also. Okay I'm going to stop now. People are probably tired of reading a long post.—*Pixie*

♦ ♦ ♦

I am a fifty year old man with Chore retinitis of the right eye which is a result of histoplasmosis as a child. I have been legally blind in my right eye since I was 29 and had laser surgery in the macular region to stop a retinal bleed. Two years ago I was diagnosed with glaucoma and the pressure has been pretty much out of control for the whole two year period. I have been on many regimens of eye drops with the current being Xalatan, Alphagan and Cosopt. The really pathetic part about this is that when they diagnosed me with glaucoma I was diagnosed as having primary open angled glaucoma and after being jerked around in a slip shod ophthalmic practice for the last two years, I recently went to see a very well known ophthalmologist who is a professor at Jules Stein at UCLA and he told me flat out that I had CLOSED ANGLE GLAUCOMA and that the drops would do me absolutely no good at relieving the pressure and if I had continued to do what I was doing for any length of time, I would just go blind as my eyeballs were ready to pop out of my head.

I'm just wondering, if an ophthalmologist misdiagnoses a person and they end up losing vision because of the misdiagnosis and the fact that I have been taking medications that are contraindicated for closed angle glaucoma, would you recommend that I have a legal representative look into this situation? It scares me to death that the only thing that prevented me from going blind was the notion that the doctors that I was seeing were not doing their job. I ended up having bi-lateral iridectomies the day after I saw this new doctor and he said it was the only thing that would prevent me from going blind and or losing more vision. The other doctors never mentioned any options like this and completely misdiagnosed the type of glaucoma that I even had. What would you do? I really could use some feedback here. Thanks,—*A Very Lucky Guy*

Hi everyone. I was wondering if those of you who had your eye removed due to eye cancer could share with me your symptoms, etc. before you were diagnosed. Mine started with a flashing light type thing in a corner of my vision, and over the year progressed to a blind area that eventually became larger and larger. My doctor never saw it, even when a quarter of my vision was gone in that eye. During my anger phase of recovery after having the eye removed(by then no vision left anyway) I took my records to a lawyer, and it looks like there is a case, which is upsetting me all over again, I feel like it is all my fault that I didn't know what was going on inside of my body. Was wondering what others have experienced.—*Mary*

Hi Mary, My experience wasn't too much different from yours. I went to my regular eye doctor in October, 1991 because I felt like there was a thin black line at the top of the range of vision in my right eye. It was like if I looked straight ahead, there was the edge of a baseball cap up there. After checking me out, the Dr. said he didn't see anything wrong. I went on my merry way, not completely satisfied with this answer, but he was the doctor, so I trusted him. Then the light flashes started. I only saw them when I went to bed before I fell asleep. It was very weird, but I pretty much ignored them. Had I known then that light flashes are a symptom of a detached retina, I wouldn't have been so blasé about them. You know what they say about hindsight!

Then, one Sunday in August, 1992, I was at the gym and all of a sudden, this black line above my eye became more pronounced. I don't know if something I did at the gym caused the retina to detach a little more, or whether I just became aware that something was different. Anyway, I called the eye doctor the next morning and when I told them what was going on, they had me come right in. They did a range of vision test, which I thought was a waste of time, because when the Dr. finally examined me, he saw the detached retina, but never mentioned a tumor. I don't think he saw it. They immediately arranged for me to see a retina specialist at Wills Eye in Philadelphia that day, telling me to go prepared to be admitted as a detached retina needs to be operated on at once.

So I packed a bag, got my cousin to drive me over, and after being examined by the retina specialist and hearing the doctors saying amongst themselves "This looks like MM. Has anyone said anything to you about a tumor?" they walked me over to the oncology section, telling me not to be frightened! Ha! You try not to be scared. This all happened on that one day. After being examined by what seemed to be a hundred other doctors (really residents, since CM is so rare, they wanted everyone to have a look) they told me what I had, choroidal melanoma. The tumor was producing fluid, which was causing the retina to detach. Three days later, my eye was removed.

This is kind of a long way of telling you that I also thought of seeing a lawyer about my situation. When I realized that I had the first symptoms of this nine months prior, and the ophthalmologist didn't catch it, I was really angry. Maybe if I hadn't been so consumed with getting taken care of, I would have looked into it. I did ask the doctors at Wills if this could have been caught earlier and they said that special lenses are needed to find CM and he probably couldn't have seen it without them. How true this is, I don't know. Plus, I felt somewhat to blame because I did nothing to find out about the light flashes. So I just let it go, which wasn't easy.

Obviously, you have to do what is right for you. However, if you lost a quarter of your vision while you were under his care, and he did nothing, like sending you to a specialist, I think you should pursue it with the lawyer. And you shouldn't blame yourself for not knowing what was happening. You did the best you could at the time, and you can't go around kicking yourself because you know more now. If that were the case, I probably wouldn't be here now, as I fell into quite a depression after all of this. It was only after the help of a good therapist that I learned to live with it. I hope my story has helped, if only to let you know that your experience was probably shared by others like me. I wish you the best of luck. Keep us posted on what you decide.—*Nancy*

Hi, Mary. As I live in the UK my story is probably very different to yours. I had no idea there was anything wrong with my eye just thought I needed my glasses changing. When I was having a routine eye test my optician said she thought there was a problem and referred me to my own general practitioner. He referred me to the eye dept of a large hospital quite near me. The specialist looked in my eye and I had lots of tests and he told me straight away he thought I had a malignant melanoma in it. Well you can imagine the shock I even had to have chest x-ray in case cancer had spread, luckily it hadn't. He referred me to the eye infirmary where it was confirmed I had cancer. I was admitted 3 days later and had my eye removed the next day. It all happened so quick I didn't really have time to worry about it. I can only praise indeed the way I was treated from the first visit to the optician up till today. I have been very well looked after and have no complaints at all. All I can say is thank goodness for the national health service in the UK. Hope to speak to you again.—*Anne*

◆ ◆ ◆

I'm so very glad I found you all! I'm 53, lost the sight in my right eye due to detached retina. Have gone through seven surgeries. My retina doc here in Kansas is THE BEST. My doc just told me two weeks ago that the sight will not be returning to my eye. I still have the eye. Is there anyone out there who is in their 40s or 50s who lost sight in the last two years or so? I'm trying to find someone who can relate to emotional reaction I'm having. Please write back! Thanks and thanks sooooo much LostEye!—*Molly*

Hi Molly, I lost my vision 2-years ago when I was 42. Mine was a little different circumstance than yours. I had a detached retina due to a large choroidal melanoma. I kept the eye for 2 years after treatment, but then I started having severe migraines and was diagnosed with neovascular glaucoma due to radiation damage. I recently had enucleation and looking forward to getting my prosthesis. I think the vision was secondary to me because of the cancer. I'm also an artist and sight is so important. I'm very thankful that my untreated eye is hanging in at 20/20. I wish I can help more. I was sad, but because of the cancer very thankful to be alive. I wish you all the best and just realize it will be an adjustment, but it is definitely doable. Hugs,—*Sherri*

Hi Molly I had my eye removed in April2002 as I had a malignant melanoma and like Sherrie I am glad to be still here. I was 53 when this happened and it has taken me a long time to get used to it. I have never gone back to work but I worked in every big engineering factory and even my employers thought it would be too much for me to handle. I am going into hospital on 11th for another operation which will be my 4th. I know exactly what you are going through but believe me it does get better. If you need anything this is the group to be in hope you get the help you are looking for.—*Anne*

Hi Sherri. I am having some plastic surgery done to try and make my artificial eye fit better and not hurt so much. They are taking some tissue from inside my cheek and grafting it to my lower lid to make it a little bigger. I don't know the exact details (probably better that way). The doc said my mouth would be more sore than my eye. My eye will be stitched closed for 2 to 3 weeks till the graft takes. Not really looking forward to it just hope it makes some improvement to my appearance. People tell me I shouldn't worry that it doesn't look perfect but its not them going through it is it. The only people who really understand are people like you and everyone on this site. I just want to look "normal" and if this can happen then I am willing to go through operations. Speak to you soon,—*Anne*

Dear Anne: I totally understand how you feel. If this surgery will help your self-esteem, go for it! I'm getting a little worried as my upper lid is sagging a lot and hoping the prosthesis will make me look more normal than I do now. I have to go to a lot of meetings and meet new clients and it's been hard wearing these glasses. Since it's raining here I can't wear sunglasses and these glasses are clear in one-side and frosted on the other. It brings lots of questions of course. I do it with a smile on my face, but when I get home I feel drained somewhat. In the scheme of things, I know this is just a bump in the road. I'm wishing you the best and can't wait to here about your results. Here's to a speedy recovery too! Many hugs,—*Sherri*

Sorry to hear about your ordeal Molly. After the neighbor kid decided to shoot my 12 yr old in the eye with a pellet gun last may, he was first seen by an eye specialist in Topeka. While my son is only 12, he obviously was forced to suddenly get used to the idea of, and the peculiarities of going from monocular, to binocular vision. He still has issues with bumping into things on his left side, but aside from that has gotten along just fine. He still races BMX bikes in National Events, and plays just like you would expect a 12 yr old to do.—*John*

Hi Molly, I am 45 and lost my left eye due to an airbag accident almost two years ago. It has taken me awhile to adjust, physically and mentally. I used to get frustrated more often (due to difficulty pouring things, shaking peoples' hands, banging into things, etc.) but now I have pretty much accepted that this is the way it is and I need to just go on from here. It's helped to try to focus on what I can do instead of what I can't do. In a way this accident has actually helped in the self-confidence department! At any rate, hang in there and know that you are not alone.—*JYS*

◆ ◆ ◆

I recently lost vision in my right eye due to an "eye stroke"—went to bed one night feeling fine and woke up blind in the right eye. A week later I had to undergo carotid artery surgery. It has now been 18 days since I lost my right vision. I wear glasses—blindness took my dominant eye and it has been tough. I am very depressed—don't know if I'll be able to cope with this. Doctors keep telling me to be patient with myself—they keep saying in time I will be doing everything I did before but I have this feeling of dread that I will never feel the same again. Questions I have are 1) is this feeling normal 2) will my mind adjust to this situation 3) any suggestions to help this funk 4) will I stop focusing on what was and accept what is 5) will my weaker eye take over and become stronger. I thank you for any insight you can give me.—*Don*

Hi Don, firstly I am sorry to hear that you have lost your vision, but as all of us are testament to. You DO get over it. Answers to your questions: 1) This feeling is totally normal, but like the Dr's have said, be patient with yourself and you will find that eventually you'll be capable of everything you did before. except perhaps watch those 3D movies through the funky green and red glasses! 2) Yes, give it a little while. Keep practicing pouring out of jugs into glasses, going up curbs and catching balls and stuff. The depth of vision issue can be a problem at first, but don't believe all you hear, you'll adapt pretty quickly. Remember to be kind to yourself though, and if you spill something, remember, it can always be cleaned up later, so go easy on yourself. 3) See above and read through old posts. 4) Eventually yeah, but like I said, give it time. It is normal to compare how you see now to how you saw things before, and you will get frustrated from time to time, but its normal so don't worry. 5) I'm really not sure about this, but to be honest I don't think so. I think that the weaker eye only gets stronger through practice in the cases of children with "lazy" eyes (amblyopia) when they are patching the dominant one to try and make the weaker one do all the work. I think the ability for this to happen diminishes somewhat with age. Ask your doctor to be sure though.

I think I've answered your questions for now, we're all here to help each other out after all! Take it easy,—*Elizabeth*

Hi Don, I also lost vision in my dominant eye due to an "eye stroke". In my case, the clot formed in my heart (I had 2 previously unknown congenital heart defects), and blocked the flow to my retinal artery. This happened about 3 years ago, at the age of 35, and I've since had the heart repaired.

I never felt too down about losing the eye—at first I didn't think I'd drive, golf, jet ski, or live the same way, but once I realized how very lucky I was, losing the eye seemed minor. Don't get me wrong—it IS tough at times—but think of this as a blessing in disguise. You can get medical help to reduce the risk of having a full-blown stroke that could leave you severely disabled (or dead). As far as getting used to things—the first night without my right eye I spilled milk (completely missed the glass) and got so frustrated with eating that I gave up. I would stab at something, and miss the food completely. Everything seemed difficult the first few weeks/months. Now—unless I'm reminded somehow, I honestly forget that I have vision in only one eye. At the time of my stroke, my non-dominant eye had quite poor vision—it has drastically improved since. Now I wear glasses for protection—not because I need them (like before). Take care of yourself—get to the root cause of the stroke!—*Jessie*

15

Accidents

Each year, many people lose their eyes due to accidents such as fireworks and car crashes. Sadly, children seem to be the most susceptible to losing their eyes to accidents. The loss of an eye due to an accident is usually immediate, meaning that at least one does not have to endure the prospect of losing an eye as do cancer patients. On the other hand, there is no time to mentally prepare one's self for the loss.

LETTERS AND E-MAILS

I just wanted to write to thank you for your very supportive web site. I lost my eye when I was 14. I was in a local park with a couple of my friends, when one of them pulled out a BB Gun. I was shot in the left eye. I was rushed to the hospital, where they proceeded to try to remove the BB, but to no avail. I was in the hospital for a week. Everyday they would check me to see if I had any vision at all. Finally at the end of the week they determined that I would never get any vision in my left eye. I then had to make the decision to remove the eye, or leave it alone. It was a tough decision, but finally my family and I decided that I should have it removed. This is what the ophthalmologists there had recommended. Two weeks later I was back in the hospital to have the eye removed.

That period in my life was so hard. I was so scared of what I was going to look like with a prosthesis. I thought everyone would know by just looking at me. I was just a freshman in high school. I thought no boy would ever want to date me. I went through a rough time. When I was finally fitted for my prosthesis, I could not believe how great and natural it looked. My ocularist did such an awesome job. No one could even tell! I was so happy.

Today, I am a 22 year old woman. I work full-time, and go to school part-time. I have a son, and I am planning my wedding for September. Obviously this terrible incident has not slowed me down at all and I found the greatest man ever who wants to marry me, glass eye and all.

Of course everything is not always fine and dandy. I still come across those young children who look at me and say "What's wrong with your eye?", but don't we all! I am just grateful that I have my right eye, with perfect vision I might add! I would really like to talk to people who have gone through the same type of experience. So if anyone is interested in writing, please do. Thanks again for this resourceful website!—*Jill*

Dear Jay: I just found your web site and thought it was very well done. My name is Linda. I run my own small business out of my home, have four children and have a wonderful husband. I am a member of the PTA, a girl scout leader, a Sunday School teacher. I also have one more thing. A piece of coral where my eye used to be.

You see, one year ago this week I was at a hockey game and one of the players slap shot the puck from center ice, only it did not hit the glass as it normally does and did not defray into the audience. Instead it made a direct hit into my left eye. It completely lacerated it 90% around and crushed into tiny pieces all the bones in the orbital eye area and more and has done some permanent nerve damage to the nerves around the eye and down to my lips.

I was rushed from the arena medical facility to a trauma center, who could not handle this extensive injury only to be rushed again, via ambulance into New York City.

I have had nine surgeries in the last year. The first was 4 1/2 hours in the middle of the night on the evening of the accident to do emergency repairs and stop the bleeding and try to reinflate my eye and get pressure back into it. Surgery number 2 and 3 were back to back one and half weeks later to make another attempt at repairs—however it was at this point that they realized the true extent of the bones being crushed, into the nasal passage and the eye itself being non-repairable. Surgery 4 and 5 were also back to back two days later, the day before Mother's Day. Four being the actual enucleation itself and the fifth being the replacement of crushed bone with plates and the placement of coral covered with the sclera of donor eye where my own eye once was and reconnection of muscles and veins to the coral. Surgery 7 was to add density to a sagging lower lid and add volume for aesthetics sake. Surgery 8 was to repair and shorten muscle in the upper lid because the eye muscles are not holding up due to damage and are almost closing the eye and finally, surgery 9 was to further do work on the upper lid muscles again. We do have surgery number 10 to look forward to but hopefully that will be the last for a while.

My face looks absolutely normal and outside the pins and needles sensation over my lip, I am fine. I too, go on with my life as normally as possible, understanding however, and appreciating the sight I have left in my other eye more. The joy of looking into my children's beautiful blue eyes and knowing I will see them graduate High School and College, see my sons hit a home run or even just strike out at their little league games and see my daughter wear a wedding gown. I watch them with new meaning to the words, growing up before my eyes or eye, as the case may be.—*Anon*

I found the stories on your website inspirational, as it was three years ago, my husband was mowing with a brush-hog, I realized that an extension cord had been left out, I ran outside, and as I bent over something hit me in the head and knocked me over. That something turned out to be a 2or3 lb. piece of steel off of the machine itself. It was a direct blow to my right eye and the skull around it. I begged the doctor to leave my eye and try to repair it and he did. but, in a few weeks he realized as did I,that the damaged eye would have to come out and I would be getting the ever-dreaded "fake-eye" I can remember wishing that I would have just died from the head injury. Isn't that sad? I suppose that I felt that way because losing a part of my body was overwhelming, especially my best and most expressive feature. I had a very skilled and understanding physician, and a gifted ocularist who I believe was a blessing. and my friends and family were and continue to be very supportive.—*Anon*

Thank you for your web site. My 18 year old son was hit in the eye with a paint ball in July. He had been accepted into the Navy; however, that was not to be. He has gone through 6 surgical procedures trying to save his eye, but unfortunately this has not worked and his eye has gotten significantly smaller. Next week on he will have his eye removed. This is something he wanted and said no more surgeries. Your web site has given me some insightful information and reassurance. The letters of the younger people have been encouraging. My son has had the time to adjust to vision in one eye so that is one thing he won't have to adjust to. Now it will be time for him to think about a plan for life since his life has been on hold for over a year. As a parent it is so hard to see your child go through things like this but I know it has made us stronger and God has been with us through all of it. Thank you again for your web site.—*Bobbi*

At thirteen years of age my left eye was severely damaged by a home made explosive device, the surgeons patched it up, but it never regained sight. Having sight in one eye has never been a problem I managed to become a relatively successful racing cyclist and I reverse a truck through a gap just a whisker wider than itself.

The left eye however grew uglier, misshapen, bulging and cloudy with intermittent periods of extreme discomfort. I thought that I would rather soldier on rather than have part of my body removed and thrown away. The unknown was pretty scary, but once that I had discovered your web site I knew that my life would be improved if I could just be brave enough to let go. In a few years ago, I had the eye removed, it is all behind me now, I have no discomfort at all and for the first time in twenty years look normal again. I have three small children, and they have not been troubled at all by me having an artificial eye.—*Andrew (Bath, England)*

Thank you for your website! I am a 28 year old woman. I lost my left eye when I was 16 due to a gunshot wound. At that time, I was very depressed. I felt like I would never be able to do the things I did before or that no one would ever want to be with me. When I got my artificial eye it was a turning point for me. It looks so natural and my muscles were not damaged so it moves. Its just a little slower than my good eye. I am still at times self-conscious about my eye, but overall my life is as normal as anyone with 2 good eyes. All I can say is that you get use to it with time. I have no problem driving or parking. I just use my mirrors a lot and take extra care when changing lanes. I still do run into people sometimes when I'm walking but its not a big deal.

Most people never know that I have a artificial eye at all. In fact, a lot of people don't believe me when I tell them. For anyone who is going through the pain of losing an eye. Be strong it does get better.—*Anon*

I had an accident just over 12 months ago my eye was lacerated, leaving me with my poor left eye which is fine with glasses for long distance, but need to take them off to read small print. I have no 3D and I don't see one thing or the other! My confidence totally has gone. I do still work and drive, but miss so many simple things. I was very frightened about sympathetic eye syndrome. I also have so many floaters in my left eye it does make it difficult, So glad to find your web site.—*Ian*

Thank you for this website. I just lost all sight in my right eye due to a golf ball hit teed off near me last week. People are amazed at my optimism (and my wife's) and it's nice to see someone else with the same view. I'm still adjusting, but it's good to know this info. is out there. God bless, and take care.—*Anon*

Wow! This site has been so uplifting for me. My 30 year old son lost his eye in an accident last year, and he is afraid that he won't be able to move to another state to take a new job, because he won't be able to get a license. I'm going to give him this address. It is so helpful to hear from others who have the same challenges and fears. Thank you.—*Brenda*

I have just recently found this website, and wish I had visited it at the time that I lost my eye. It was very informative and answers many of the questions I had before my surgery. I lost my eye in a work accident that involved my eye and a nail enough said. It has been 2 years since I lost my eye and everything is back to normal except now I wear my safety glasses at work. And to answer one of the sports related questions it does affect my basketball game Which I wasn't to good at before the accident, but now I know what a blind side pick is…ouch. Thanks for your time and the site.—*Tim*

I really enjoy your website. I lost an eye in a mountain biking accident several years ago. The optic nerve was pulled from my eye due to severe head trauma. I would like to offer a suggestion. The way I dealt with learning how to maintain depth perception was shooting basketball following the injury. I did this for about six months. I really felt that it helped in learning to read how near or far an object was within 20 feet.—*Ryan*

Since I lost my left eye in a gun accident I have spent numerous hours searching for means to improve my depth perception & your web page is unquestionably the best I've come across. You mentioned that you have a ping pong like object attached to the muscles in your eye socket. I don't have this & it may be because all socket muscles were destroyed in the accident. However, due to your web page I am now armed with the information to ask my ophthalmologist. Thank you for a very informative web page.—*Bob*

You don't know how good it feels to know there are others like me in the world that I can talk to about this. I lost my eye in an accident (exploding car battery) years ago.—*Michael*

I will have my right eye removed next year. I was blinded in an accident in almost 30 years ago and lost all vision. Now I have been battling glaucoma, headaches and many infections. As of this past week my doctor stated there was not much to do anymore and just get the eye out. We have had this discussion before and now I want it out. I'm going to a highly rated surgeon recommended by my insurance carrier. I have had the opportunity to see him once before and have no second thoughts of the surgery. I have spent a lot of time on your web site and it has been very helpful and has made me content. After the surgery does it really only take one day for the artificial eye to be implanted? I know I will have many more questions but that one is important with time lost at my job.—*Chuck*

Great to see a site that is so positive. I lost my eye in a shooting accident fifteen years ago and had very little contact then with other people my own age who had the same thing. Good to see that there is a resource now. I will pass on your details to my eye specialist who is sure to recommend it to others. Keep me in touch with any good developments.—*Toby*

I lost my left eye in twenty years ago but I now play table tennis in my local league! I am also a phenomenal pool player with only one eye and one arm, my left arm having been paralyzed in the same accident that took my eye.—*Mad Dog*

My husband was hit in the right eye with a golf ball and so far has lost all sight in the eye. That evening he had emergency surgery to repair the deflated globe including 18 stitches in the globe but so far he can't see any light in the eye. He is living on pain pills and there seems to be a great deal of concern about a condition that could occur in the good eye due to this trauma. It's called sympathetic ophthalmia but the doctors can't give us updated statistics on it. It could show up in weeks, months, many years later or never. Depending on his pain level and what the eye will eventually look like, we might end up having to remove the eye in the future. I would like to know if other people were faced with this dilemma regarding the good eye. We need all the advice we can get right now!—*Helene*

Thanks for answering me so fast—my husband is scheduled for an ultrasound tomorrow to see how extensive the damage is from his golf ball accident and surgery last week. He has so much pain right now and is living off of pain pills. Aside from getting rid of this pain, will he better off with leaving in a bad eye (provided the pain in time will go away) or removing it? Now I'm reading about some phantom pain people experience? We are still in a state of shock here from this freak accident and can't believe how life can change on a dime. There's talk about a condition called sympathetic ophthalmia which could affect the good eye in time. What do you know about this? One reduces the risk by taking out the bad eye from what we have been told. What's facing us will be whether to leave in a bad eye or take it out and I guess if he could rid of this pain, then maybe we could wait to see what a bad eye looks like over time. I guess I've never seen anyone with a bad looking eye. I've never seen anyone with a glass eye either. Any advice you could pass on to me would be greatly appreciated. I need to find someone on this website that had a bad eye taken out due to an injury or one that is living with a bad eye.—*Helene*

Back at 1993, I had an eye accident, due to foreign bodies, they had to operate twice to remove them, and the result was a soft eye. I know that the vision is impossible, at least now, but is there any new techniques that can bring back the eye to the normal size?—*Tarek, Egyptian*

At the age of 8 I had an accident and am blind in my right eye since then. Now, at 33, I can't even remember how many operations I've had.

Over the years the cornea of the eye has become clouded, here and there even completely white (my left eye is dark brown). I had been wearing a tinted contact lens for quite some years, but as the eye has become more and more fragile, I had to give that up a couple of years ago. At that time I decided I would be able to live with a small, red and ugly eye. But even after all these years I hate being stared at and I wish more and more people could just deal with me like a normal person.

On Monday I got my cornea tattooed. Unfortunately, the result is not satisfactory and the only possibility left would be to have the eye taken out. As I have been suffering from a severe glaucoma for 13 years (headache, acute attacks from time to time), I wouldn't have to worry about that again, either. A tough choice as I have to decide it myself. It would definitely be easier if the eye definitely had to be taken out due to medical reasons.

Anyway, I would like to thank you for your website which has given me at least a little idea of what I had to expect if I end up losing the eye.—*Ulrike*

I so glad to see the web site you are developing. I agree whole heartily with every thing you had to say about the effects of losing an eye. At 17 years old, I lost an eye due to an automobile accident. I live a very productive, happy, successful and full life. I have worked as a nurse for thirty years, and have been able to help others threatened with the loss of an eye or other body parts. I would be happy to contribute in any way I can.—*Suzanne, RN*

Hi, Jay: Interesting website. I lost my left eye due to trauma in1985. Most of what you have said about driving, depth perception, field-of-view, etc I have found to be true also. I lost my eye removing the back door from a '58 Chevy station wagon. The steel rod that it was mounted on sprang out and hit me in the face. I don't recommend this to others. Hurt quite a bit.—*Tom*

MESSAGES

On Halloween me and a couple of my friends were trick or treating and some local jerks, 3 of them, were driving around looking for my big bro to shoot him with a paintball gun for taking a parking spot at school. Anyway, they were driving around they saw me so one of them shot a couple of shots at me with the paintball gun and one of them hit me in the top left side of my right eye, I have had 2 surgeries one of them a laser to keep my retina from detaching all the way but that just slowed it down, about 1 week later I had to get a cryogenic treatment in which the use nitrous oxide to freeze the retina in place, it's a last resort, to were they stitch the retina to the eye. Anyway I have lost my peripheral vision in the right side of my right eye almost no depth perception. I can no longer dive deep depths. I used to free dive 30 ft but now I can't even go 6 ft under water. When I fly I have to get all drugged up. Now the good news. The person that shot me is in juvenile hall and they will keep him there until they think he is ready to be a nice person. They can keep him there until he is 21. Then I am suing him and the other passengers, their car insurance, etc., BUT THAT WONT GIVE ME BACK MY VISION.—*Chris*

I am so relieved to find people who are positive about their situation. First, I found out yesterday, that I have a total detached retina, and that surgery will not help. I have some vision, but the doctor is very adamant about not regaining any vision. It was my own fault for not going back to Wills in PA. I am meeting with a surgeon on Tuesday, but I know that he is going to tell me to opt out of trying to repair it. My first detachment was successful. I have a condition called Stickler's Syndrome. I guess that I just have to accept this, but it is so hard. I know that because of this, someday, my eye is just going to have to be removed. Thanks for listening!—*CD*

If your retina has not died they might be able to reattach it. When I was shot with a paintball gun part of my retina had died instantly and then it was slowly falling off but they caught it and lasered it on then froze it on but it might be a little scary and a little painful. Sorry about you eye, CD.—*Chris*

That is terrible about what happened to you. I have been blind in one eye for 8 years now. You will get your depth perception back to some degree at least, because your brain learns to compensate. Trust me. I can anything I did before I lost my eye, except for using 3d glasses, but that is not an important part of life. I wish you the best in all you do. Me and everyone here on this board will be there to help you in any way possible. And just to mention again about the depth perception. Before I lost my eye, my depth perception was as good as it gets, and now with only one eye, I bet it is still 90 percent of what it was, and some people with two eyes don't have that good of depth perception. I know at first it is weird but it will come to you, it seems I just woke up one morning and my depth perception was great, and has been ever since. Well, I will sign off for now, let us know how things go. PS: oh yeah, a good way to get good at getting around with one eye is to get yourself some safety glasses, and go run around in the forest if you have one near, trust me, you will learn to use your one eye.—*Anon*

Wow. What an excellent idea. Put on safety glasses and run around in the forest. I've NEVER thought of it like that, but that is exactly what I did when I was a little kid. We had a magnificent forest around our house—it's a mall now—and my friends from down the street and I were ALWAYS back there, running around like maniacs.

My step-father, a man of many faults, did some excellent things after my accident to help me. They never said, "We put the basketball hoop in the driveway because we wanted you to get used to having one eye" at the time, but a few years ago, he said that was why he did it. We played a gazillion games of HORSE, and since I had an older brother, I learned to take shots to the head (!) and learning to shoot baskets in the bizarre ways kids playing HORSE do, it must have got me working on my depth perception.

Driving the Los Angeles freeways will terrify any reasonable person, and I always use my "Seattle-rain-inspired" following distance on the freeway. I've only had two auto "incidents" due to my eye situation. One was running over the backyard cyclone fence in an old Dodge van when I was 17 (and in a hurry, not paying attention to see it was only partly opened) and last semester I scraped the bumper of a colleague's mini-van. A Lexus, of course. It was a finger-nail sized scrape, and she didn't care. Whew! After I mowed down the fence, I called into work sick and tried to repair the fence—I remember sweating and grunting trying to unbend the galvanized steel posts that were bowing as if taking a curtain call. I really didn't want anyone to know, and I repaired it pretty well. That night, though, my mom asked me what happened to the fence and I burst into tears so that she thought something horrible had happened. I finally put it together that I was so upset because it actually was something that happened because of having no vision in my right eye. She said she believed me, a big thing when you're 17, because I'd never used my eye as and excuse for anything in the ten years I'd had it at that time.

You know, there is something about this gathering of "LostEye" people that really sets me to babbling! Our own "Jarrod" is having his surgery today, I think, and I'm thinking of him. Six days to go for me. Since mine is a "re-do" of my implant, I won't be dealing with all the things those who've experience enucleation recently have. I'm mainly afraid of the reason they enucleated back in the sixties—because of the chance the healthy eye will get sick. They've assured me this doesn't happen anymore because of steroids, but old fears die hard. Kind of like no matter how old you are, you can talk yourself into being afraid of what might be under the bed. I'm not as worried that they'll do something to my healthy eye, since my right eye is already prosthetic, but I think I will do the magic marker thing anyway, just to chill me out. I did that when I had "female" surgery two summers ago. I wrote on my stomach "If you give me a hysterectomy I will SUE YOUR ASS!" because I insisted that unless I had cancer, I absolutely didn't want them to take my uterus. They didn't, and the surgery residents/students who worked with my surgeon got a huge laugh out of it. Apparently I became a question on the final. I was so drugged when they came to see me, all standing around the foot of my bed, that I could have said anything.

My friend is going shopping and to lunch with me on Monday, to spoil me with some goodies for my recovery and to distract me from thinking myself into a place of abject fear. Retail therapy, baby! Love and hugs to all.—*Alicia*

Hi, Alicia! Just found this forum and I'm so grateful. I had my eye removed from an M80 hitting me in my left eye .Not good for a 15 year old to go through. Well, I had one of the best doctors. He did a great job but after all these years I think after reading about all the new technology I should look into a second surgery for maybe the orbit to help my eye move a little better. I still have to do some research. Well, thank you for sharing. I really need to have support from time to time.—*Lucia*

◆   ◆   ◆

In a racquetball accident last week I lost the sight of my dominant eye. Has anyone else had this happen? How long will it take my brain to understand that the eye that is seeing something is the one that now needs to lead? The dominant eye wants to tell me to see blank while the other one sees. I also seem to have had nerve damage that makes my face numb under the eye to the middle of my nose to the middle of my upper lip. Anyone else have this and if so did the feeling come back? Also—one more question, I was a good golfer—how much will this affect my game? Thanks—it was nice to find this site (no pun intended) and read thoughts from others.—*Orsteve*

The regional retina specialist said that the best he thinks it will get is 20/400 with correction. Right now I don't see anything. The dominant eye is the one that does most of the work on focusing for reading and under 20 feet. It is something that is more known in target shooting, pool playing, etc. The weaker eye is kind of along for the ride. This makes it confusing right now because the stronger one (OK used to be the stronger one) is telling my brain to see nothing. What this feels like is when you "space out"—you see something but you are not seeing it in a pure way. It is hard to describe. As far as patched, it is up to me. It doesn't make a lot of difference but I get some light into the eye around the outer edge and that is enough to give that eye some confidence that it is seeing what I should see. Again, hard to describe.—*Orsteve*

Orsteve, I lost vision in my right "dominant" eye 20 months ago. Prior to the loss, the vision in my right eye was perfect, while the left eye was very blurry. Within a few months, my left eye strengthened—to the point where I no longer need to wear glasses (though I do simply because I can't afford to lose my remaining eye). I also had the flashes—though I tried from day one to accept that I'd never see out of the right eye again (had a very, very slim chance of getting some vision back). It was as if my eye and brain were trying to "communicate". The flashes went away after several months.

I'm right handed, and do have a tough time shooting pool and playing darts. I'm an avid golfer—was on the course 18 hours after I lost my eyesight. Anyway, it does affect your game, but I have confidence that within a few years, I'll be back where I was. My depth perception is a little off, and my short game is worse. I don't like to look for lost balls, as changes in the terrain are hard for me. It is frustrating at times, but when I remember that I can still play the game. And now I have an excuse for a bad shot! Best of luck.—*Jesse*

◆ ◆ ◆

Hi Everyone, I am in my thirties. I lost my eye when I was very young due to an accident with a pen. I have had a prosthetic since then. This is a very neat forum.—*Scotty*

Hi—Just found this website and I think it's great. I lost my eye when our airbag deployed in an accident, when we hit a deer. This happened about 1 ½ years ago and I am still adjusting to loss of 3-D vision and very limited peripheral vision. Most troubling problem? Bumping into people on my bad side!!—*JYS*

JYS, that's a most unfortunate occurrence! Let me ask you something, I have always had the fear of such a thing happening with the air bag, I mean so fearful that I would like an air bag to be removed or switched off, cause I would rather die than lose my remaining eye! Here is the question, due you think it is common place for such an event regarding air bag deployment?, or due you think your case is unique or rare? I'm very sorry that happened to you, maybe you could file some sort of law suite?—*Jarrod*

I think my situation was very unique, and I have been told that if there hadn't been an airbag, I might not be here today. I also know that more recent car models have adjusted the force so that airbags aren't as powerful as they used to be (or so I have been told). At this point, I don't think I would want to go through the hassles of a lawsuit.—*JYS*

You know, I was very concerned about this very thing when I bought a car with airbags. I read the online-available research at the time and decided to disable the airbags in my car. There were many instances of eye loss as a direct result of airbag deployment. More than instances of death or cases of "dead if not for the airbag." I would like to read the current research.—*Alicia*

JYS I'm curious about how tall you are? I've heard that mostly women and children 5ft and below get hit with the airbag causing the eye injuries. I'm very sorry for your loss. Regards,—*Michael*

I am about 5' 6", which is pretty average—not particularly short. I have two kids, and believe me, I am going to wait until they are tall enough before they can sit in the front seat!—*JYS*

JYS wrote. Hi—Just found this website and I think it's great. I lost my eye when our airbag deployed in an accident, when we hit a deer. This happened about 1 ½ years ago and I am still adjusting to loss of 3-D vision and very limited peripheral vision. Most troubling problem? Bumping into people on my bad side!! A-men to that! I also have a hell of a time catching something that's thrown at me!—*Mike*

◆ ◆ ◆

Here's my story: Back in 2002 I was involved in a pretty scary fireworks injury. I was standing over a "mortar shell" type of firework unaware that it was loaded and lit when unfortunately it exploded. I was hit with a 2" diameter explosive from about 2 feet away and it was traveling about 40-50 mph. With my horrible luck it lined up directly with my right eye upon impact. The explosive hit me in the glasses which shattered. It left me with a 3 inch cut under my right eye, a cracked orbital socket, and my eye literally "popped".

My first surgery consisted of my eye being sewn back together and filled with nitrous oxide in an attempt to make it round again instead of flat. Second surgery was an attempt to re-attach my retina but unfortunately it has since fully re-detached. At this time they also discovered that my optic nerve was severely damaged. I also had surgery to repair my lower eyelid which turned in towards my eye (can't think of the correct terminology for the procedure). Peace.—*Mike*

Hi Mike, Thanks for posting—I'm glad you still have your eye but make sure that you get polycarbonate lenses (or at least plastic) for eye protection even if you don't need any correction in the good eye. One time recently I had something hit the lense of my eyeglasses in my good eye and thought "I'll keep my glasses on always unless I am sleeping." If you need to have your eye removed then these folks are the ones you will need.—*Jeff*

◆　　◆　　◆

I came across your website whilst looking for an eye patch and wish I had found it sooner. I lost the sight in my left eye during an accident at work in 2002. Basically, I was a truck mechanic, and whilst undoing a bolt a metal plate was released under spring pressure and went through my spectacles, cutting open my cheek and eyebrow, but most importantly, my eye was penetrated and instantly lost the sight in it. I lost my HGV driving license, so being a trained HGV mechanic I was unable to return to that line of work as I am unable to road test vehicles. I was also learning to fly at the time. I got 31 hours in my log book and had completed several solos. My flying license has been temporarily revoked and I am unsure if I am ever able to continue to gain my private pilots license.

I am left with a "phthisis bulbi" (Shrunken eye) http://www.ocularists.org/shell.htm. I have gone through many emotions and fears since the accident. Many of the symptoms I have experienced I was not warned of which caused me great anxiety, and as result, slipped into depression. I have just returned from the eye hospital where I needed to go to get my remaining eye checked. I have many questions to ask anyone who has experienced a similar fate and many experiences and advice I can offer anyone who is going through a similar experience.—*Speed-Bird*

I had an accident in 2003 which resulted in the loss of vision in my left eye. I also have had multiple reconstructive surgeries to fix my damaged orbit and surrounding bones. I did not have an enucleation, but I have still had to deal with many changes that have occurred. My ocular plastic surgeon has informed me that as soon as all my bone grafts are finished and healed (when my reconstructive surgeon gives him the OK) then I will be going to see an ocularist who will fit me with a scleral shell.(Don't think I spelled that right) Cosmetically my non-seeing eye looks hideous. It is smaller than my other eye and the color is definitely not like my right eye at all! I really hope that this will solve some of my insecurities about how I feel and look. I am really getting tired of wearing sunglasses everywhere I go. I just want to feel and look somewhat normal again. I still struggle day to day with what happened to me. Some days are definitely better than others. I honestly did not think that after all of this time I would sometimes still feel the same as I did back in 03. I have been a member on this website since 04 and this is the first time I have been able to reply to anyone on this website. Maybe there is hope for me yet! Good luck to you and remember, You Are Not Alone!—*lilcmh*

I have been coming to this site for quite a few months and I just joined so that I could reply to you. It was something about what you said that made me want to truly talk for the first time since my accident. I can relate to how you feel and I just wanted to let you know that I understand what you are going through. I had an accident in 2004 which resulted in the loss of vision in my left eye as well. I to have had multiple reconstructive surgeries to fix my damaged orbit and surrounding bones. My damaged eye is pretty terrible looking and I am also very uncomfortable with the appearance of my face and my eye. My eye has shrunk and it really just looks dead.

I really don't know what to do to resolve the issues I have with how I look and I hate having to hide all the time. I just want to feel and look like I use to look. I ask God why this had to happen to me everyday. I struggle day to day with just getting out of bed and just doing normal things like taking a shower. I lie to my family and friends and pretend that everything is ok when it really is not, just so they don't have to worry and give me pep talks.

Though I continue to improve and my family says that I look good, I know or think that they are just saying that to make me feel better. I am continuing to take one day at a time and praying that more than anything else I find the ability to accept what I will probably have to deal with and look like the rest of my life. You were very brave to finally write in and I would like to thank you for helping me to find the courage to finally write as well. I would like to wish you Good as well and to let you know that You Also Are Not Alone!—*Johnson*

I had a serious injury to my right eye when I was barely 2 years old. My dad lit an illegal firework on the 4th of July and it exploded, injuring 3 people. I got the worst of it, losing 20% of my eyelid, puncturing my iris, and catching my clothes on fire. I have a large scar cutting through my eyelid and my iris/pupil is very distorted.

It has been 29 years since this happened and I still am having a hard time accepting my eye. There have been many days I did not want to get up and live the day, especially after glancing at myself in the mirror and seeing my dead looking eye staring aimlessly! I sometimes wonder if I have that dysmorphia where all I see is an ugly monster some days instead of me. I ask the same question "why me, God?" This seems to have made me so unhappy. All I ever wanted was to have 2 pretty eyes I could wear makeup on and actually look people in the eyes. I am angry that I never had a time in my life I looked normal, and this accident was not my fault. I have never had anyone to talk to about this because how could they understand when they have never lost an eye?

Today was the 1st time I have visited this website and I found it very relieving to find others who have gone through the same thing—-But most have overcome and seem so strong, and to see so many famous historic people who have overcame is very inspirational for me—I need a change in the way I perceive myself. I think it is ridiculous that I have held on to this "complex" for so long, but when it is literally staring you in the face everyday it is hard. Even if nobody reads this, it is relieving writing this and talking about my problems in an appropriate forum. Until today I have never heard people come so close to my heart and feel the ways I have. We all have our ups and downs.—*Chandra*

Chandra while you may feel "why me", over what happened to you, imagine how your father must feel? If it were me in his position, I don't think I could handle the guilt of knowing that a moment of stupidity, cost my little girl her looks, and ½ of her eyesight for life. You WILL make it thru this. My son lost his left eye last year due to a pellet gun injury (note, I did NOT say accident). While it may be the zest of youth that is on his side, he has NEVER let his monocular vision keep him from doing the things he loves to do. Remember. It could be worse.—*John*

It is so nice to finally speak out to people who actually do understand. I have felt so much relief since I found this and have been reading the posts. I am not so crazy after all! Other people feel the same things as me! Losing an eye or eyesight is a tough thing to get through, but just knowing other people have had a tough time dealing with it too brings me relief. I know I will feel better about myself and heal, which I have doubted before. Thanks so much!—*Chandra*

Hi, Chandra, I also lost my eye as a baby (due to a tumor). I can relate to so many things that you said in your post. You said, I still am having a hard time accepting my eye. I understand this feeling. There are days that I still feel down about it. I have always hated to have my picture taken because the pictures always look so bad and I feel so embarrassed by them.

You said, All I ever wanted was to have 2 pretty eyes I could wear makeup on and actually look people in the eyes. Boy, I know this feeling. As a little girl, I used to pray to God at night that in the morning I would wake up and have two normal eyes like everyone else.

I have never had anyone to talk to about this because how could they understand when they have never lost an eye? I never talked to anyone until I was 18 and even then it was like the floodgates opened and I cried and cried while I talked to a friend about it. Even though she was sympathetic, I knew she didn't really understand since she was beautiful and had two eyes. It still helped to get it out finally. Each time I was able to discuss it, it was a little easier.

I need a change in the way I perceive myself. I think it is ridiculous that I have held on to this "complex" for so long, but when it is literally staring you in the face everyday it is hard. Yes, it is hard. My brother was born with a serious heart abnormality. I used to envy him because, at least he didn't have to wear his "defect" on his face for all to see. The truth is, my loss of an eye is minor compared to what he has been through—several heart surgeries, a major stroke from a clot that broke away from his artificial heart valve and went to his brain, years of rehabilitation and he still can't talk well, uses a cane to walk and can't work anymore. I don't even think he is still able to read even though he doesn't admit it. His shallow wife even left him saying, "he's not the man I married." So, I have seen the reality that not being what the world calls "perfect" and "normal" for me is certainly better than a lot of other things. And, even though God didn't "fix" my left eye, He still gave me my right one and a beautiful world to see with it so I am thanking Him for that.

Until today I have never heard people come so close to my heart and feel the ways I have. Yes, I just found this forum myself and it is literally the FIRST time I have been able to communicate with people who are in this same one eye boat with me (and I am 48 years old!) I have never actually spoken face to face with anyone else who gets it!

We all have our ups and downs. Yes, they are part of life. Sometimes I think that having this thing to deal with has made me a better person than I would have been otherwise. Maybe I would have been the kind of woman like my X-sister-in-law who couldn't love an "imperfect" man. Maybe I would have been all hung up on myself for being beautiful and missed the really important things in life. My eye has also been a really good instrument to filter out the people in my life who would be so superficial as to not like me because of it. The people who love and accept me anyway are the people worth knowing in the first place.

And about how we see ourselves—we have to see our total selves, not just our eye. We are beautiful in so many ways that matter more than some physical part of our body. I knew a women once that had all the looks of a gorgeous model. She was striking and heads turned to look at her when she walked down the street. But when she opened her mouth, she would spew out the most hateful angry filth you can imagine. She also drank a lot and smoked. (sorry to those of you who smoke. I pray that you will be able to quit.) After I got to see this side of her, she no longer looked beautiful to me. It was so odd how it seemed her appearance actually changed because of her behavior. And, remember this, physical beauty does not last very long. If we live long enough, we will get old and wrinkled and saggy.

So Chandra, I am glad we both found this forum. Please allow yourself to feel what you feel when you get sad. (My Grandma always said "Crying washes your brain.") But try to see the bigger picture. You are so much more than just an eye! Whatever you look like on the outside, (and that is probably a lot better than you think), it is really the person you are on the inside that counts. Love to All!—*Mini*

Mini, thank you so much for your personal reply to my post. Everything is so right with what you have said and I am glad you can benefit from my expressions in this forum as I have benefited from so many others postings of personal feelings. It has brought so much healing to my mental state—I realize I have a right to feel the way I do, but I can not let it diminish my life in any way what so ever. I love reading old posts and one I have really taken to heart is the one where someone wrote about how children can not help but to notice and make comments about our differences, but when adults choose to purposely hurt us because of our personal tragedies—well it was something to the effect of "to heck with those selfish people, it's not me that is horrible, it is them". It is so true. I too believe I am a better person than who I could have been had my injury never happened. Everything happens for a reason and I trust in God. I will say it again—it is nice to talk to people who can truly understand what I am going through. I don't think my mother or father even fully understands how painful certain events have been for me. Thanks again for all the support,—*Chandra*

◆ ◆ ◆

I lost sight in my right eye when I was 2 years old, due to an accident. My parents decided on no surgery hoping that in the future something could be done. When I was 10 I developed severe headaches, I'm told because of high pressure in the injured eye, so it was removed. I live a really normal life, I have never really been hinder with having vision in one eye only. I'm glad to find this site, I never really talked with other people with the same condition.—*Patrick*

I am interested to know if your headaches went after having your eye removed. I also have high pressure in my eye and suffer from headaches but have always been told it was migraine and nothing to do with my eye. Welcome to the board by the way.—*Penny*

Hey there, everyone! Like Patrick, I'm also new to posting here, but I've been reading the boards for a couple of years. I've had problems with both of my eyes since I was born. Nearsightedness, astigmatism, displaced lens, lazy eye. My right eye was far worse that the left (I was legally blind in it) and when I was fifteen I had a retinal detachment from a volleyball accident. My doctors didn't repair the detachment because I wouldn't have viable sight anyway. The detachment left me with a disfigured eye (my left is blue, my right turned black then yellowish), pressure issues, terrible migraine-like headaches for two years and tolerable headaches from then on.

When I was eighteen, I had the first of six laser surgeries to my left eye to prevent impending detachments there. I've also recently been told that my soft contact lens was not letting in enough oxygen to my cornea (I wear a-17.00) and had to switch to RPG hard lenses. I'm finding them difficult to wear and am tempted to go back to the soft ones. Has anyone had any experiences with RPG lenses?

Sorry. Back from my tangent. After ten years of dreadful headaches and a year of feeling like there was crushed glass in my right eye (calcium deposits, as it was), with the encouragement from reading this site, I had my right eye removed in 2004. The fitting of my prosthesis was successful and I haven't had too many issues with it.

Penny, I just wanted you to know that my headaches disappeared after the surgery. I woke up from the anesthesia and the first thing I was aware of was that my eye/head didn't hurt anymore. Well, it ached from the surgery, but I could tell the difference. I haven't had the headaches since!

I know this is long, but I also wanted to thank all of you who have been sharing your stories! It's been a big help to me before and after my surgery!—*Adeline*

Patrick, I'm not TOO far from you—I live in New York. I, too, am curious to hear if your headaches are cured now! I've had headaches since the day of my accident (shot in the eye with a bb gun). The bb is lodged permanently near my brain and it's inoperable, so I have to endure the pain daily. It's worse when it's more humid out and the atmospheric pressure is great. I also get migraines often enough too!!—*Chris*

Chris. I know how you feel. My injury was past the eye socket. I had internal bleeding inside my brain. It was pretty scary. I too suffer from migraines.—*Michael*

Are you on any headache preventive meds? What are you on when you get a migraine?? (I should start a new thread about meds!). I'm on Nortriptyline to prevent headaches, although it doesn't work anymore!! I'm on Maxalt for migraines, which usually works, but I can only get 9 pills a month and sometimes I have more migraines than pills!—*Chris*

I still get bad headaches, but not like the pain I remember from that time. I don't think the headaches I get now are from my eye. But I don't really know. I'm not good about regular visits to doctors.—*Patrick*

Welcome, Patrick, I am also new to the postings here. I was diagnosed with high eye pressure 2 years ago and was put on eye drops. Last year I was diagnosed with high blood pressure and now taking daily medication. I went back to my eye doctor and now I don't have high eye pressure. I'm just wondering if the 2 could possibly be linked. I used to take pain meds for migraine headaches, but I found out that taking the pills only triggered more headaches when the pill wore off. So I stop taking them. Since then I just take Excedrin Migraine when I feel a headache coming on. This has just been my experience and it works for me. May not for you. Anyway, nice to meet you.—*Brenda*

Chris, I am been prescribed Vicodin for the pain. I not only have the headaches, but muscle pain in the temple on my blind side.—*Michael*

Thanks Michael. Thirty years ago doctors only advised you to take aspirin for pain. Only recently did I go to a neurologist and got put on Rx's. I don't think that my doctors would give me anything stronger than the Nortriptyline and Maxalt, although there are many times where I know I could benefit from them! Maybe I'll mention it to them! Thanks.—*Chris*

Chris, there is a lower dosage Vicodin that they can prescribe. Even the smallest dose can make the pain subside. Sometimes the higher dose Vicodin will keep you from sleeping. I found that out real quick.—*Michael*

Thanks Michael! I'm writing it down and I'll bring it with me ASAP! I also wrote down info about Topamax. I've heard good things (and also bad!) about that Rx too, although it's used to stave off headaches daily. I'll see what the doctor has to say! Thanks again!—*Chris*

◆ ◆ ◆

Hi! My name is Anthony. About 6 years ago a devastating accident happened to my cousin" at just 7 years old at the time. We were camping out in the forest, for the night, just having an awesome time with our families, and just living life. Until late that night when me and my cousin went to sleep and while we were sleeping a tick came up and went into his eye and ate his eye out. Sadly we rushed him to the hospital and the doctors examined him but there was nothing that they could do for him. So till' today he's 14 now, and he still has no eye site in his left eye due to the accident.

But he's a really great cousin and full of life! He was telling me things about his eye site about how he said that his Eye muscles take over his eye coordination but he told me it doesn't bother him and that he still feels like he still has his normal vision. But. He told me the other day that he could not wait till he got his license and I was just wondering if you guys could answer a question for me "Will they let him get his license"? (live in California). Well thanks for listening to my story! All comments appreciated. Do you guys think that in the near future that their will be a cure or something to bring back your eye site in the blind eye so you would have 2 eyes again?—*Anthony*

I am blind in one eye and grew up in California. I was worried when I went to the DMV, but they gave me no problems. As long as you see good in one eye, you can drive (I heard not big rigs or buses though?) I came across this same info earlier today on the web. Good luck!—*Chandra*

◆ ◆ ◆

Getting rid of the gross red eye is the first step. Last summer I was mowing my grass when my lawn mower shot a rock out of the bottom and crushed my entire left eye. They tried putting it back together with a total of 21 stitches and three surgeries. Three months later they decided to take my nasty red eye out. In place they gave me a coral implant and a oval prosthetic to go over top. Thank god, big relief to finally get rid of the pain of a foul eye, but the week after you get your eye out will be the most painful time in your life(not kidding). But don't let that get you down because the advantages far out weigh the disadvantages. With the prosthetic, people hardly notice the fake eye unless I say something. With the new technology available today, having a prosthetic isn't that bad. Mine actually moves with my good eye. I always hated when I met someone new, how the only time they made eye contact was when they were staring at my left eye. After awhile you get used to it because it is just instinct to be thrown off by messed up eyes, I know I was before my accident. All of my friends have been real supportive and that helps. Friends and family will be the most important things to you during this horrible process. I may never get used to it but being bitter isn't going to grow me a new eye, things can always get worse.—*Willy*

Hi, I felt I had to post to you. I just had my eye removed, I took Vicodin for four days, the pain was okay if I watched myself. It wasn't bad, I had my spleen out years ago, that was way worse!!! If you need to talk email me.—*Mary*

I had a red, ugly, achey eye before due to a failed retinal detachment surgery in the 6th grade. I've had an evisceration done recently and my eye feels great. Unlike an enucleation (where the whole eye is removed), the evisceration procedure leaves the outside of the eye and only the inner contents are removed. I now wear a scleral shell that has great mobility and very natural.

◆ ◆ ◆

Hey Everybody. I am 16 years old and I lost my eye in a power tool accident. It was October of last year. I just got my artificial eye today. It is nice. The lady did a great job on it. If anybody has any tips to prevent something or such. I would be happy to get some hints or help from anybody. I never really had a chance to cope with it. I had to be strong for my mom and never got a chance to let my feelings out, if you know what I mean. Well, thanks!—*Pim*

I was a little younger than you when I had my accident. Are you a guy or girl? I'm 43 and a woman, and going through that was pretty tough on a young girl. I know what you mean about being strong for your mother (or parents). I didn't think twice about such things until recently, so it's good that you're somewhat in touch with your feelings.

My advice is to talk things out with someone if you're bothered by anything regarding the loss of your eye. It's a lot for a 16 (or 15) year old to deal with on their own, and you may be more comfortable talking to someone other than your parents. I'd also suggest that you read all you can, here and elsewhere. You'll get a lot of good suggestions. Keep well and let us know how you're doing!—*Chris*

I have been talking to a counselor-psychologist since it happened. Things are good. I've coped, and I think I got it taken care of for the most part. I mean I have talked to so many people about it. And it is really weird to think just how many people do have prosthesis. I didn't know how many people had them until I hurt my eye. The people started coming out of the wood works. "I am blind in one of my eyes too" they say. It just surprised me, because I never really noticed. And these are people that I am around all the time. It just never occurred to me.—*Pim*

Wow! I'm really glad that you talked to a counselor and that you now know people who have a prosthesis! That's great! The only one person I knew (other than myself) was the boy who shot me. I haven't met anyone else since then who has had a prosthesis, except for the people I meet when I go to the ocularist! Anyway, stay well, and keep posting!—*Chris*

I'm already liking this site A LOT. To answer your question, I am a male. I forgot to answer it in my last reply. Its hard for younger people to deal with the lost of an extremity, but I've always been around older people so in my short time of being alive. I have become more mature than a lot of my peers, and I do believe that this has made me even stronger as a person. I've had many people I can talk to, like my counselor. My mom and i have always been close, so I can pretty much talk to her about anything. I've also got a girlfriend that I can talk to whenever I need to. She has been a tremendous help to me over the past 3 months, and probably will be for a long time. My prosthesis is settling in now. It is starting to look a lot better in my eye. The day I got it, It was pushing my eye lids out a lot. I went to lunch right after my appt. and everybody was staring, but it didn't bother me. Thanks for talking to me. See ya!—*Pim*

◆ ◆ ◆

Hi all, first of all, let me say that I am SO HAPPY to have found this site. Thank you! I'm 35, an American working overseas. Long story short, I'm one of those walking LASIK disasters you might have heard about. I had LASIK in September, 2002, that left me with a severely scarred cornea and very painful dry eye. PRK in June, 2004, removed some of the scarring but made the dry eye worse. I can see with my left eye. sort of. the quality of my vision is terrible and doctors can't figure out a lens prescription for it due to the scarring and astigmatism. My nearsighted, not operated upon right eye is corrected with glasses, no problem there, but the difference in vision between my eyes gives me headache and eye strain.

The last resort at this point is a lamellar cornea transplant, and I'm willing to try it BUT, that may actually make the difference in vision between my eyes worse. If the transplant works perfectly, I might have -5.0 or better in the left eye and -9.75 in the right. So the headaches, dizziness, and eye strain could get even worse if a transplant is successful. And I hear that the pain of dry eye (which sounds like nothing until you've had it, as many of you probably know) could get worse and certainly won't get better.

There's also a cosmetic issue in that I'm horribly photophobic now (even bright white walls are hard to look at) and I spend a lot of time wincing, not meeting people's eyes, etc. From what I understand, I'd look less "in pain or drunk" with an artificial eye than with my injured biological eye. Again, I'm willing to try the cornea transplant. But I'm also eager for feedback. One of my fears is that I'll get the transplant, it will technically be a wonderful success, my quality of life will plummet, and I won't be able to find a doctor to take me seriously when I say "Please take this out!" It's not like I'm in constant terrible agony, but the constant discomfort is really wearing on me. So, that's me. Any recommendations or advice will be most heartily appreciated. Looking forward to meeting everyone,—*Ya'ara*

Hi all, so, in reading through some of the threads, it sounds like "dry eye" is a problem even when the eye itself isn't there any more.—sigh—I'd been entertaining fantasies of NEVER HAVING A PAINFULLY DRY EYE AGAIN.—*Ya'ara*

Hi there, well all I can say is enucleation is not an easy decision. It took me years to finally agree to have my painful blind eye out. Having a prosthetic is not a whole lot of fun either. I wear mine only 1/2 the time as it is a pain in the butt. But then my situation is not the norm. Lots of people have no problems with their prosthetic. Make the decision that is right for you and know that there are a lot of us to support you through. I couldn't have gotten through my surgery and all the crud afterwards if not for everyone here (my surgery was in Jan of this year). All the best to you,—*Starr*

Ya'ara, I'm sorry to hear of the problems you've been having, it sounds like LASIK wasn't the best choice! But I guess that its one of those things you do and think "it'll never happen to me". I'm really sorry that you had to be "the one"!

Anyway, I'm also contemplating enucleation of my blind eye at the minute, but for different reasons to you. I know what the pain of dry eye is, and to be honest I don't think the dry eye pain associated with corneal disease and the dry discomfort that occurs with a prosthesis are anywhere near the same. And, where artificial tears may not work so well for a real eye, if you keep your prosthesis well lubricated and have some tears naturelle on standby then you should be fine.

Its a HUGE decision to make, and one that you should not rush into. I know the argument of your Dr may be to get the corneal graft done and THEN decide, but to be honest its become apparent to me that with eyes, when the Dr says a possible outcome to you. It more than likely going to happen! Therefore I think you really need to talk this over with you Ophthalmologist and see what they say.

But remember that once your through the adjustment period after the enucleation, and you've been fitted with your prosthesis, life should pretty much get back to the preLASIK era (just watch out for door frames. especially when you've had a few pints! lol) and after all, that's what you want! Feel free to ask as much as you want, and do keep us posted.—*Elizabeth*

Hi Ya'ara, you might try an eye patch on your bad vision eye just to see how much that affects the other eye. I would only do that on a temporary basis. I have 4/200 vision in an eye that had cancer removed and I patch that eye because of the distortion. Wal-Mart has inexpensive patches, I got a really nice one from Lenfante.com, it is made out of ultra suede. My eye is real and looks normal but I have to patch it to try to cut down on distortions in the other eye. Best wishes,—*Barry*

I agree with the suggestion to patch the bad eye and see if that improves your quality of life any. That way, if you decide to go the enucleation route, you will know more of what you're getting into and what kind of effect it will have.

It's a big decision to make. Honestly, if I'd had sight in my left eye, I'm not sure I could have done the surgery. Even if it were bad, I don't think I'd want to give it up, but then, I've always had monocular vision, so I'm a little jealous of those who have two eyes to begin with.

Some people have all kids of problems with their prosthesis, poor fit, dry eyes, no movement, etc. Personally, I've not had any. I had some dryness right after the surgery, and then even a little too much watering for a few months after that, but now, and for many years, things have been normal and great. The eye stays in my socket and only comes out once a year for its annual polishing, and everything is fine.

I'm going for a new prosthesis on Thursday, because this one is 10yrs old and doesn't fit properly anymore. Hopefully, it will go smoothly as well.—*Kelli*

Thank you all so much for your replies. I feel a bit more centered reading what you have to say. I have trouble wearing a patch because I also wear glasses (I seem to be contact lens intolerant my vision gets too cloudy to function). I hear that one option would be a dark/opaque contact lens, the sort of thing used by kids with amblyopia who don't like patches, but darned if I know where to find one here. (I live in Romania.)

I'm curious to know what effect my bad eye has on my good eye. Apparently sometimes the good eye becomes stronger to compensate and sometimes it deteriorates out of sympathy or something? Boy, if my right eye is getting worse because my left one's shot, I'll be mad. Anyway, I'll be in the States in July for a conference, and will see a specialist then. Until then, I guess I'll just keep reading here and hoping for insight. Thanks again,—*Ya'ara*

Ya'ara, the only time your bad eye will effect your good eye is in the case of Sympathetic Ophthalmia. This is a condition which occurs when, usually after trauma, the Uveal Tissue of your damaged eye has been "annoyed" (very scientific I know, but you get my drift! lol) and then the good eye will react out of "sympathy", usually by presenting with Uveitis. This is a serious condition, and requires enucleation of the damaged eye, to save the sight of the good eye.

Contrary to popular believe your seeing eye cannot get "Overstrained" due to just using it, and therefore any prescription changes in that eye are said not to be due to the loss of the fellow eye.

As regards patching whilst wearing glasses, have you thought about just blanking out the lens on your bad side? Examples of some stuff that has worked for different people I know include: Clear Nail Varnish, Frosted Glass, and also (less expensive than a proper frosted lens) the frosted paper that you can get from art and craft shops. Cut it to fit the lens of your glasses.

These are just things I know other people have used. I'm not sure If I'd be happy with any of them on my specs, but I know when my double vision was at its worst, I was happy to try anything! Hope that helped,—*Elizabeth*

PART V
COPING

16

Introduction to Coping

Those having sight in only eye will usually live 99% of their lives like everybody else. But there are, of course, certain special issues that must be coped with such as the loss of some depth perception. These issues include job-related concerns, sports and related activities, driving, and others.

LETTERS AND E-MAILS

Hi, my name is Andrew and I lost my eye last November from an air pistol wound. I asked the paramedic if I would ever see again from my right eye and he said "it is very unlikely." This memory will never fade, I was actually in a very bad way, the pellet had split my eye ball in half, I don't know how I done it but I stayed conscious through out it all. I wasn't upset that I would never see again, I was upset because it ruined my career. All my life I dreamed of becoming a soldier, to serve my country and to make my family proud. I had been in 2 training courses firstly with the Royal Anglicans and then with the Royal Marine Commando's. I thought my life was set. As I sat on my hospital bed it was like a dream, I was covered in blood and had no pain killers for about half an hour now. I could see the worried faces but all I could do was sit up in my bed looking around. Finally they gave me morphine and as it just started to take effect I saw my family come through the door and my mums face drop and the tears well up in her eyes. I told them not to worry and that I would be fine but she was taken away by a doctor who I later found out was telling her that I may not survive through the operation as the pellet was in a very dangerous place, I knew this anyway, I don't know how but I knew my chances were slim.

But I managed to survive somehow and I am still walking around with the pellet in my head, I have had five operations to try and make my eye "presentable" but so far no luck. But at the end of the day I have added another chapter in my book, I survived and have not looked back even 1 day. I'm not sure why I am writing this, I think it is just my story to say to others who have lost an eye that there is light, there is hope, don't look back on what could have been, look forward and never give up on life. Because of this I have decided I want a career in helping people, I don't know exactly how but this is a step. I hope that I have inspired you even a little bit to look forward to a good future.—*Andrew*

My husband fell from a ladder two weeks ago and has undergone 2 operations. He had a ruptured globe and a detached retina. He is having a difficult time using only one eye. He gets sick to his stomach trying to watch TV. I find he is spending most of his time in bed. The surgeon at Bascum-Palmer tells us that everything looks good but they cannot tell us if he will ever regain sight. Does anyone have any suggestions as to how he can overcome the problem of getting "seasick" from using one eye to see? Does this usually go away and, if so, how long does it take?—*Pat*

I'm very glad you have had so little problem adjusting to the loss of your eye. It has not been as easy for me. Sammy Davis may have done it in two weeks, but for me it's been five very difficult weeks. I am not a complainer, rather I figure that as this is what I have to live with for the rest of my life, I'll just get on with it. Even a number of greeting cards I received had hand-written notes saying, in effect, that if anyone can adapt to this, I'll be able to do it in fine fashion. But it is the most difficult challenge I have ever encountered.

One reason is that where I live (Ohio), no one, not doctors, rehab or therapy facilities, has any idea how to guide a person through the adjustment process. If I were blind, they would put braille labels throughout my home and teach me to walk with a white cane, but since I still have vision in the other eye, they don't have a thing to offer. They all said, "You'll get used to it eventually." Finally, a nurse at a retina specialist's office suggested an optical practice that works with vision training. I had a consultation today and learned a lot of techniques that will be helpful, not only to "do" better, but also to help keep me safe. She also said to expect the process to take about a year. The lady could empathize with me as she also has lost an eye. She thinks she may be the only one in the state who does what she does. She also said that several doctors, including that specialist, refer patients to their practice, even though he had told me earlier nothing was available.

Even living with my husband's loss of one eye 45 years ago did not begin to prepare me for my own loss. His was gradual (over a year or two), while mine was sudden. I watched him struggle to cope and regain skills, but he says you never get good depth perception back. As a farmer he has learned to back a truck or wagon into a barn, keep the combine on the row, and changed his "shooting eye" and can still hit a varmint ground hog from 50 yards. But it has not been easy for him, either.

So the bottom line is. speak for yourself, but be careful about being too optimistic where other people's situation may not work out as quickly or easily as your own. They might get discouraged if it doesn't go as well for them. Thanks for the web site. I'll check it for new information every once in a while.—*Anon*

Jay, we have communicated previously about the loss of an eye and I am wondering if you have experienced a loss of balance, especially after a couple of glasses of wine. I have experienced this phenomenon and it truly worries me. Your response would be greatly appreciated. Thanks much,—*Bob*

I was shot on August 18th and I was shot in the face at close range and I lost my right eye during the process. The doctors said that if I haven't been wearing my glasses I wouldn't be here today. I am also living proof that living with one eye can be hard at times when you can't find work in your home town, or get any help from your state.—*Connie*

I lost sight in my right eye about nine months ago (temporal arthritis). Now I am experiencing awful side effects. Perception and balance is not good. I cannot walk without the aid of a walker and just standing alone without holding on to a counter top is inviting a possible fall. I can no longer drive the car or leave the house unassisted. Can you offer any advice or encouragement for my situation and will I ever be able to cope to a somewhat normal degree again? Very truly yours,—*John*

Nice site, Jay. I went through enucleation surgery about five years ago. I'm amazed at your words. How you function, that is. I can't say that I have had any complications but I find the whole damn thing terribly annoying. The depth-perception issue is probably the worst handicap for me. I'm always knocking stuff over! Anyway, thanks for the site.—*John*

Hey, I'm glad u made this website, Because like you I lost my to, but not to cancer. I'm 19yrs old and lost vision in my eye due to an accident. My left eye is still physically there but instead of being hazel its completely blue with scars all around. Luckily my right eye is ok. I wish to learn ways you have coped with one eye. I'm young and want to be famous. I have lots of musical talent and a great mind, but I am having lots of trouble getting my confidence back since the accident. Thanks again,—*Zubair*

Hey, my brother lost the sight in one eye shortly after birth and the eye cannot be repaired now due to improper development of the optic nerve. However, from childhood he has played a variety of fast-paced sports and found his niche in tennis. He won the Southeast Regional championship in his division a few years ago.

Now at 31, he's trying his hand at coaching. Do you know of any other one-eyed tennis players? Is he as amazing as I think he is? Do you know anyone studying such a phenomenon? Thanks,—*Ruth*

Thank you so much for writing what you have on people losing their eye. It has helped me on both a learning stand point, and in some ways, an emotional stand point. I recently lost my eye, only 2 months ago. I was diagnosed with a mass in the back of my left eye. This mass turned out to be an infection which we found out to be a very rare bacteria that has only been seen a handful of times before. This being true, it has been very hard to accept the loss of my eye, in regards of this only being seen a handful of times before. I have had to accept that I am now part of the handful that has only been seen a few times. This has not been easy. Although it has only been two months now since the loss, I think I am adjusting fairly well. I have seen it written many times in my research of people who've lost an eye, that "life will not change all the much" and have been very happy to see that this statement is pretty true. I was not ready for the changes that did happen, but have adjusted to them fairly well I think. I was also glad to see that the changes are not all that many. Unfortunately I have not gotten behind the wheel quite yet. I was one of the very few, according to my doctors, that have continued pain after the eye is removed. This was a problem in getting back on my feet and back to a normal life. But thankfully the pain is going away and is less every day. This has allowed me to get back now to a somewhat normal life and one that I'm sure will get more normal every day.

Again, thank you for your writing, especially for the information on the fitting of a new eye. This information was some of the best I had seen in all my research. I have done research on the loss of an eye virutally ever since I found out I would lose my eye completely. Thank you for all you've done. Keep the good work. I am hoping to someday be added to your list of celebrities who have "made it" inspite of the loss. I am living in Los Angeles now and maybe with a little luck I'll make your list someday. Sincerely,—*Michael*

MESSAGE THREADS

I've been to Canada in the winter, and, it was beyond FREEZING (I took my fur coat to wear!), yet the air wasn't as dry as in New York. How do you deal with the cold in your eye? I wear glasses, so I have somewhat of a layer of protection, but I find that my eye gets so dry due to being out in the cold and wind. I've just been laying off the eye makeup, and dousing myself with eye irrigant. Any other suggestions?—*Chris*

Actually there is nothing you really can do. Here in Manitoba it is the coldest across Canada as far as the Provinces go and also gets the warmest here in Summer. I have tried drops and even an eye patch on our really cold days. But someone made me and interesting eye protector. Basically it is like a band that goes around my head that protects my ears but has a flap on the left side that covers my eye! It works great, I get some strange looks but on the high wind-chill days I could care less what people think. I get such a huge headache from the cold hitting my eye and when temperatures are so bad exposed skin freezes in a minute you really have to be careful!!—*Ski*

◆ ◆ ◆

Hi everyone it is 2 years since I lost my eye to cancer and I feel as if I am coping worse now than when it first happened. I am so nervous when I go out (NEVER ON MY OWN I MAY ADD) that I have recently got myself a white cane to carry around so other people know there is something wrong with my sight. I have started bumping into things and tripping up curbs and steps are a real nightmare now. I was wondering if this happened to anyone else and how did you get over it as I feel I am not coping very well at all,—*Anne*

Anne, sorry to hear that! How's the site in your "good" eye? It's important that we keep on getting checkups to make sure that our "good" eye is healthy. If it is, then I'm sure you're just feeling very nervous about only having sight in one eye right now. I think that we all go through that "scare" period, when in sinks in that we're only seeing from one eye. I, myself, never walked with a cane, but I know I'm pretty careful about some things (walking around in the dark, driving to some places, etc.). I think that some of us DO have some limitations due to having monocular vision, but we're all individual that way.

I'd just make sure that your remaining vision is in tact, and if you NEED to walk with a cane, and if you need to be more careful right now, then so be it. You went through a big loss, and it's bound to affect you at some point. But, you'll be okay. Lots of us can only see out of one eye, and we're functioning just fine! Stay strong!—*Chris*

Hi Anne, I suppose I'm more fortunate than you in that I lost my eye at age 8 so had a better to chance to adjust but I don't think you should feel you need a white stick.

I think there was someone called Brady who wrote a book called "a singular view" about such things as depth perception. I was never told anything about monocular vision and wondered why I could not play tennis in secondary school.

But walking around should be OK. Are you worried about bumping into people? I think sometimes people will just think you're clumsy. But so what? I don't know what the learning curve is for adults losing an eye but I would hope you must be through the worst. Don't let it get you down.—*Chil*

◆ ◆ ◆

This is the third message I post within three days, and I think it's about time I explain why I'm here. First of all, let me apologize for my English grammar. I'm 21 and I'm a student. I was born with my left eye almost blind (family thing and it also seems that I had a hemorrhage in my optical nerve). I had surgery very young, but it went wrong and didn't help at all. I had my eye patched after that, for what it had seemed to be ages, but for probably only a few months. The patching was supposed to help the lazy eye and also straighten my eye, which was turning outward. It didn't improve my vision of course, and that was the last attempt. My eye now looks pretty straight and I'm so use to live with one good eye that I don't even mention it.

But recently, I had trouble to get a driver license (see post below in this forum). After two attempts, I had to back up, at least until I find a solution. Since law in my country theoretically allows monocular drivers to get a license, it's more prejudgments that I'll have to fight. And that totally killed my confidence. Suddenly, at 20, I realize that having one eye wasn't a normal thing, at least for most people. I felt the need to talk about it, something that I've never done before. Hence some research on the Internet, and here I am. I started to worry about it, and I don't want to lose this confidence.

I've been learning Chinese for 10 years, went backpacking everywhere in the world, all Central and South America, China, New Zealand, Australia, I work, draw, speak 5 languages, well I think I prove to myself that I could do anything I wanted. But I don't want to spend my life proving other people. During the time my eye was patched, I was basically blind. As I'm a book addict, I had to find a way to be able to read again, so I learned Braille (great way to cheat in classes after all!). Of course, I never reached a high stage in this reading method (I believe it takes years), but I had made me feel good at the time. When a teenager, I had quite a lot of blind friends that I had met during my Braille reading attempt. At the time I found it perfectly normal, looking back I guess I was looking for something. But we had a great time together. Of course, each of my friends had his way to live with this, but I learned a lot. We were doing anything we wanted to, going to the movies, swimming pool, playing board games. People were never mean to them but ignorant most of time.

I've tried to mix my friends many times, building a bridge between the two world I believed I belong to, between blindness and perfect vision, but it was harder than it seemed. But I like to remember that those guys were wonderful, and certainly not "disabled". Just different. I think, thanks to them, that I never feared blindness. Saying that I would be comfortable with it is too much, but I remember how we can adapt. I saw myself as someone "normal" for all those years and suddenly, by being denied a driver license, I doubt again. I'm also scared that my eye is turning outward again, as it happens more and more, and not only when I'm tired. Well, at least I'm glad that for the first time in my life I can actually share my fears instead of hiding them. I took some time to read the posts on this board, and I know we are all in different situations, but we're all fighting for the same thing.—*Zhu*

Interesting post. Thanks for sharing! I have to say that when I first came here, some things were hard to absorb. Just reading about people with one eye was tough, and realizing that my case was pretty bad was hard for me to accept.

What I STILL don't accept is that there is always the possibility for us with monocular vision to go blind. Guess I NEVER think of that! I'm careless too often (don't wear my glasses). I've had close calls over STUPID things (had bleach splash up in my "good" eye; had a wire hanger fall very close to my eye; got hit with baseballs and all types of balls in my good eye; had my children accidentally hit my good eye, as well as my bad eye.). Anyway, we all should be very careful and have respect for our only remaining vision. Your post was a reminder of that for me, so, thanks!—*Chris*

◆ ◆ ◆

Hi folks, I was surfing for information about eye infections and found an article on monocular vision (it is unrelated to infections). I am amazed at how those of us with "one eye" are portrayed by this article. It's like we can't do much independently and have real trouble with everything from crossing the street to threading a needle. I know everyone takes time to adjust, but from reading parts of this you'd think we were clumsy all the time! There are other parts that are interesting, but on the whole I think it is really misleading! Have a read and share your views. Love n Hugs,—*Elizabeth*

I read this article till the point where disgust overcame me, maybe about half of it! I think it is the biggest bunch of Malarkey to ever be written! I would like to email them and tell them the truth! I'm sick of stereotypes! People with only one eye can do this, and not this. And not just that scenario! I'm sick of every stereotype! Is it false that people with one eye have decreased peripheral vision. Absolutely not! But it's not that much! I don't have to jerk my head back and forth to judge distance! I don't need special mirrors! I can drive just as good as anybody with two eyes, and by Hell, if I want to pilot an aircraft, get out of my way, cause I can learn how and accomplish the task just as good as if not better than Ten eyed Bob! I can thread a needle, and drive through Chicago traffic, I past my drivers test with no practice., I can see every color in an rainbow, I can tell you the distance between any amount of cars at any distance as good as anyone! They can kiss my friendly neighborhood ass! All their little article is going to so is just discourage someone who is about to loose and eye, or has just lost one! Someone should give them a lesson in accuracy! Please excuse any foul language, that's my personality, and if anyone was offended, I offer my deepest and most sincere apologies.—*Jarrod*

Oh dear, I found this article quite informative and totally non offensive. I didn't feel there were any stereotypes about people who only have sight in the one eye and I didn't think it called us useless. I think it raises several points that are true.

There IS a slight reduction of peripheral vision and we DO have depth perception issues which can cause us to bump into things (hence being seen as clumsy lol) and can cause us not to perform well in certain sports (tennis is bad for me). As for driving while do-able it can pose difficulties for some people (I'm always further over to the left due to my field of vision).

I'd also like to say while it does say that we have difficulties with these tasks it DOESN'T say that we can't do them and DOESN'T undermine us as individuals.

One quick note to Jarrod, I think that it is better to be realistic, with people who are going to lose sight in an eye or have just lost sight in an eye, and inform them of the problems they may face. I don't think it would upset or discourage and it does say that within a year most patients do adjust to changes in sight. I think if anything they should be prepared for what they may face.

Would like to get others input on this. It doesn't matter how you feel on the inside, it's what shows up on the surface that counts. Take all your feelings and push them down. Then you'll fit it, be invited to parties and boys will like you. Then happiness will follow.—*Traci*

Dealing with the depth perception was kind of rough at the beginning. Pouring too much oil into pans. Trouble seeing things real close. Bumping into people on my blind side. As with anything you adjust. I did for 5 years driving $250,000 pieces of heavy equipment. I did it so well my employer told me I don't consider you handicapped". One fellow employee told the boss "I'd rather have Tommy loading dump trucks with one eye than anyone else with two". I was not going to let the loss slow me down. The guy who wrote that letter doesn't know the will of a survivor expecting more from themselves!—*Tommy*

For myself, depth perception is great! Like Alicia said, I cannot watch a 3-D movie in full effect, but I can see those 3-D images in the newspapers! The ones you have to stare at for a while to see.—*Jarrod*

I agree with some of the points, and although depth perception is something you do adjust to with time I'm sure there are those of you like me, when you are tired or upset or whatever, doorways and busy crowds etc etc can be really bothersome! But I have to say, I think there are some points which are really out of town, (the bit about on average monocular drivers have 7 times more accidents than others!) and if the contributors had monocular vision themselves, or lived full time with someone who did they're attitudes may be different. Its great to see so many reactions to this, I didn't really think anyone would take much notice! Love n Hugs to y'all,—*Elizabeth*

Having lost my eye in an accident at age 8, nobody told me or my parents of the implications of monocular vision. Playing compulsory tennis in senior school the games teacher accused me of not even trying because I could only hit the ball about one time out of ten. I found it really hard to thread a needle and still do.

I think the most disabling thing would be if one couldn't drive and the only affect it has on my driving is that I turn the radio off driving around big roundabouts or navigating strange city centers. Oh and my parallel parking is rubbish and I don't trust myself to judge the speed of oncoming vehicles so I have to leave a bigger gap. I think it's useful to be able to read the research but then get on with life, as all of us have done.—*Chil*

◆　　◆　　◆

Hey guys, thought I'd just let you all now. I am going to be in a magazine called "best magazine" which we have over here in the UK. I shall be featuring in an article about my eye. The whole basic idea of the piece is women who have things wrong physically with them but still feel beautiful (which I do, coz I am :p). If just ONE person picks it up and feels better about themself then I would feel so great. This is a real big step for me because I'm basically saying to 1 million readers across the UK, this is me, this is what I look like and I love myself. Hope you are all ok—*Traci*

Thanks for the kind words guys. I will have to set up some web space somewhere so when the article is printed you can all have a look (Yay, you'll all get to see how I look) I am going to mention this site in my article and how there are many diff support groups out there for most things and you can always find others in the same boat. Hope everyone is well.—*Traci*

◆ ◆ ◆

Hello everyone, Just wanted to hi I am 31yrs old lost my right eye when I was 14 but that has never slow me down I own two motorcycles that I love to ride and I gave a shot at riding bulls a few years ago but then found out my wife was pregnant and gave it up. My current job requires me to climb telephone polls and it pretty cool. Anyways just want to say hi and think this site is pretty cool.—*Fred*

◆ ◆ ◆

I came here looking for information about improving my driving abilities. I've been one-eyed ever since I can remember. The problem with that is I was always told about my limitations by my parents and teachers. As a kid I didn't know any better and so I just believed it. I thought I was really handicapped. I'm now 47 with a newly completed Master's degree in library science. I'm corrected to 20'40 in my right eye and have an unrestricted drivers license (except for glasses). I can see by many of the other letters that a good support system is a must. Without one, I suppose one could feel completely alone, full of doubts and experience a huge loss of confidence. I didn't have one and have spent my life trying to recover from all those implanted false beliefs from childhood. It is as if I'm still learning to cope with monocular vision. You all are doing a good job here. Thank you,—*Mark*

◆ ◆ ◆

First off, I want to thank all of you for posting here. I've been reading the last day or so and learning so much. I lost the vision in one eye a few years ago—surgical efforts to restore it weren't successful, and am still working on adjusting to the consequences.

This may be an old topic, so forgive me for going over old ground for those who have been here awhile, but does anybody know of any sources for devices that aid in coping with monocular vision? Little lifestyle things can be challenging for me because I'm very nearsighted in my other eye. For example, I haven't been happy with the way I've done my eyebrows since this happened, and would love it if there were such things as mirrors to help me with this. Just little things, but they sure would help! Thanks again for being here. the discussions help me very much.—*Janet*

Hello Janet, I am also nearsighted in one eye. I use a lighted makeup mirror that has magnification on one side and the mirror over and I get a regular mirror. I would be lost without this mirror with its huge magnification capabilities. I can see the tiniest of hairs so plucking my eyebrows have never been a problem for me, and its a breeze putting on eye makeup.—*Brenda*

Brenda, I use a magnified, lit makeup mirror also. I even take it with me when I travel, and I'd be SO lost without it! My "good" eye has a slight vision impairment (20/100), so the mirror helps see when I apply my eye makeup. I also am a nut for checking for hairs and such (that mirror makes you addicted to checking your face a hundred times a day!).—*Chris*

◆   ◆   ◆

I've lost sight in my one eye for about three years now, but I still have trouble putting on make-up. Especially mascara and eye shadow. Do any of the girls have suggestions and tips that I could use? Thank you.—*Mir*

Mir, do you still have the eye, or did you get it enucleated? When I first had my prosthesis, I didn't wear makeup. A wonderful ocularist (a woman in Manhattan) showed me how to apply the makeup to make my eyes look more balanced.

Alicia is an expert with theatrical makeup, so maybe when she comes back from her Seattle trip, she could help you some more. In the meantime, I'd think that whatever makeup you used before should still be good to use now. I use a soft eyeliner, creamy eye shadows and I can only use a few brands of mascara or I get an allergic reaction. Good luck!—*Chris*

Hi Mir, I have "permanent cosmetics"—my eyeliner is tattooed on. The cosmetician talked me into doing my eyebrows as well and I'm glad I did—they look great! Next year when I go to the States I plan to let her tattoo my lipstick, and then I'll never have to worry about make-up again. I know it sounds strange, but it looks totally natural. Also, if you want to change your look, you can put makeup on over the tats and no one knows. I'll upload a picture if I can ever figure out how.

My advice: Don't waste your money on semi-permanent cosmetics that fade after 3 or 5 years. Call the local tattoo studio and ask where you can get yourself done for real. If you're going to pay the money and go under the needle, it might as well be permanent. BTW, it doesn't hurt (much) because they use numbing gels, etc.—*Ya'ara*

I would love to see a picture of your tattooed eyebrows and eyeliner. I have seen several pics online, and it does appear to make a big difference. I just wouldn't want my eyes to look like "cat eyes". I prefer the softer look. I have also considered "permanent cosmetics", but I was concerned that she may screw up on my bad eye. That would really be a bummer. I surely don't need more attention drawn to my bad eye.—*Brenda*

I still have my eye, but I have no vision out of it. I can do that eye ok, but I have lots of trouble putting makeup on my good eye. The permanent makeup is a good idea. The other person would do it for me, and it'd be done and over with. Thanks, I'll have to think long and hard about that one.—*Mir*

Pictures of permanent cosmetics are often taken very soon after the tattooing, so they look a lot more strident than they will after they heal. I looked like I had thick wet gross eyeliner for about five days, but now it's pretty subtle. I'm going to get my lips done next spring and am dreading the first few days, when I'll look like Julia Roberts on silicone and won't be able to move my mouth. oh well, we must suffer for beauty!—*Ya'ara*

◆ ◆ ◆

Hey, I was just wondering if any of you wear a contact on your eye, I've talked to several eye docs over the years about this and they all discouraged it, my vision isn't really that bad but is corrected.—*Patrick*

Hey Patrick, I had been interested in getting a contact & wearing a patch (& chunk the glasses), but docs don't want to risk anything happening to your good eye. The cornea has no blood vessels so it is your tears & blinking that largely provide for it's good health. Contacts somewhat restrict the benefits that blinking & tears normally provide. Using a contact puts your good eye at a risk, & while it may be marginal, I think most doctors would see it as an unnecessary risk. Infections & irritation are more common. Wearing glasses is a good way to protect your good eye as well as the damaged one also. I know it's a disappointment, but there is some good reasoning against it. I hope you can find a healthy solution that will make you happy & comfortable. Blessings,—*E*

Patrick, E's information is pretty dead on accurate. The only reason I wear a contact lens is because my prescription is so high that I can't see as well in my glasses (I won't even drive unless my contact is in). Even though I wear a hard lens now, I did wear a soft lens for about 7 years. It was very comfortable and I had no problems with infections because I cleaned it religiously. If you really want to try a contact, ask your doctor about daily disposables with a high oxygen permeability. They should be available, and safe for your cornea, if your prescription is low. If you wanted, you could even wear the lens on a part-time basis. Best of luck!—*Adeline*

Hi, all. I've been wearing a contact lens in my good eye since high school (early 80s and lost my bad eye which I was born blind in 1987). None of my eye doctors (including my retina specialist) has ever said anything to me about increased risk of anything bad happening to the eye. Because of my prescription, I do have a daily wear lens and it is replaced about once a year whether or not my prescription changes. We looked in to disposable lenses for me, but they don't make them for my prescription.—*DJ*

◆　　◆　　◆

Hello I just found this site whilst browsing the net. I'm 32 and have been blind in my left eye since birth due to a coloboma and detached retina. I have been reading the forum and have seen posts where people have been suffering the same problems I have. I was always told that having sight in only one eye doesn't cause problems, however my experience disagrees with that. It is reassuring to see other people experiencing stuff. Means its not all in my mind.—*Natty*

Hello, I am just realizing, and this is after many years living with one eye, that the stuff that bothers me isn't all in my mind. I have just been away for the weekend and firstly found that the airport is a difficult place to deal with. The huge space, the loads of people, and lots to watch out for. Then walking in a strange environment at a new place with steps and curbs that need to be watched out for. I find that I get tired out far more quickly than I used to and just want to sit sometimes and stop thinking.—*Marmalade*

I just posted to the job interview thread, and then realized I don't seem to have introduced myself yet. I am female. 53 years old wife and mother and music teacher (private lessons, several instruments). I have eclectic interests, including needlework (I wonder how vision loss will affect that), Tae Kwon Do (black belt and assistant instructor), reading (I belong to a book club) and more.

The optometrist has been observing my nevus for several years and at the last regular checkup (end of July), noticed that the nevus appeared to be darker, so he took a few more digital pictures and another look inside the eye. I had another consultation last Friday with an ophthalmologist who visits the office once a week. He told me I have CM and should be seeing an ocular oncologist within the next few weeks.

I have yet to see the oncologist and have a final diagnosis and recommendations for treatment, but from what the ophthalmologist and optometrist were discussing, it sounds as if the tumor is growing and is close to the optic nerve, so, like Jay, I'm probably not going to mess around with radiation, but get straight to the point and go for enucleation. Of course, I'll need to see what further imaging (ultrasound & angiogram) shows and hear the diagnosis, prognosis & treatment recommendations before I make a final decision.

Because I still don't know exactly what I'm up against, I'm merely gathering all the information I possibly can, so that, hopefully I can ask some intelligent questions and understand the answers a bit more clearly. Not to mention make an informed choice.—*Judith*

Judith, Welcome to Lost Eye! I too had a nevus which was being monitored by my ophthalmologist for the last two and a half years or so. I went for my check-up in June, and they determined that it had grown and was indeed a melanoma. They said that the eye needed to be enucleated. Mine was right near my center of vision, so my vision had been getting worse and worse over the past couple of years. I had my surgery at the end of July, and just this past Thursday, picked up my new "eye". There are lots of people hear that can help you through this. Best of luck to you and keep us posted.—*Renee*

17

Coping With Depth Perception Issues

When you are about to lose an eye, you will be told that you will lose some depth perception. The key is "some", which for most people turns out to be "very little". Oh, yes, it will become more difficult to do some things, such as thread a needle. It will also become more difficult to play some types of sports. But for the most part, the loss of an eye will probably not significantly affect your depth perception or your life.

How do you get depth perception in the first place? Because your eyes are a couple of inches apart, each of your eyes sees a slightly different image, shadows, etc., and your mind has learned to compare the two and make judgments on distance. Depending on your age, your mind has probably made millions of judgments and over the years has been trained to recognized distances.

Outside of about 20 feet, the couple of inches between your eyes doesn't make any substantial difference, and so in gauging distances outside of 20 feet it doesn't matter if you have one eye or two. A guy with one eye sees the world outside of 20 feet the same as the guy with two eyes. It only really matters for stuff closer in, and the closer in the more significant the difference.

Again, you get depth perception because your two eyes are a couple of inches apart and see a slightly different image which your mind compares. If you only have one eye, you only get one image unless…[gasp]…you move your head slightly from side to side so that you get a couple of different images from your one eye for your mind to compare. This allows you to, essentially, mimic with one eye what you would see with two eyes, and thus alleviate the close-in depth perception problem.

Where this simple and effective trick does not work is with an activity which is fast-paced, such as sports. You will simply not have enough time to move your head around and get different images if, for instance, you have a tennis ball coming at you at 90 mph.

So, what can I tell you about sports? Not much, because I have not yet had enough practical experience playing many sports with just one eye. I can tell you the obvious, that some sports will not be affected at all by your one-eyedness. These will include jogging, swimming, water-skiing, snow-skiing, snowboarding, surfing, etc. Some sports, such as tennis might be significantly affected. Other sports may or may not be affected, depending on the position you play. For instance, I doubt that your one-eyedness would make much of a difference if you play the pitcher in baseball (the plate is outside of 20 feet), if you play in the post position in basketball, or if you play on the offensive line in football.

Remember that your brain will have to re-train itself to cope with your single vision. You can help it out by practicing your one-eyed depth perception, such as by laying on your back and repeatedly throwing a tennis ball straight up in the air and catching it as it comes down (be sure to wear safety goggles when you do this).

There are some things which might cause you trouble at first, which are solved if you just do them a little more slowly than you did before. An example is shaking somebody's hand—don't feel uncomfortable slowly extending your hand and letting the other person grasp it (I haven't found this to be a problem at all). Steps can be weird at first, and of course you need to be careful of the blind spot, caused by your nose, on the side on which you lost your eye.

Other problems can be solved by just proceeding slowly and cautiously at first. An example is pouring orange juice. If you hold the pitcher a foot above the glass you may or may not hit it. What you should do is lower the pitcher (or raise the glass) until the lip of the glass almost touches the pitcher, and then pour so that it is a "sure thing". After a while, your mind will learn to compensate for your one-eyedness and such things as pouring will once again become second nature to you.

Driving, and particularly parking, may pose some depth perception problems. After my eye was removed, my girlfriend placed a board on the garage floor to indicate to me when to stop my car. However, I've learned that it is easier to simply find a familiar spot on the wall next to my door, and to learn to stop when I have lined up with it. Like everything else, parking with one eye will simply take some practice, but you can expect to get good at it over time.

MESSAGE THREADS

Since loss of sight in the right eye, I am experiencing perception and balance problems. Cannot stand or walk without the aid of a walker. Cannot drive the car. Cause of sight loss (Temporal Arthritis). Help! Any helpful suggestions for my dilemma will be appreciated. Cheers,—*Jayne*

Hi Jayne, I have no sight in my right eye, and balance is definitely a problem. For an attempt to improve my balance, I try to have my eye that can see to be closer to the side foot, then to the center of my body. I can see out of my right eye, I try to center my body closer to my right foot, then to the center of my body, this helps to improve my balance. I hope this is of help,—*Doc*

◆ ◆ ◆

Hi, I am new to this forum. I am a 36 year old female, blind in my right eye due to amblyopia. My three sons have inherited the condition that lead to my blindness, strabismus. I am doing everything possible to ensure that they do not go blind in one eye from this condition. It has affected my life to some extent. The eye with age has changed a lot. It turns into my nose, even though I have had two eye surgeries. The pupil in the eye is much larger than the pupil in my good eye. Driving is ok, except for parking, and I do not drive in big city traffic.

My 7 year old son has been undergoing vision therapy, and we do a lot of it at home, and see the therapist once per week. Through doing the therapy with my son, I have learned a lot about my own vision. For instance, I have learned that my "center", is actually one inch to the left of my nose, where a two eyed persons center would be at their nose.

I am very interested in the subject of perception as related to one eyed vision. Has anyone ever read the book "The Man Who Mistook His Wife for a Hat?", by Olive Sacks. Do a search on Google. I have not yet read it, but again, I am intrigued by how the lack of an eye can greatly change perception. Hope to learn and share with this group.—*Deb*

Hi Deb, I haven't read that book yet but will give it a look-see. After 38 years of having normal(2-eye) vision, I had a very hard time with depth perception after losing my eye to cancer. My mind was playing tricks with me and when I would reach for objects I missed much of the time. I was usually off by a couple of inches. Learning how to fill a glass with liquid was probably my hardest "redo" to learn over. It's been 7 plus years now and I don't have any problems that I know of. My brain has compensated? for my singular vision. I still hate parking the van though. Scary! I'm a special education teacher in a vocational setting. I've been a mechanic all my life. I still work with my students and with my hands everyday. Is it tough? Yes, but I'm still alive and kicking. Welcome to the site. There are many great people here to help out in any way. Good luck.—*Ron*

About the whole monocular vision perception. I've only had sight in one eye since I was 13 (30 years ago), and I can BARELY remember having a tough time with the change. Maybe at first my depth perception was off a bit, and the most challenging thing was facing stairs or steps, but that's about it. I did also find myself looking into my nose a lot. Guess that's normal. As far as driving a car, no problem, but I limit my abilities. I don't drive in the city, nor do I drive in heavily populated areas, and driving at night is more of a challenge. We had another thread about that topic. Anyway, welcome again. It's always good to get different opinions on topics!—*Chris*

Hi! As a person that has one eye vision and has a child with amblyopia, I had to respond. First off, my child is 14 and we went through surgery and patching when she was 4. The doctors thought she was cured. For two years she kept telling me that she couldn't see well out of that eye. This was during my time of a cancer diagnosis and treatment that took the vision of my right eye. I took her to the eye doctor to make sure that she didn't have what I have and the amblyopia popped up again. The eye doctor said that she could lose her vision and we are contact lensing that eye. He was surprised that her previous doctors said she was fixed and took a look at her previous records. He apologized that the operation didn't take and that even though she was followed for years after, nothing was caught.

I'm the one with a little depth perception annoyance. I say annoyance, as I do everything as I did before. I do spill things now when I pour, hate to parallel park, but usually can and also drive long distances in the rain, fog and night. I'm just very thankful that my untreated eye is still 20/20. I am blind in the right eye and steps can be a problem(annoyance) I fell a couple of times, when I first lost the vision, but not at all lately. It just takes awhile to get used to. I wish you all the best and many hugs,—*Sherri*

Hi Deb, I was born with Optic Nerve Hypoplasia in my left eye, however doctors didn't give my parents this diagnosis until I was about 4. At 2 I had quite a pronounced squint and the hospital treated me for Amblyopia by patching my "good eye". However my mom realized something was up when every time she would put on the patch I would have a bit of a temper! I was referred to the eye specialist unit in Belfast where they immediately told mom I had little to no vision in that eye. I had my squint repaired and had no problems until about age 14, when one day I had a fierce headache which I thought was a migraine and so I went to sleep it off. When I woke up my eye was pointing at my nose and wouldn't budge! I went to the hospital where I had a CT but nothing showed up and they were unsure as to what happened. Over the next few weeks I started to get double vision which was worse some days and then others it wouldn't be so bad (this turned out to be related to the degree that my squint happened to be at that day!).

So back to the hospital where they said that my muscle had obviously snapped, hence the headache, and I was getting double vision because my eye had moved off its "suppression area". I was fitted with a prism to my glasses and eventually had surgery last October to try and correct my squint, which didn't work. I was fitted with an Occlusive Contact Lens/Painted Scleral Shell, 6 weeks ago, (4 years after the problems began!) and its GREAT! I have no double vision when its in, I can drive again (I had my license suspended because of the double vision, which was probably the hardest thing to deal with!) and It doesn't look that odd. The only problem is I have to use artificial tears because the shell clamps on which can be quite painful! As for depth perception I didn't have problems as a child, because I was always used to having no sight there, But when I started to get diplopia my depth perception changed and steps and pouring out from the kettle became quite an annoyance, but I overcame that pretty soon. The only depth problem I have is with sports like badminton and tennis which are fast paced, and others like cricket and baseball where the ball might be dropping from quite a height, it can be hit and miss (excuse the pun lol) as to weather I will catch the ball. Like Sherri said above, it just takes time to get used to, but eventually its no problem!—*Elizabeth*

◆   ◆   ◆

Hi can anyone help me to stop walking into people on my blind spot. This happens a lot I forget about only having one eye till I walk into someone or something. Thanks.—*Tony*

Tony, I always hold my arm, on my blind side, about 6.8 inches from my body. This keeps people at a slight distance from me & gives me a little time to react if someone is there. Don't get me wrong. I still run into people but less frequently. Good luck.—*Rich*

Tony, how long have you been monocular? You'll get used to it. I often joke with my husband, that his senses are much worse than mine are, and he has vision in both eyes!—*Chris*

Hi Tony, I always figured even if I had both eyes I'd still be a klutz but my blind eye makes a darn good excuse for me! I usually try to walk with people on my good side whenever possible. For me I always bump into doorframes in new places until I get to know the layout and am forever reaching more than once for doorknobs because I miss! I am so used to bumping things/people I hardly notice. It was worse when I was a kid, neighbors called the Children's Aid on my parents due to me having so many bruises on my legs & arms. But I was a tomboy and refused to let my blind eye keep me out of the neighborhood rough housing and tree climbing with my siblings. I was always a scabby/bruised kid. Now I'm just a little more cautious and stay out of trees.—*Starr*

Hi Tony, Another thing that helps me is to look down a lot while walking, it helps with ground changes and you find a lot of coins too!—*Tommy*

I've never had a problem with it, but very rarely I will miss something on my right side. I usually keep my head turned toward my blind side out of habit, but not to much that it looks ridiculous! I have unusually good peripheral vision, I have about 130 degrees visual field. Just try to keep your head oriented toward the blind side, or frequently look that way.—*Jarrod*

18

Coping With Jobs And Careers

Losing an eye typically should not interfere with one's job or career goals. We have even had commercial airline pilots lose an eye and resume their career. Where losing an eye may have an effect is where the job is such that there is danger of losing the good eye, and in certain job occupations where full peripheral vision is a must.

There are also concerns about whether having one eye will hurt chances of getting a new job (it usually doesn't), how job interviews will go, and in getting along with co-workers. These problems are almost always much larger in the mind of the applicant than they are considered by others. Indeed, many employers will consider the fact that the person has overcome a disability to be a tremendous strength, so long as it does not adversely affect their job performance.

LETTERS AND E-MAILS

I am 23 yrs old from southwest, VA. I am married, have a one year old child, and am a part time college student. I have been legally blind in my left eye my whole life, due to a childhood cataract and abnormal lens in the eye. But looking at me you can't tell. This has never really slowed me down though. I got my driver's license at 16, finished high school, became a beautician, married, had a child, and like I said am attending college again. Just because you have one eye doesn't mean you can't do the things you want to do. I'm sure losing your eye suddenly is more of a shock than being born this way, but having only one good eye can be kind of depressing no matter what. You just got to say "this is how it is; and I'm going to make the best of it!" Take care all,—*Tabitha*

Hello, Love your website and hope you can direct to one specifically dedicated to jobs for people with only one eye. My husband lost is left eye in Vietnam and has been discriminated against during job interviews because of this. Specifically, from the FAA, not for a pilot position, but for airport security. I was hoping you could send me in the right direction to help him fight this kind of discrimination. Again, your sight is inspiring.—*Doris*

Hello, my name is Michael and I now live in Texas. I had lost my right eye in 1984 at the age of 14 due to a stray gun shot. I have earned my CDL and got one of the few federal waivers to operate a tractor trailer interstate. I had also been appointed constable for the city that I lived in Massachusetts, and I have completed the Texas Department of Criminal Justice Academy for Correctional Officer and have been on the job for 4 months, in the single most dangerous and hostile prisons in the state.

Even after proving myself with every tasks that had been thrown at me. I have been trying to get into a Police or Sheriffs department position and have been told that I was not eligible due to my eye loss and also the fact that they felt that it would hinder my ability to function effectively in that position. (I have 3yrs Constable Exp.). I am trying to find out if there is anything that I may be able to do, and if not. Is there a department in any state that does not have this weak closed minded hiring criteria? I am sorry the length of this letter as I know that you are very busy and probably receive a lot of mail just like mine. I would greatly appreciate any assistance that you may be able to lend me and my family. Thank you,—*Michael*

MESSAGE THREADS

Hi All, hope you are doing well with beating the hell out of the challenges thrown you way. Just a recap on me, I lost my left eye when I was 4 yrs old. this year at the age of 25 yrs, I would be completing my MBA from a prestigious college. Doing a quick SWOT analysis, I found that I would be weaker in an analyst kind of job, where I need to study lot of information and analyze lot of data. I also discovered that I have strengths in conceptualization, execution and people skills.

Thinking about future, I understand that I have to adopt learning styles keeping in mind my physical challenge. By learning style, I mean how do you assimilate new information, and approach the new skills learning opportunity. Could you tell me what are your unique learning styles that you have adopted to succeed in your respective career? Waiting eagerly for your reply. *Cheers,—Prab*

◆ ◆ ◆

Hi All, I just wanted to know, if anyone of you has consultancy or managerial career despite your handicap. I have lost my left eye when I was 4 year old. Now I am final year student in the top most management institute in my country. And I have to choose a career. I wear specs with power. 4. I feel very afraid that how I will fight in competitive world out there, if it is just based on no. of hours you can work, the no. of books you have read and sitting long hours in front of computer, all needing healthy pairs of eyes.

I fought all my life to get the best deal in life. But now once my college life gets over, there will be no competitive exam to prepare for, where one can do some smart preparation and get through. And that really scares me. I am very ambitious, and can not accept anything but the best. But I don't have the imagination to think through this problem and choose a career where I can reach to the pinnacle despite this handicap. Your advice would be really appreciated. Cheers,—*Prab*

Dear Prab: I don't know if it counts as "managerial" but I've had a career as a teacher since I was 23, and I'm now 41. I lost my right eye at age seven. It is a miracle that my left eye has better-than—perfect vision, since everyone on both sides of my family has poor vision. I'm currently a Senior Lecturer (like a Professor, but not on the tenure track) at the University of Southern California. I'm also a theatre director, lighting designer, makeup artist and have done just about every job associated with theatre at one time or another. Since 1995, I've become a soap maker with my own small soap and toiletries business. In the past two years, I've written and published two books on soap making.

I think what I'm trying to say is that I've never felt held back professionally. I've never considered myself a person with a disability. My looks have never been what I'd hoped, and that inhibited me as an actor, but luckily there are things in theatre I like better than acting. I was in a dance company when I was 21, but I had a back injury that ended that. You appear to be highly motivated, intelligent and sensitive. With your training in management, there appears to be nothing to stop you from achieving at the highest level you desire. I'm sure there are many others here who will have similar stories of full lives. Take care,—*Alicia*

I wholeheartedly agree with Alicia-I don't consider it a "disability". I've been a paralegal for over 20 years and it never slowed me down, even with TONS of reading and typing to do. I never even thought twice about it. Don't let anything stop you from fulfilling your dreams. Good luck!—*Anon*

Hi, I absolutely agree. Do what you really want to do and do not consider yourself as a person with disabilities. When I was a little girl my parents treated me like a disable person. They were keep telling me: oh, you can not do that because of your eye; you can not go there because of your eye and you should not try this because of your eye, etc., etc. Now, I am 28 years old and I know they were wrong and somehow they destroyed a small part of my dreaming soul.

Thanks God not everything and now I am enjoying my life and I am doing what I really wanted to do. Good luck.—*Anna*

Hey! I have been clinically blind in my left eye my whole life, due to a childhood cataract called Posterior Lenticonus. Surgery is risky, so my parents and I chose not to operate on the eye when I was younger. Honestly, I'm kind of glad we didn't. Had we operated, I may have lost the eye entirely. But anyway, I have never let this slow me down! I'm 23 yrs. old, finished high school, became a beautician, married, have an 18 mo. old daughter, got my driver's license, and I'm going back to college again. I guess since I was born this way, I don't know any different. But I don't feel any different either. My mom and step-father who raised me, never treated me any different. Mom always told me I could be whatever I wanted if I put my mind to it. However, she did discourage me from high school sports such as softball, and basketball, because she was afraid I could injure my good eye. But I was in band! So anyway, don't feel bad if you only have one good eye, you can do anything you want, as long as you can see at all to do it!—*Tabitha*

I'm a project manager in a large (40,000 employee) company in the US. Specifically, I'm a Six Sigma Black Belt and Lean Master. I lost sight in my right eye in June of 2002, and I do not consider myself handicapped in any way. I still travel, run projects, teach classes at my facility, and most people I work with don't know I have one eye. Rather, they know, but don't discuss it. I'm never judged by my "handicap", only by my performance. I have just learned to compensate. for instance, I get to meeting early so I can grab a chair that allows me to see the whole room. It's only a "handicap" if you treat it that way.—*Jess*

◆ ◆ ◆

I wanted to talk to some one out there who is an artist or knows an artist with one eye. I am really struggling, I did do a lot of portraits as my job, just discovered your website. Lost my sight in right eye—which luckily I managed to stop them from removing after a car crash. Still need surgery to my face if they will do it, really trying to move on.—*Sarah*

Hi there, I just happen to be an artist myself, though I'm not a painter. I do drawings, and I'm good at it. I lost the sight in my right eye when I was 16 years old and had a lot of work done to my face as well. I remember wondering if I would be as good at drawing as I was before, so I gave it a whirl. It turned out the very first drawing I did was a portrait of Angus Young on the Let there be Rock album, and it was as good of a portrait as I have ever done. When one does art on paper of a canvas, it is really two dimensional, even thought there is the illusion of 3 dimensions! So, you see it the same, with one or two eyes. You should be just as good a painter as you ever were, if not better. I hope I have helped you, feel free to email me if you have any questions.—*Jarrod*

Hi! I lost my eye a year ago and I am still getting used to the lack of depth perception. well, my husband was born with vision problems, and he has never had depth perception. he is an unbelievably good artist. we were talking after reading your post and he wanted me to pass on to you—not having depth perception should improve your artistic ability because you will see things as they really are as compared to being fooled by foreshortening effects. so keep your chin up, you will do great!—*Mary*

Hi Sarah, I have a degree in painting and have painted for many years, my subject matter is realistic and figurative. An accident took my fovael (or sharp focus) vision in one eye when I was less than two years old. 5 years ago I lost the rest of the vision in that eye which is now being rejected by my body. I'm trying to just "deal with it" for another year, until I finish graduate school, although it is not pretty and the pain and pressure is escalating. After I graduate, I will have the dead eye removed and get a prosthesis. I feel lucky to have that option as I read the other posts on this forum.

Having vision in one eye affects artwork in many subtle ways, but none that should cause an artist to stop working. The condition does not decrease my facility in painting or drawing, the problems with perspective and to some degree with color, can be overcome with a bit of persistence.

My experience has been that art is the main thing that keeps my world exciting and beautiful. My vision is best when I work, and the work makes me sing inside. I forget about the lack of depth perception that makes me clumsy, tripping over uneven pavement or knocking drinks over on people. Art is about vision, and our visual difference should make our art better. We are unique visual creatures and artwork is the one place where that difference can fill us will joy. Keep on Truckin,—*Sleepy*

◆ ◆ ◆

Hi, I just want to say that I really like this forum, it's nice to know there are others like me in the world. I was born in 1980 w/an early childhood cataract in the left eye called Posterior Lenticonus. Surgery was very risky then, and still is, so I have never had the eye operated on. I am legally blind in that eye. I see 20/20 in the right eye w/lenses. I am a 23 yr old married female w/a baby. I completed high school, got my drivers license, got a cosmetology license (beautician), and am attending college part time for a second degree. So just because you may have one eye, that doesn't mean it will slow you down! So I'm a one-eyed beautician too!—*Tabitha*

Hey, Rick, I lost my eye 30 years ago, when I was a 13 year old young girl. I went on to finish my schooling (making the honor society each year, having only missed one year of school & being home-tutored that year). I went on to go to a good New York University, and became a paralegal.

Seeing from one eye didn't slow down my reading or my desire to work. I never stopped and gave it a second thought. Only once in a while did I need a little surgery here and there, and it somewhat slowed me down, but I always got back up and had a job to go to, until I settled down, married and had children and decided to stop working (well, being a mother IS a full-time job in itself, and the most important one you could find!). Hope that helps!—*Chris*

Hi Rick, I'm a high school vocational/special education teacher. Funny thing is I remember when I was in high school, my voc-ed. teacher had one eye too.—*Ron*

I lost site in my right eye at the age of 10. I was shot with a bb gun by another individual with that happening I ended up with a detached retina the eye wasn't removed though. I am now 30 and it's never slowed me down a bit. I've been a volunteer fireman for 8 years, also go out of state to fight wild land fires, My full-time job is working for the University Fire And Rescue Training. Although my self esteem was low for quite sometime. I never let it keep me from doing something I enjoy.—*Kyle*

Kyle, I, too, was shot with a bb gun (30 years ago). I wanted to know how close you were to the gun, and how it is that you didn't lose your eye. I guess I was at pretty close range-maybe a foot away. The bb entered through my eye and ended up close to my brain. There was NO way to save the eye. Besides that, they called it pretty much a worst-case scenario. I lost the eye, and the prosthesis has no movement due to the damage. I also needed nearly 30 surgeries to repair a lot of things, and my body rejected most implants, etc. Anyway, it was strange reading another bb gun accident! Wonder how many more of us there are out there! Take care, and I hope you continue posting here.—*Chris*

◆ ◆ ◆

Hi, I just discovered this site because I was searching for help with my struggle with discrimination over monocular vision. I lost the sight in my left eye when I was 10, and my other eye has adjusted well with prefect vision. I am an ordained Lutheran Pastor in Nova Scotia Canada, a volunteer fire fighter—I drive the trucks and fight the fires, Scuba diver, and wood worker. I recently applied to the Canadian Military to be a chaplain. I completed all their requirements and ranked number 1 in a nation-wide ranking of people applying for the positions of chaplain. but I was denied because I have monocular vision. While I understand some positions need binocular vision—but a chaplain. I am fighting it through the Canadian Human Rights Commission. They have taken up the case. I wonder how many others out there have run into the same problems and if they were successful.—*Paul*

Welcome to the board, Paul! My goodness, with all of the other things you do, you would think the military would be happy to have you! I agree with you that you don't need two eyes to be a chaplain. I have never experienced any problems like this. However, a while ago someone from Singapore posted that they were denied a driver's license because they are monocular. Must be a governmental thing. I wish you lots of luck with your case. Keep us posted.—*Nancy*

Paul, first of all, welcome to the board! I'm really sorry about your experience with the Canadian Military so far! Is there an attorney you could contact who could possibly answer your questions? Maybe there are restrictions on applying for the military. I remember that the military in the U. S. had special provisions for people with extremely bad eyesight (that used to be a possible way out of serving!). Anyway, maybe someone could help answer your questions. Good luck, and if we could be of any help, let us know! P.S. My husband's an attorney here in the U.S., and I'll ask him about it as soon as I can!—*Chris*

Hi Paul, I am the Singaporean who was mentioned by Nancy. I was denied a driving license in Singapore due to monocular vision. I tried couple of ways to seek help but all turned out to be unsuccessful. I had also tried to get help from a vision-loss organization but they failed to help. Well, it is pretty hard to change the law, but I am willing to fight until the end. Don't give up,—*Paul*

I tried to join the Royal Air Force's Nursing Corps, but was turned down because apparently I would be unable to fire a weapon to protect myself or my patients should the need arise. I feel this is a pure crock because, after all, when long range aiming. don't those with two eyes close one to shoot a weapon? I asked the RAF recruitment officer to come play a game of Time Crisis on the Playstation2, or come pheasant shooting through the forest so he could judge my shooting abilities for himself, he politely declined lol. I know a few people with monocular vision who are EXCELLENT shots (I know it isn't a very girlie pastime but I quite enjoy it lol) and so for discrimination to be this ingrained into the state. and then to see how I couldn't join a UK ambulance service, I did get quite annoyed. Time has helped me move on, and at least I have other opportunities. I hope you have got somewhere with your fight through the courts and I'd love to hear how you are getting on now.—*Elizabeth*

◆ ◆ ◆

Is this a dreaded thing or what? Have ya'll ever been to a job interview and knew that you was the best fit for the job, but somehow never received that phone call? The whole interview goes well and seemed to have all the correct answers after hours of practicing in front of a mirror. Here comes the dreaded #1 question. tell me about yourself. Eye contact is the key and he seems to look at you and you can sense he notices something different, but he can't seem to grasp it. You do your 2 minute spill, and maintain that eye contact as if he was not staring. I know that this subject is not a medical problem, and maybe I posted this under the wrong thread. I was just wondering if others have had the same experience and how you coped with it.—*Brenda*

Hey, Brenda! I just came off of a round of (successful) job interviews recently and I definitely know what you mean. Even though I spent two years doing Human Resources, I still get jittery. Before I go into any interview or important meeting where first impressions are key, I just try to remind myself of all my positive attributes and then I try to project that confidence during the meeting. I also try to be very animated during the conversation—moving my head, gesturing. From the recruiters perspective, it indicates interest in the position, and frankly, I think it helps to distract from any physical imperfection, whether it's an eye or something else.

I've also been in the situation (especially before my disfigured eye was replaced with the prosthesis) where I've been "overlooked" for promotions/jobs. While logically I know that I wouldn't want to work for a company or people who are discriminatory, it still hurts to feel rejected. Best of luck for any upcoming interviews!—*Adeline*

I totally know where your coming from but don't you just find in general that when you are talking to someone new and you make eye contact you are always so aware of the eye and you always get the feeling that they notice! It can be quite difficult at times. I wish you the best of luck in interviews, I wish I could say try not to think about it. but it is kind of impossible (for me at least).—*Traci*

I notice that myself. When I go out at night to a store. I'm not wearing my shades. I get double takes all the time. I thought it was me at the beginning, but I've noticed that I was not imagining it.—*Michael*

Hey there, I too know the stress of meeting someone new and dealing with the issue of getting and maintaining eye contact. Sometimes I think people are just in shock when they see 2 eyes that do not line up or look normal so to speak—people just do not know which eye to look at or cant figure out who you are looking at. One trick that seems to work for me is if I quickly look back and forth at both of their eyes (searching for eye contact)they seem to figure out which eye to look at. People want to look you in the eye when speaking to you—and this technique helps me give them an opportunity to make eye contact with me instead of just looking away while I speak(which I had done for years).—*Chandra*

What a great sense of humor! My brother lost his eye in an accident about 20 years ago and likes to tell one-eye jokes. Once someone asked him to keep an eye on a package for him, so he pulled out his "glass" eye and put it on top of the package. He was recently hired by the RCMP (computer job, I think) after passing all their interviews and security checks. So, whenever you go for a job interview, be confident and hold onto your sense of humor.—*Judith*

19

Coping With Activities

The loss of an eye typically should not affect one's hobbies and activities. People lose an eye and continue to follow their normal pursuits, and start new ones. So get out and enjoy life! Just be sure to protect your good eye while doing so.

LETTERS AND E-MAILS

My husband has had only one eye for over ten years and he has adjusted very well. He plays pool so much better. We have adjusted and even laugh a lot about it because life goes on.—*Lisa*

Many thanks for this awesome website. I lost vision in my right eye while mowing my lawn. A few hours later, the doctor confirmed that 1) I had a retinal stroke, and 2) my vision would never return. Yours was one of the first websites I encountered, and its positive tone truly helped.

Over the course of the next few months I went from fear of losing my other eye, to great relief as I realized I lost my eye, but still had my life. I've since had a hole in my heart repaired (the culprit of the blood clot. never knew I had it!), and am pretty much back to normal!

The day after I lost my sight, I had an 8:00 am tee time in a charity golf tournament. It was a struggle (my depth perception was off!), but I managed to play 18 holes and didn't whiff the ball once! Sure, my depth perception is still off, but the loss in vision has not changed my activities at all. In June, I didn't think I'd EVER drive again. I now drive in the rain, in the snow (we get quite a bit here!), long distance, I jet ski, golf. Nothing has changed.

Just a big thank you. I believe your attitude determines how well you cope. I chose to not feel sorry for myself and to get on with my life. Thank you for some encouragement along the way!—*Jessie*

MESSAGE THREADS

Hi all, I am just guessing how many of this forum are avid cyclists and whether monocular vision has any negative impact and whether there would be any tips to share. I used to cycle a lot, but these days I must bring work home for weekends, so not much anymore. But I would like to get back to it. The time my left eye was removed I still had time for cycling, so I it did not take long after enucleation when I was back on the saddle. I cannot recall exactly, but I maybe I did not even have a prosthesis as yet. In beginning, say my first 50 km trip, I felt a little unstable or unconfident, hard to describe. Strange, because I had been cycling before the enucleation when the eye was already blind. However, these feelings moved away.

There are some concerns, however, which I would like to hear others' opinions. I am a little farsighted on my right eye and I do not seem to see ahead that well if I am using sun glasses without a degree. I am hesitant to by sun glasses with degree since mine is with a progressive lens. So I just use those sun glasses for protection against the sun.

Another thing is the sun. Here, near the equator the sun can be really bright. I am not sure is that the reason, or the heat, but sometimes on my way back home I begin having a migraine. I do not get any head ache, but I get the visual effect. It moves a way when I rest a bit and have something sweet to eat, like ice cream. It might also occur for the reason that I start early in the morning and never eat anything until I get home; and maybe because of the heat. Or combination of all the input. But it could be that one eye has to work more and also to take the brightness of the day.

One more concern is that if I fall or fly off the bike, could the impact throw the prosthetic eye out from the socket? Would it be safer not to wear the eye when cycling, for this reason. I have never cycled without my eye, but this thing is in my mind. Any comments?—*JPH*

My son started racing BMX in the fall of 03. On May 1st of 04, he had won the required number of races, to be advanced from Novice, to Intermediate. On May 8th, he was shot in the eye with a pellet gun, and is now permanently blind in his left eye. All he wanted to do for the 6 weeks he spent face down in bed, was to get back on his bike, and that is exactly what he did. Two days after being released by his eye surgeon to resume normal physical activities (the damage was done), he went to a Regional race, and made the main event. He still races, and has learned quickly to cope. Instead of being able to use his peripheral vision to know if somebody is on his immediate left, he listens for them, or watches the ground for shadows.

I am sure it causes him some problems, as he gets nervous in traffic, but he hasn't slowed down much (if any), and still enjoys BMX racing as much as he did before his injury. He has been back on his bike for nearly a year now, and has not had a crash yet, that can be attributed to his vision. Remember. It could be worse.—*John*

Hiya folks! I was actually talking about this topic with a few mates the other day, as to weather we would get bikes to commute to and from our hospital placements. The general consensus was that if two eyed people get knocked of their bikes by crazy bus drivers in London every day, then I don't really stand a chance! Anyway, the tube is handier and you don't end up all sweaty when you arrive at work! lol. I think its great that Alan is so good at his BMX racing, he's brilliant!—*Elizabeth*

My left optic nerve was damaged in an accident, so the vision in the left eye is rather reduced (I still have some vision in it). One very good investment was a rear view mirror mounted on my bicycle handlebar, which allows me to see if anything is going to overtake. so when I want to turn left, I first look in the mirror, then turn my head around (I have to turn it more than before to see clearly) to see if it's really free.

I still hope that some day it will be possible to repair an optic nerve, because the eye itself is well, as the eye doctor has confirmed. Anyway, to JPH I would really suggest to get optic sunglasses because it is essential to see sharp in road traffic.—*tk4*

◆ ◆ ◆

I have been training boxing for a time but are a bit concerned about the risks involved when you only have one eye. I know there are protection that covers you head and eyes quite good, so you avoid any direct contact to the eye, like a poke or a thumb. But I don't know if you still could get an eye injury by heavy contact to the head, like a blow to the head, or as in wrestling getting your head slammed to the canvas sometimes?

Is it only direct trauma to the eye that are hurtful, or could you risk a retina detachment even if your eyes are protected? Like a blow the chin for example? Maybe it's better for me to stop playing in such sports, or do anyone else have any experience with being one-eyed and doing martial arts?—*Daniel*

I was told by my surgeon to never go bunjee jumping as even it can cause retinal detachment! Id really think twice before taking part in Kick Boxing, Regular Boxing, Tae Kwon Do, Karate or any of the like. To be honest I just don't think its worth it!—*Elizabeth*

I guess the best thing to do is to talk to an eye doctor about this. I also heard about bungy jumping and retina detachment, but I guess this must be very rare, maybe for persons who are prone for retina detachment? I lost my left eye by a retina detachment, but that was due to a direct hit to the eye with a hockey stick.

The protection equipment I was thinking about is some form of goggles designed to protect the eyes, and also a padded headgear with protection for the head, nose and chin. So direct hits to the eye will be no problem, but maybe the hit of a boxing glove or kick to the side of the head/chin is enough to cause a retina detachment even if the force is somehow stopped by the padded headgear. Maybe the eye specialist can see if you are in the risk zone for having retina detachment easily, don't know if they can se that by examining the eye?—*Daniel*

Do you still play hockey, Daniel? I do sometimes, I work as a carpenter, I am also the captain of the local volunteer fire dept. I guess the decision about what to do or not do has never really been an issue for me, I try not to be stupid about things, wear safety glasses a lot. You need to live life I say.—*Patrick*

Hi Patrick, no I don't play hockey any longer, but probably could with only one eye, some professional hockey players still perform good even if they have serious eye injuries to one of their eyes, so I guess you can play hockey even with one eye. But I like an active lifestyle and for the moment runs and lifting weights quite much.—*Daniel*

I have been in wado kai karate for four years now, three of which I have spent without the vision in one eye. it has been a little difficult, especially with kicks. I would think that you should definitely wear protective equipment because a strong enough blow could probably detach a retina. light sparring would be alright, and if you set ground rules with your opponent first, like no head shots, things would work out alright. but I agree with almost everyone else here that you shouldn't let the loss of an eye or loss of vision stop you from doing what you want.—*Mir*

I agree with Irishangel. The risk just isn't worth going blind. My son is a black belt and a participate in wrestling, and I personally know there is intense contact in these sports. I have seen numerous guys taken off the mat to emergency rooms with broken ribs, broken nose, etc. I couldn't imagine letting my son be active in these sports with only one good eye. I agree to live life to its fullest, but I'd like to be seeing what I was doing and not live with the regrets of some foolish decision I made earlier in life. Again, just my opinion.—*Brenda*

◆   ◆   ◆

Hello everyone, just ran across this excellent forum and felt compelled to post. I lost total vision in my right eye 23 years ago due to an on the job accident. While unloading a truck for a retail store I accidentally stuck my right eye with blade I had in my right hand to cut package straps. Total, immediate loss of sight. Reconstructive surgery and cornea transplant failed to recover vision due to scar tissue. I remember having dreams associated with loss of balance such as trying to cut grass but I could only push mower in a circle. Probably just another form of the brain trying to adjust. These dreams faded after several Months.

Growing up, I always was fascinated my airplanes. So it came to be that after my accident I started tossing around the idea of flying. Ultralights were very popular at the time of my accident but I wanted something more substantial around me as well as the desire to carry family members along. I got my third class medical in the late 1980s and soloed shortly thereafter. I didn't follow through with certificate until later years due to financial reasons. Finally received certification with a Statement Of Demonstrated Ability (SODA) in March of 2000. One of the highlights of my life. Like walking on a cloud, literally. One of the things I pride myself in is making solid consistent soft landings. Contrary to popular belief, landing an aircraft is runway perspective and not depth perception. In fact, if you rely 100% on depth perception by focusing on a point on the runway, more than likely you will hammer it down hard whether single eyed or two eyed.

The same thing applies in driving. The next time you are on the expressway, try focusing on a spot a few feet in front of the car. You will wear yourself out as well as make more adjustment to steering to keep it between the lines. This applies whether you can see out of both eyes or not. Anyway, just wanted to post my thoughts to let those who might feel hindered by loss of sight in one eye to not give up and certainly don't let others discourage you. I am also red green color blind but this was overcome on the SODA as well. I had more people tell me that it couldn't be done than those who encouraged. My biggest advice: Protect the good eye at all costs! Wear protective lenses regardless of the situation. Enjoy life. The Lord has purpose for everyone.—*hpyagl*

♦ ♦ ♦

Has anyone played golf before they lost their eye and then went back to playing? I played a lot of golf before my operation and just wondering what pitfalls are waiting for me when the snow melts.—*Guy*

Guy, I lost vision in my dominant eye in June, 2002. in the middle of the golf season. The day before my retinal stroke, I had a 43 in my ladies' league (was averaging mid-high 40's). The loss has added about a stroke per hole to my game. Things to watch out for: 1) depth perception. I have a tough time judging distance to the pin, and never had that problem before. 2) sun. Seems to bother me more. WEAR GLASSES. 3) I've had a few run-ins with flying insects. Last year I was ready to tee off, and a bug flew into my good eye. I freaked for a minute as I couldn't see. Glasses will help! 4) don't touch your eyes/face. never know what kind of dirt of chemicals you pick up. 5) I rarely look for lost balls. Many of the courses I play have thick woods. I can't always see the branches. 6) The ground. Watch out for little dips/holes/etc in the ground. they can be hard to see. 7) putting. Analyzing the green is harder now. Take your time.

You get the picture. just be sure to protect your good eye. I received a gift, a range/depth gadget, but I find it hard to use. Be patient with yourself. your game will improve with time. By the way. I was out playing in a charity tournament the next morning. 18 hours after the stroke!—*Jessie*

Thanks Jessie. That was great. I will need some practice when this snow melts. I like to play a great deal. I get out about 100 times a year. I am very nervous about my first shot this Spring. I guess the fear comes from not knowing if I can ever get back to the same level that I played at before the operation. I have lots of support from everyone around me. My Family tells me to work on my game as hard as I want. I can't wait, but I can. You know what I mean. I just got a nice pair of Maui Jim glasses for the golf course. They are real nice. Thanks again for your reply. We should play this summer.—*Guy*

Guy, don't get too worried about that first shot. You might psych yourself OUT of a good one! I think the key is to play often. You just lost a reference point, now you need to find a new one. I noticed a huge improvement last year. not in the score, but definitely in the quality of the shots. I'm hoping to play a lot more this year, but of course that depends on the weather. Last summer was very wet and cold.—*Jessie*

Hi Jessie, you were right about last summer. Cold and rainy for most of it. I plan to play and practice a lot this year. I want to get back to the level I was at when the season ended last year. It may be hard, but I have a bunch of friends and Pros willing to give me any help and support I need. I can't wait. By the way, just got my new eye today. It looks real good. I look like me again. My ocularist did an amazing job.—*Guy*

Guy, congrats on the new eye! I'm lucky. so far, I still have my "real" eye, and I'm thankful for that. Anyway, with luck the weather will break soon for both of us. Still cool here. 20's and 30's, but the sun has been shining lately (we seem to have cloud cover from November until March. Right in the middle of the Lake Effect bands. makes for a long winter!).

Take advantage of all the tips your friends can offer! In all fairness to me, the stroke per hole that I've added may not be the fault of my vision loss (or at least not 100%). I've also had wrist surgery on both hands, and was in quite a bit of pain prior to that. The wrists are completely healed this year, so I'm hoping to regain some of what I lost. Have a good one. congrats again on the new eye!—*Jessie*

Hi Guy, I have been blind in left eye since either birth or early childhood, due to a poorly formed or deteriorated optic nerve. I've always golfed with just one eye. Recently I switched to putting left-handed as I can see and read the line better with my good right eye. I've considered going left-handed for all shots, but I learned to play with right handed clubs and the vision thing doesn't seem to hamper my long and medium shots. Good luck with your game.—*JK*

Got out and played this weekend. Shot 86 for my first round. Not very good at all, but all things considered not too bad. I played on Sunday as well and shot 78 and missed a few makeable putts so my score could have been better. It was a much better day and I felt better about my game. I know it will take some time to get back to where I was. Looking forward to playing more and more.—*Guy*

Well before I lost my eye I used to be able to drive a golf ball pretty accurately and my putting sucked. About 5 months after I lost my left eye, I was in a Texas scramble tournament, the first time on the golf course after my eye loss and could not drive a ball straight for the life of me, but putting I was making 35 foot putts! Could not believe my putting! And the best part was WE WON 1ST PLACE! I still golf, not as good as before but I love the game. Now billiards, that is another story all together!—*Ski*

I never realized much difference in playing except on and around the greens. I was a 4 handicap when I lost my eye and lost my right eye (my dominant eye) which I found as an advantage as a right hand player. Jack Nicholas used to tape his right eye closed when he practiced to develop his left eye dominance which is crucial for a right hand player for hand eye and alignment, because you will find difficulty in reading greens and depth perception. A little trick helped me a great deal. While sizing up your shot, keep your head moving a little forward and backward and side to side. This lets your brain see the small differences in depth and greatly helps in seeing undulation and distance.—*TBone*

◆ ◆ ◆

Throughout my life, I have dealt with a certain amount of adversity. Despite being born blind in one eye, I realized that in order to achieve my goals in life, I needed to work hard and believe in myself. The skills I acquired along the way were instilled in me by my parents. I feel very fortunate that they taught me the values of education through athletics. They believed that athletics would give me the dedication and discipline needed to excel on the field and in the classroom. They always stressed that education should be the number one priority. As a result, I soon came to realize that with perseverance and good study habits, anything is possible.

Looking back on my career in the National Football League, I feel a great deal of pride knowing that there was no obstacle too large keeping me from achieving my dreams. Sincerely,—*Wesley*

20

Coping with Driving

The first thing you should know is that—at least in the U.S.—you are not going to lose your driver's license. Pretty much all of the states allow one-eyed drivers, so long as their eye is correctable to close to 20/20 vision. You probably want to check with your state's motor vehicle department for any special restrictions or rules, but by and large your state probably won't care that you only have one eye (unless you try to drive a big rig or a school bus).

Sadly, as you will read, some foreign countries will not issue driving licenses to those with only one-eye. This is unfair and, frankly, stupid. But it is the law in some countries. Mostly, it seems to be in the Far East.

The next thing you should know is that outside of about 20 feet, everybody sees the world as if they only had one eye. This means that your driving will be pretty much unchanged for everything that you see which is more than 20 feet away from you. But you do have to watch out for two things:

First, and most importantly, you will not have the same peripheral vision as you did before, because of your nose. This means that you will have somewhat of a "blind spot" on the side of your lost eye. It will take a couple of days to get used to this blind spot, and you will need to learn to turn your head more frequently from side-to-side instead of merely relying on sideward glances from your remaining eye.

Second, within about 10 feet you may have a slight decrease in depth perception. This means that you must be especially careful in parking, and you should avoid "tight spaces". I've found that it is easier to back into spaces, using my mirrors to position my car within the lines. Although at first this can seem slightly difficult, with time it is easier to do than pulling straight in, and your chances of dinging somebody when you pull out are much lower.

I suggest that you mount some "fish-eye" mirrors on your side rear-view mirrors, to help eliminate those blind spots. You might also try one of the large wide-angle rear-view mirrors.

I also suggest that in the future you select vehicles with excellent fields-of-view and few blinds spots. After my surgery, I immediately sold my sportscar and instead purchased a Jeep Cherokee/Ford Explorer-sized SUV which offers excellent visibility and is very easy to corner and park. I would also avoid, at least at first, large automobiles because you might find them difficult to park.

Obviously, you should take greater pains to protect your good eye while driving since if something gets into your good eye you won't have many choices except to slam on the breaks until you can get it cleared.

Except for these two concerns, your driving should be about the same. I suggest that you get out and drive as soon as possible after the loss of your eye, to psychologically reassure yourself that you will retain the same mobility as you had before your loss. For me, it was a big mental step towards recovery to get out and drive myself to work and back, and figure out that I can still go where I want to go when I want to go there.

But don't be careless—for your first several trips please take someone with you to help you with the blind spots and measuring close distances while parking (this is more for your confidence—you'll find in the first 20 feet that you don't need any help and will be just fine).

Some states will actually give out handicapped placards to those with one eye. Some one-eyers make the application, while others refuse to apply for them on the basis that they are perfectly normal and can simply park further out and walk if they can't find a space they are comfortable getting into.

LETTERS AND E-MAILS

Dear Jay, I found your website recently and wanted to thank you for your wonderful work. I am certain that you gave courage to a lot of people like myself. I've been looking for such a support like this for a long time!

I was practically born with a single vision due to a lazy eye and my left eye never developed an eye sight. Although my case is bit different from most of the people in this website who lost a vision suddenly in life, I had a fair share of pain being a one eye blind.

I moved to California from Boston recently and I had to go through confusion and humiliation at DMV. California DMV told me that I have to renew my driver's license every two year, instead of every four year and I have to take a road test every time I renew my license. I was shocked by the fact that I had to take a road test every 2 year for my life as long as I live in California. When I was in Boston, they honor my good eye vision and I didn't have any condition to drive.

In October 2002, when I went to DMV to renew my driver's license I was told that this rule has changed and that I don't have to take the road test anymore and this one is the last one!! I was excited but my heart sank again when I learned that I still have to come to DMV every 2 year to take the eye exam and my license is valid only for 2 years instead of 4 years!

I assume that you live in California. I would like to know if you have to renew your driver's license every 2 year as well and also used to take road test every 2 years until recently. I could not find any rules or regulation regarding a monocular vision driver. I appreciate it if you could share your experience with California DMV.

Thank you again for your time and for creating such a wonderful website. Good luck! Sincerely,—*Kaoru*

◆ ◆ ◆

Jay, I have recently come across your website and I have to say it's amazing! I lost the vision in my right eye 3 years ago, and I would say I'm pretty much adjusted to it. But I have some questions:

1) Do you know if the driving laws in Canada are the same as the U.S.?

2) Do you know of any support groups in Canada (Toronto area)?

3) What are some good websites to keep up on eye research?

The last question is important to me because I was in an accident which resulted in getting metal in my eye. They managed to save my eye and reattach the retina but I cannot see because I have scare tissue in my eye. I have in effect a blind spot in the middle of my eye. My lens was torn apart so they never put a lens in there, but they said they could if I could develop usable vision. The good thing is that I have peripheral vision still. Thanks,—*Mike*

I can't remember where I read this tip about adjusting auto mirrors, but I followed the tip and it works very well. Most people adjust their outside rear view mirrors so that they can see the area that is most directly behind them. When this is done, there is some duplication of the rear view that's shown by the interior rear view mirror. It's possible to eliminate some of this redundancy and also, most importantly, to eliminate the blind spots. This can be done by merely adjusting the outside rear view mirrors more outwardly. Check the inside and outside mirrors during the adjustment to see the improvement in visibility.—*Anon*

I have one good eye, no useful vision in the other. I play sports, racquetball, baseball, and other hand to eye coordination activities. I have no problems driving a vehicle. I want to start flying aircraft. Do you feel there will be any difficulties in this? I feel confident that, I can perform with one eye. Thank you—*Marcel*

Hello my name is Matt, and I am 22 years old and currently a student at Illinois State University. I came across your site today and think the information is excellent. Although some of the things I read such as on depth perception and driving I tend to have much more difficulty with than you. Unfortunately, I know what you are going through. May 23, I was struck in the left eye by a bungee cord. I had pulled it too hard and the hook straightened out causing the bungee cord to snap back at me. After weeks and weeks of examinations I learned that I had a detached retina, and severe damage to the optic nerve(which obviously is irreparable). Luckily, after many pressure tests to my eye I was extremely fortunate that my eye could actually be saved. Cosmetically it looks pretty much normal besides a cataract that I have developed within the past 8 months from the trauma.

This accident has taught me quite a bit about what I take for granted. I start everyday and think to myself how fortunate I really was, it could have been a lot worse. I now am a vision major at Illinois State University and someday hope to help others just like you and I. Thank you again for all of your effort on this website, it is people like you that go the extra effort and make a significant difference in society and peoples lives. Take care and best of luck to you. Sincerely,—*Matt*

I had brain surgery and now have double vision. I have a contact to block the vision of one eye so I would be driving with one eye. The thing is I haven't driven regularly for over 3 years. I know I'd have to get my license renewed, but will it be more difficult and dangerous for me to drive? Thank you!—*Cristina*

I am 27 years old and blind with one eye. I lost my one eye when I was just one year old. I never felt any depravedness throughout my life. One year before I came to Saudi Arabia and join Ernst & Young. Here the life style was some what different and your life without a car is incomplete there is no public transport then I was very uncomfortable. Today I decided to search Google for an expert view either I can drive a car or not, and the result was favorable by visiting your site which is very informative and supportive. Now I am feeling very good that I can do any work and I am not disabled. Thanks for your support and effort and for your kind information. Kind regards,—*Zaman*

Hi Jay, I have been legally blind in my right eye since birth. I live in LA and have a CA driver's license. I read the Driving: One Eye page with interest, and I was wondering how you got a handicapped sticker. I have trouble sometimes, especially in reverse. Like you, I think being able to access handicapped parking would help. By the way, I have a Subaru Forrester with a huge windshield and rear window. It has virtually no blind spots, which helps immensely! Thanks,—*Penelope*

◆ ◆ ◆

Jay, Thank you so much for getting back to me. I am so happy you started your web site. I plan to introduce myself in the forums very soon. In my 35 years I have never met anyone else with one lost eye and I am really relieved to find a support group. By the way, you rock for getting your pilot's license!—*Penelope*

I was glad to find your site, my son wants to drive but has very poor vision in one eye, due to a true lazy eye, it cannot be corrected with glasses. I didn't think he would be able to. He really just uses the one eye. Thanks for your info. I am sorry you had to lose your eye, but you have a great attitude and are helping others cope.—*Pat*

My daughter was born with a blind right micropthalmic eye. She is now 16 and wishes to get her driver's license. I am having some difficulty in teaching her. She has a hard time staying in the middle of the lane and often drives too far on the right. Also, lane changes are difficult for her. I'm not sure what to do to help her correct this. Do you have any suggestions? Thanks.—*Patricia*

Hello Jay, I have been checking out web sites and came across your. You have some really GREAT info. I was diagnosed with Carotid Cavernous Fistula in March and suffered damage to the nerve in my right eye which caused me to become cross eyed and forced to wear a patch. The most difficult part has been deep perception and driving. I am doing good, but it's still a little scary going out there on the great black asphalt. I am also a librarian, this makes it double the trouble. The one good thing that came out of this is my best friend and I have started a business making eye patches. We figure since I had to wear them I might as well have some fun with them. It makes me happy when a child comes up to me and instead of looking at me like I am the boogie man, they say "Wow, that's a cool patch." I giggle and say Thank You.—*Wendy*

I want to applaud you on your website. My husband has just been diagnosed with a large choroidal melanoma in his left eye. There is tremendous stress and worry about his future. The information on your site about driving and depth perception really helped my husband greatly. Thank you so much.—*Sherrie*

Hi, Jay-interesting website. I lost my left eye due to trauma 1985. Most of what you have said about driving, depth perception, field-of-view, etc I have found to be true also. I lost my eye removing the back door from a '58 Chevy station wagon. The steel rod that it was mounted on sprang out and hit me in the face. I don't recommend this to others. Hurt like hell. Have a happy.—*Tom*

Jay, I am Matias from Argentina and I haven't my left eye since I born and I'm so sad mostly because I think I could never drive but your page really help me.—*Matias*

I hoped u fine, I am graduated student studying biomechanics in Iran. I research in "Driving with One Eye" and special rear view mirror for those lost one eye. Can u explain these mirror and position of them at car. I need your help. The best regards,—*Reza*

I would like to know if there are sensors for the left side of a car? I am blind in my left eye. So any type of whistles bells or lights to help me drive with confidence would be appreciated.—*Robert*

Hello. Your site is a very good one. I'm 18 and I have yet to get my permit or license because I've only been able to use one eye for most of my life. I have corneal scarring and we don't have the money to get a corneal transplant for me yet. I was wondering, will I still be able to get a permit/license with basically only one functional eye? I live in California and have about 20/30-20/40 vision in my good eye. All help is appreciated and thank you for making such a great site, thanks.—*Jason*

Hi my name is Nicholas I lost the vision in my left eye due to an illness, the optic nerve was severed. I really was enlightened by your site. I live in Massachusetts and I do drive, it has been quite a learning experience. I'm glad to finally see that there are people who are in the same situation as me. Take care—*Nicholas*

I was wondering about my nervousness about driving. When I drive, I can't tell how close I am to the car that's driving parallel to me. Its very frustrating and I am constantly worried that I am driving on the other side of the lane. Even checking my side-view mirrors doesn't really help. I still worry about it. Is there anything that I can do to learn how to tell how far my car is from another car when I drive in parallel to it? Thanks for listening.—*Ley*

MESSAGE THREADS

Hi, I can try & give you an answer to your two questions: 1) Each state set their own vision standards. For example, in Massachusetts a regular license is issued for 20/40 or better vision in the better eye and a day license when vision is 20/70. Most state require either a vision test or if there is a question then a doctor's statement. So, most people with only one good eye can pass the vision requirements. 2) The IRS deduction for blindness applies to legal blindness, which is either a very restricted visual field or 20/200 or worse in the better eye with correction. Most people with one eye are not legally blind. You can take it only if you do not itemize & meet the requirement. Good luck,—*Jeff*

◆ ◆ ◆

I was in a room, with 5 other people, but between us all, there were only 7 eyes working! (I was tempted to enter for the World Record of getting the most monocular people in a room at once, but as most of you guys are across the pond maybe that wouldn't work! lol) 5 of us were monocular, 3 had lost sight in their left eyes (myself included) and 2 had lost their right.

The conversation got around to who had the hardest time driving. Those of us with left eye loss, said that roundabouts, looking over your left shoulder reversing and cyclists coming up on your inside were difficult, those with the right side loss said that lane changes and the natural blind spot in a right hand drive vehicle made their life more difficult. So what are your views?

Remember we are driving Right Hand Drive Vehicles, on the Left Side of the Road, whereas you guys in the US are the other way round. So I guess what ever you find difficult, I just swap around to fit in here. Confused?! LOL. Anyway, its just a wee fun question to compare notes! Love n Hugs to all,—*Elizabeth*

◆ ◆ ◆

Just prior to my accident, I was about to purchase a pickup and horse trailer so I could transport my horse to shows. I'm feeling good about my driving so far.(I had my eye removed on 1/19/05) but I'm wondering if pulling a trailer would be a stretch for me? Anyone have experience. Especially at night?—*Jan*

I have towed a 26 foot travel trailer to Florida from Virginia several times and north to Wisconsin and just about every place in between with no problem whatsoever. Although I just had my enucleation in November, I have been totally blind in my right eye for 15 years. I have become so accustomed to using my mirrors with the little birds eye mirrors, I almost never turn to look behind me. I say go for it. It won't take long before it is completely natural. Good luck,—*Shaggy*

Lost the use of my right eye, and have been pulling trailers ever since. it took a bit to get adjusted to the depth changes, but I haven't had any problems so far, and I pull several trailers during the week as part of my work. I have two SUVs and have been able to tow trailers with them both. Lost use of right eye during a traffic accident. Doctors are trying to rebuild eyelids to regain some usage, but till they work out a way to build or transplant just eyelids.—*Froggy*

♦ ♦ ♦

Jan, I have found towing trailers to be no problem at all as long as you have good towing mirrors on each side of the cab. I imagine this is the same for driver though. I never had towed anything prior to the loss of my right eye at 19 so I don't know any different. Got pretty good at backing boats down extended ramps when I lived in Illinois.—*KC*

♦ ♦ ♦

Hi! I'm new here, and take the chance to ask a question I hope you guys will help me with. I'm blind in one eye (from birth—actually, it's more like a really bad lazy eye) and recently got my drivers' license. Thing is, although I was really proud to pass the test, I'm a pretty bad driver, and nobody seems to understand why. Basically, I'm scared, and it has to do with my blind eye. or should I say my blind spot. My blind eye is the left one, and I find it really tricky to get on the freeway/highway, or simply to turn. I know it's because of my eye cause I drove in New-Zealand and in Australia, and found it much easier! But let's be realistic, it's very unlikely that Canada will start driving on the left side (and I don't want to immigrate in OZ) I also have problem to see where I'm going. Okay, it's not that bad, but I'm always scared to take the wrong way—it's hard to see the road as a "whole". I can't explain it! I'm never going to turn into a Formula 1 driver, but I'd like to get some advice to feel more comfortable driving.—*Jul*

I started using round mirrors when I bought my used car and it just happened to come with them. But they're really good, it helps you with your blind spots, which is when a car is next to you but farther back. It does take a little getting used to though. I'm sure they sell it in most car accessory stores.—*Andrew*

I'm blind in my left eye too, and here in Ireland and the UK we drive on the left. But I find it more difficult!?! I have 2 other family members blind in one eye, one of them is blind in his right eye, (so the same situation as you only reversed, if you understand what I mean?) and he finds it easier to drive here than in the US. Strange! LOL. We all have problems with driving at first, but I think the more you drive then the more you get your confidence built up.—*Elizabeth*

Hi all, thanks for replying to my message—I feel that for once I'm with people who know what I'm talking about! Irishangel, I still think it's harder to get on the freeway when you're blind in your left eye. For me, it's mostly because even if I turn my head to the maximum, well, after all I'm human and my head doesn't rotate 360 degrees, so there's always a blind spot. It's also hard to judge the speed of other cars. I spend so much time wondering whether I have time to go or not! That's actually surprising for me, cause having only one eye never caused me troubles (maybe cause it's from birth).—*Jul*

Hi Jul, I'm blind in the left eye and understand the uncomfortable feeling of merging on to an interstate or changing lanes to the left. My advice is to give a signal/show your intention of merging/changing lanes well in advance of doing it. Then as you are going with the flow of the traffic, take your time on making the merge instead of jumping lanes quickly. Maintaining the speed, just sort of "inch" over gradually. If there's a vehicle in your blind spot(s), hopefully he will blow his horn to warn of his presence, or slow down some to allow you to get in. A quick glance over the left shoulder and rear-view mirror and side view mirror monitoring are essential too.

Another thing that I find myself doing is being conservative about changing lanes. So what if someone is driving 5 mph slower than me in front of me? Unless there's an urgent need to change lanes, I'll back off on my speed, until I am very sure there is no one in the lane to my left. There are gadgets—-mirrors, cameras—-that I've heard other people have success using. I haven't tried them, yet, but have been toying with the ideas.—*JK*

Thanks for your advices JK. One thing which actually drives me crazy, is despite I signal myself really well (I'm prob. one of the most cautious drivers around here!), there's always someone to speed so that you can't get in. The first time ever I drove by myself, I was try to get out of one of those huuuuge parking lot, and I was being really careful, cause which all those big SUV and me in my small car, well, blind spots are easy to get. Anyway, 2 minutes later, I got yelled at for going to slow (actually, the guy wanted to park—hey, some people are in a hurry to go to the store). I got off of my car and yelled back that he should distract a half blind lady while she drives, that I could cause trouble and accidentally "bump" his car. Okay, that's bad. But felt good!—*Jul*

Hi Jul, this is the blind in one eye giving advice to the blind in the other eye You mentioned sometime you are not sure if you can go, it is hard for me to do but I try to wait until I'm sure. The people who get mad are just looking for someone to get mad at anyway. If I'm merging and someone is tailgating me I slow down some so they will also have to slow down, and then I speed up to get them off my butt so they won't be there to pass me right as I merge. There are times merging will be very difficult even for people with both eyes.

I think it's helpful to look for a flow and fit in somewhere, or create your own flow by speeding up or slowing down, I try to be really careful but sometimes I do speed up pretty quick in order to merge, then you have to watch out for the person in front so they will not slow down while you are merging. I avoid rush hour when possible, and I try to never ever never ever never ever tailgate, tailgating kills!! I think if you ever drive in Nashville it is also good to pray before you start your car, the drivers are so crazy and impatient here every time you drive might be your last chance to pray on this earth.—*Barry*

I think we all have problems with merging lanes and turning out of junctions, I know I find it difficult and especially at night time. As for driving in a small car, I always prefer the SUV kind of vehicle, as then I'm up high and can see a lot of what's going on. One Eyed Queen of the Road! LOL. Off the road, I'm having problems with lamp posts at the moment and so I have a rather sore shoulder today.—*Elizabeth*

Driving is not ANY different for the one-eyed driver, it just requires moving the head around slightly more (which, as others have said, the use of mirrors can alleviate). So get out there and go, and quit making excuses!—*Jay*

Jay, I'm not making excuses—I'm trying to talk to people with the same problem as me to improve and find solution. I'm perfectly fine with having only one eye and never had any problem with it. Only recently when I started to drive I found it tricky. Sure, it can be psychological as well, but I still think driving with one eye is slightly different than driving with two working eyes. Being confident about our difference is one thing, being over-confident is another. I think I can achieve exactly the same as a person with two good eyes, but I sometimes need tips on how to do it. I'm not complaining or crying on that everyday, I was just asking for your opinion. Thanks you Irishangel—stop hurting lamp posts.—*Jul*

It is slightly different. Emphasis on slightly. The only time that it bothers me is at night on a fast freeway, like the I-5 up from San Diego where everybody is driving 90. There, sometimes it's hard to know when some black vehicle has slipped into your blind spot. Otherwise, you shouldn't have any problem driving so long as you learn to move your head around slightly more. FWIW, it's also better to buy an SUV so that you are higher up and have better visibility.—*Jay*

◆   ◆   ◆

I have been monocular for about 1 and 1/2 years after an strabismus surgery that the Dr. did not follow standard practice. Lost sight on my left eye. Driving has been my passion for over 40 years, specially long trips (1k to 3K) and of course that night driving is there. Right after a third surgery I had to travel by car (could not fly due to the surgery) to California from New Mexico and while I was not doing the driving I started to notice that at night it was a lot more difficult for me to distinguish the road, signs and approaching vehicles.

I mentioned it to my doctor and he said that it was to the fact that I needed a new prescription, something about "refraction". I got the new prescription and since then, the same. This becomes even more difficult when there is rain or snow, when I have to fully concentrate on some "marks" to have any idea where I am. I increased the light on my headlights and this had improved the situation a bit. I understand for another message that not many doctors want to deal with this issue. Please let me know your experiences. Saludos,—*Jorge*

I am sorry about the trouble you are having but I totally understand since I have the same problem. My night vision is terrible—especially in rainy weather. I don't know if this is different since I lost my eye shortly after birth. My husband says if he closes one eye, it is more difficult to drive. I now just do my best to avoid driving at night. It is limiting, though. Take Care,—*Mini*

◆ ◆ ◆

Hello, I have a question about driving with one eye, its quite simple, how many hours can you drive? I feel like I can only drive for about 2 hours, then my eye starts to hurt badly and I can't concentrate anymore (after work, where I have to read a lot that is). Are there any pain relief eye drops or pills or anything like that, for those kind of problems? Thanks,—*RB*

Hello RB, I've never placed any driving limitations on myself. Last month I drove to Michigan, which is a 13-hour drive, and I drove straight through with meals and occasional rest stops along the way. I do, however, try to drive mostly during the daylight hours when planning long trips. That prevents eye strain due to night time driving. I guess it depends on the individual. I don't see why there should be any eye pain. Now that confuses me.—*Brenda*

Hi, RB, I also find it uncomfortable to drive for long periods of time. My eye doesn't necessarily hurt, but I get more of a tension headache. I think it's because I feel constantly on guard in the car. I try to be super-aware of the road to make up for my lack of peripheral vision. Does anyone else feel uncomfortable in narrow lanes? I tend to worry that I'm getting too close to the cars on my blind side.—*Adeline*

I find that looking in the mirrors on both sides to see where the lines are. If I can see the yellow, or white lines in the mirrors. then I know I am in the middle of the lane.—*Michael*

♦   ♦   ♦

I'm not sure what fisheye mirrors are but, I have these small, round wide-angle convex mirrors that glue onto my regular side-view mirrors. They take time getting used to but are very helpful. (Actually, I never thought to get them, but my used car just happened to come with them).—*Andrew*

I found what is called the Lane Changer at the local Canadian Tire and they are apparently available at any store that supplies auto accessories. It is great! NO more blind spot and now everyone in my family uses them! By the way the Lane Changer is a mirror that you can mount over top of the rear view mirror in your car.—*Ski*

♦   ♦   ♦

I've never really thought twice about it, coming from someone who has lived in New York her whole life! I simply took the required eye exam (just looking into a machine and reading the letters) and passed. I never mentioned it. It was never asked. HOWEVER, the last time I renewed my license, they gave a new eye exam. They asked me to cover each eye separately and read the eye chart. I had to explain that I couldn't do that, and then they said, "We can't renew your license. .". I ended up going to a different Department of Motor Vehicles to renew it, and they had the old eye exam there.

I am extra careful with my driving. I turn my head a lot to accommodate for the loss of vision in one eye. I don't, however, drive on major highways here (we have lots of traffic), as I'm not comfortable. Anyway, my advice is to keep on trying to get that license. Our eyesight is limited, but we can still see. Would they discriminate against someone with any other disability there?? You can pass an eye exam and you can see, so I don't see why they'd be hesitant in giving you your license. Good luck and let us know how you do!—*Chris*

♦   ♦   ♦

Salut Zhu, it's Anna here. I am Polish but live in Australia for the last several years. I was trying to get my drivers license in Poland but finally got it in Australia. I've passed my test and got my probationary drivers license. I did not have any problems. The only issue for me is to drive during night time. I do not know how about you guys but I do not fee comfortable. And of course I have to turn my neck much more when I want to have a look what is going on my right side, but apart from that everything is fine. Well maybe except that my sense of directions is pathetic, but hey, no one is perfect. A bientot.—*Anna*

◆   ◆   ◆

Well I may have mentioned before I lost my left eye 2 months after passing my driving test here in the UK. But like most of you I adapted. since then I have drove for a living I have drove 7.5 ton wagons,vans, long cars short cars. I now drive fork lift truck at work. (and I would challenge anyone to say I cant drive as good as them with 2 eyes) I love multi story car parks. I had a bad smash last year into a wall at night but that could happen to anyone. Keep driving!—*Kevster*

Kevster, don't you find your depth perception a bit dodgy? I lost my eye before I was old enough to drive so I can't compare and you might say it was because I am a woman driver, but there's some things, like parallel parking, where I seem to have to try much harder than two eyed people.—*Chil*

Nah, I can parallel park quite easy its just a case of using your wing mirrors, I never used them before but they are essential now! See you,—*Kevster*

Kevster, I noticed you said you drove 7.5 ton wagons after losing your eye. When did you do your driving test? I have been told that I will be ineligible for parts C1&D1 on my license (since all post 1998 licenses don't have those parts automatically) and so I cannot join any UK ambulance service (apart from the West Midlands though) because C1&D1 are a must before employment. This was a major blow because being a paramedic was all I wanted to do and now I can't. Anyone I have spoken to says that's its the UK's law and they're final, so even though those with pre-1998 licenses who have one eye are allowed to drive small trucks and minibuses those of us who came after aren't. Personally I feel its discrimination but the powers that be don't see it that way nor do they seem to care! Does anyone else know of laws in the US or Canada or Anywhere where those with one eye are prevented from driving small trucks and vehicles which can carry 9-16 passengers? Anyway, The Republic of Ireland (just down the road lol) DOES allow those with one eye to apply for C1&D1 entitlement and so that's where I am headed, first to study nursing and then to hop aboard an ambulance!—*Elizabeth*

♦ ♦ ♦

When I leave a bright room and walk into a dark room, or vice versa, I have to stand there for several seconds until I can see anything at all. This is a major problem while driving at night due to the 3million watt headlights in cars now a days. Do any of you have the same problem? I asked my doc and he said, "it is all in my head, the optical nerves are connected and your brain is trying to process input from the eye that is no longer there".—*James*

James, I have some limitations with my driving. I don't like to drive in the dark, but I attributed it to heredity-my mom has "night blindness" when it comes to driving. Both she and I are able to drive at night only if it's somewhere close by. I am somewhat sensitive to lights also. I do better if a room is softly lit, rather that really bright. I also HATE fluorescent light. I just assumed that all of this was just "me" and had nothing to do with the loss of an eye. Never gave it a second thought!—*Chris*

It does get better with time. At first I had to wear double sunglasses when I went out side. Now I am able to use the computer and adjust the lighting to my comfort. Still have trouble in stores with florescent lights, but new tinted glasses have helped. So glad I have found this site.—*Sueanne*

21

Protecting Your Good Eye

You will want to give your remaining eye much better protection and treatment than you have before. First and foremost, this must include very regular visits (at least every six months, if not more frequently) to a qualified medical professional to check your remaining eye for any diseases or abnormalities.

Second, you must take other special precautions to protect your remaining eye. Glasses are a must. Before I had my eye removed, I went to an eyeglass store and purchased several pairs of wraparound prescription sunglasses, of the type you normally see in a Clint Eastwood cop movie or on Arnold Schwartzenegger. These give my eye substantial protection from accidents, as well as protect it from harmful UV rays. They are also stylish, and I don't have any problems wearing them indoor or out in all situations. Lately, I've been wearing so-called "Transitions"(TM) lenses that automatically darken when I step into light, and those are very convenient.

Even around the house you should wear glasses at all times to protect your remaining eye, and preferably use safety glasses. If your work or hobbies include wood or metal working, you must use safety goggles (you should have been using them anyway). And be sure to wear glasses whenever participating in any activity, including such innocuous activities as playing with pets.

You should probably avoid any surgical procedures on your eyes, such as corrective surgery, which have even the risk of introducing disease or abnormalities into your good eye. For most people, it just will not be worth the risk of losing sight. If you are compelled to have some form of eye surgery, have it done in one of the several well-known eye institutes around the nation, and not just by your local practitioner.

MESSAGE THREADS

Hi all, I was curious, who here wears contacts and only has one eye? I wear contacts and have 1 1/2 eyes, I guess you could say! I have good vision in my right eye w/glasses or contacts (near sighted), and poor vision in the left. I have some vision in the left eye, but not much, so I say I have 1 1/2 eyes! I had an inoperable childhood cataract in my bad eye when I was born. you can't tell though. I like wearing contacts, but always fear getting an eye infection because of them and hurting my good eye. Anyone else here have that fear? I don't wear my contacts as much as I used to, because I fear injuring the good eye. I've read a lot of stuff on eye injuries that has kind of made me nervous about wearing my contacts so often. I usually only wear them when going somewhere nice. I'm a 24 yr old married female, and mom. I also attend college part time. Anyone else here go to college and have one eye? Sometimes I feel a little down when I think of all of the other students around me w/20/20 vision not straining as they read the chalkboard or their work in front of them. It makes me feel a little different. I usually don't tell anyone else other than family about my condition. Take care all. Bye!—*Tammy*

I wore contact(s) only for my wedding. I have that fear too. Plus, I feel more protected with my shatterproof eyeglasses.—*Chris*

It is so funny, because I wear a contact lens everyday of my life. My eye doctor who I have been going to for my whole life urges me to wear glasses once in a while if I can to give the eye a break. However, he has never told me not to wear the lenses. The only thing he says is to not go beyond 12 hours a day. I wore glasses my whole life up until age 13 (I am 22 now). I hated wearing glasses and now that I have the option of wearing contacts I choose that any day. I do have glasses that are cute, but I don't tend to wear them. I am very into fashion and so I have the plastic framed glasses, but for some reason, contacts always win. I don't know why, but the fear of wearing a contact and hurting my only good eye never really haunted me. Maybe I am the only one who feels this way?! I guess whatever works for you is the way to go. Anyway, Hi to everyone and hope everyone reading this is doing well. BTW, I'm going to see my surgeon this afternoon to show him the end result now that I have my prosthesis. I am in love with him so maybe he will fall in love with me now that I am feeling and looking beautiful! Love always,—*Jodi*

I never wear a contact, always glasses. I'd be really scared of an infection in my good eye. I also don't use power tools or ride in convertibles or on horses or on motorcycles and I haven't for many years. I'm an artist and I won't risk the vision in my good eye. I'm also in college and I can't hide the fact I have one eye, it's fairly obvious. I wear an eye patch to protect my bad eye from fumes and the toxic substances I work with in the studio. My classmates have gotten used to me in a patch and we sometimes joke about it. I lost most of the vision in my left eye before I was 2 years old when I was hit with an arrow, so I've had a lifetime to get used to it. I'm in my fifties now, the eye is totally blind. The most important consideration for me is to protect the vision I have left.—*Sleepy*

I wear a contact lens in my good eye, which is my right eye. I never saw out of the eye that I lost, so I, too had a lifetime to learn how to live with only one eye. I wore glasses when I was growing up and because my left eye was smaller, the lens in that side of the glasses was always magnified. Just before I graduated from high school, my doctor and I discussed contact lenses and he agreed that it would be fine and actually, because of my prescription being so strong, a contact lens would be better for me. I, too, am very careful to protect the vision in my right eye. Eleven years ago, my retina in my right eye detached. Luckily, it was caught very early and I had surgery to repair it. I now go to the eye doctor twice a year to have my vision checked, just to be safe.—*DJ*

Hey guys, thanks for your replies! It's nice to know there are others out there like me. DJ, what caused your retinal detachment, or does your eye doctor know? Glad they caught it in time. Well feel free to post everyone, or reply as much as you like. Take care all, and good luck w/everyone's future eye appointments and eye care!—*Tammy*

Hello all. I wear only glasses now for safety whenever I'm doing yard work, regular whenever I'm outside. It's a safety thing. I stopped wearing contacts about 5 years ago. I awoke one morning, and my vision was very cloudy in one eye. It got progressively worse as I drove into work, so I ended up in the emergency room. I has sloughed off a layer or two of cells on my cornea! The night before, I was cooking with jalapeño and other spicy peppers. 2 showers and multiple hand washes later, I put my contacts in the next morning. Apparently the oils from the peppers were on my fingers, and when I touched my eye. I basically "burnt" it! No lasting damage, but since losing sight in my right eye, I guess I'm just a little scared.—*Jessie*

Tammy, they never did figure out what caused the detached retina, which didn't really surprise me. It seems I'm a complete mystery when it comes to my eyes. As I mentioned, I was born blind in my left eye (which I lost) and there are a couple of things they never figured out before I lost the eye. First, they couldn't figure out why my eye grew to stage 2 (which I'm told is growth and control of movement, which I had), but never continued to stage 3 which would have been final growth and sight and they also couldn't figure out how I contracted glaucoma in an already blind eye. It's fun being a mystery.—*DJ*

◆ ◆ ◆

First of all I just want to say hi. I've just come across this website! Ok I've been blind in my left eye for almost five years due to an assault. After an initial period of readjustment I learned to drive and returned to playing sports etc without any major difficulties. The problem I have been having recently though is that I have had a few near misses on my good eye whilst playing sports—I had to receive stitches in my eyelid recently! Does anyone know where I can get my hands on any good goggles or glasses for sport? (in Ireland)?—*Gerald*

◆ ◆ ◆

I've been monocular most of my life. My corneal graft is now shot to pieces and I will lose the eye. Recently, though I have been thinking of ways to insure my good eye. This has proved more difficult than I though, so any help greatly appreciated!—*Simonfish*

Gee, I hardly EVER worry about my "good eye" until I have a near-accident of some sort (being poked; bleach in the eye, etc.). Only then do I think, "I should wear my glasses ALL of the time for protection," but I never follow through. When you stop and realize that we'd be blind if anything happened to our "good eye," it's very scary. Lemme know if you get anywhere with insuring your eye. Very interesting.—*Chris*

When I was a kid, the schools always sent home insurance forms for parents and mine always insured me for "extra" in case I lost my good eye. A bit strange maybe but they were trying to ensure that if another accident happened, I'd be okay financially. Now, as an adult I have wondered about insuring my good eye and like someone posted before, it only occurs to me seriously when I have done something to bugger up the good eye (I once put my steroid meds for the blind eye in my good eye. it was early one morning what can I say! and wound up with a hugely dilated pupil for a week and I could not tolerate any light!). If anyone from Canada/Ontario has insured their good eye could you please post the details? Thanks—*Starr*

◆ ◆ ◆

Hi all, I had a scary infection on my good eye a couple of months ago. It was very deep infection and caused some scarring on the cornea. The scarring reduced my vision for quite a long time, but it was temporary and I am OK now. The reduction of the vision was that worried me, I had to use a magnifying glass for reading and I did not see far too. I was so worried that I can never see properly although the doctor was confident that my vision returns to normal, however with caution that the scarring may alter my cornea so that I have greater degree of astigmatism. The best advice, I think, came from my ocularist as she recommended a thick lubricant which may have helped to heal the cornea faster. She also said that I should patch it for night for speedier healing, but I did not do it because I was worried that I get a huge shock when I wake up from sleep not seeing anything.

The worst part was when I first went to A&E in the early evening. The first doctor I saw put a patch on and called for a specialist whom I had to wait for hours to come. There I was, totally blinded and very dark thoughts in my mind; I could not even go to toilet without being assisted. I have become a bit paranoid after this episode, I cannot see people sneezing and coughing or infectious looking eyes in public places; I move away very quickly. Has anyone else got a fright like this?—*JPH*

That was a horrible experience. I suspect that we should all be wearing glasses with plastic lenses to offer some sort of protection.—*Chil*

PART VI
PERSONAL ISSUES

22
Mental And Emotional Issues

The loss of an eye brings with it many intense mental and emotional issues. It causes feelings of vulnerability and "Why Me?" It causes feelings of inadequacy, and embarrassment in dealing with family, friends, and others. It causes problems in relationships with spouses and companions, especially as it relates to intimacy. It can also cause deep depression and anxiety.

Most people have a natural desire to be strong and to be seen as strong by the people they deal with. This strength usually leads them to a sense of normalcy, which is emotionally what those who have lost an eye desire the most. Yet, deep down the feelings of vulnerability, inadequacy, and anxiety will continue to percolate, and they can eventually wear a person down and cause them to break inside, if not outside as well.

Thus, it is very important that those who have lost an eye take affirmative steps to deal with their mental and emotional issues. Sometimes these issues can be discussed with close friends and confidantes, while other times the help of a qualified mental health specialist may be desired. There is no shame in seeking professional help, as the loss of an eye is a very traumatic and permanent loss, and the sooner that such help is sought the better. Don't let these issues build up inside you! Let them out!

One of the biggest benefits of our lost eye.com discussion board is that it gives readers a chance to talk about these issues with others who have experienced the same thing. Some countries (but, sadly, not the U.S.) have support groups for those who have lost an eye, and those support groups can be valuable resources in coping with these issues.

LETTERS AND E-MAILS

Hi, I'm a 25 year old Aussie and 4 months ago I had my right eye removed due to a childhood injury which resulted in long term acute glaucoma eventually causing my right eye to become a painful blind eye. I'm still struggling to come to terms with this loss and am still very self-conscious about the appearance of my prosthetic (which probably looks fine to others). If anyone has any advice, or any inspirational thoughts to help me through this it would be greatly appreciated.—*Belinda*

I lost my eye at birth. All of the things that you have discussed have been natural to me. I feel myself lucky. Anyhow, I am 21 now and I just recently had my bad eye removed for a lovely prosthetic to take it's place. It has definitely been a transitional period for me which is not yet over. I had the enucleation last month and will receive my new eye just before Christmas this year. The best present I will ever have! I just wanted to drop you a line because I think your site is wonderful. The site is a great support resource for other people who are scared and don't know where to get the correct info. I applaud you.—*Minta*

I lost the sight in one eye after an accident when I was 9 years old; I'm now 47. I have had quite a successful professional career (I'm in rocket propulsion), but have never been good at making/keeping friends. Someone once told me that it was a "fact" that because people with only one eye have a reduced field of vision, that our "survival instinct" means that we are less secure and less trusting of the world around us. That makes a wonderful piece of "bar-stool" psychology, but I have never managed to find any professional opinion that supports it. Have you ever heard or seen anything that supports that idea? Regards,—*Barrie*

My niece had surgery to remove her eye on February 12. She has not accepted her fate and is having a really hard time with the fact that she sees herself as some kind of freak and feeling very sorry for herself. In short, she is in bad shape. Is there a support group in the US Maryland area? I don't know what else to do for her. She cries all the time and I know this will continue to affect her quality of life. Can you recommend something I can do for her. I bought her the book A Singular View and all the material I could find on the web but nothing seems to help. She is 27 years old and feels her life is over. Any advice would be appreciated. Thanks,—*Fran*

My husband is facing an eye removal within the next year. This is the result of having cataract surgery with uveitis that had not healed properly. He has been doctoring with glaucoma since then, had to have a shunt put into his eye which has the pressure controlled. His vision has gone from good to nothing over the last 3 years. Having the eye removed will help eliminate some of the medication he has to use each day and hopefully decrease infections. Naturally, he is very upset about this removal even though there is no vision in the eye. At 68 years, it is hard for some of us to accept change and I know he is going to have some depression. Your forum is enlightening and reading what others have gone through made me feel better about this surgery. He doesn't use the computer so any messages sent will have to be to my address. One thing you can tell everyone about depression after surgery is that it is normal because your body is grieving a lost part. If you think of it, even having babies cause depression because the mother has lost a part of herself. An old family doctor told that to me and it really has made a lot of sense when dealing with depression after surgery. Thanks again for your excellent information.—*Dolores*

Hi, I am female, now 34 years old. I'm from Philippines and I also lost my one eye on my sophomore year. Until now I am too shy, I am always cant make to looked on my friends and to other people eyes while were talking, I am afraid they looked my left and say something in my back. Please help to overcome this fear. Thanks a lot and more power.—*Annette*

Hi. I had my eye removed at 19 years old I am 22 years old now and have a hard time dealing with it. It gives me a low self-esteem and I feel like every one notices. I always wanted to act and model but I have pretty much given up on that. I am very adventurous and before I had my eye removed I started skydiving, I want to bungee jump but I do not know if I am able to or if my eye will fall out.—*Nat*

Hi as you can see my name is Gregg. I am 28 and I come from Dublin, Ireland. I was born with an underdeveloped left eye and wear a prosthetic eye the match is great but the feel of it is hell! I never knew this website existed and I am really impressed that it does lately I have been feeling very depressed by my paranoia that everyone is staring at me,I could really do with someone to chat to as I am a bit of a drama queen and really in the whole scheme of things my life is very good and I am and should be grateful for an abundance of things, but I am only as strong as the next time I hear the name one-eye! Yours—*Gregg*

Hello to everyone. I had my eye removed in 1993 due to a rare form of glaucoma. After five years of surgery and constant pain I made the decision. I am a registered nurse and have a post grad dip in applied psychology. Doing assignments in monocular style nearly sent me screaming from the computer! The subject of grief and loss is HUGE with the loss of any part of your body. The eyes particularly, as it is one our most precious senses. The grief we experience is called disenfranchisement. Mourning made much harder because it is not treated like other losses. There is no funeral no goodbyes and when you feel sad there is no grave to visit to put the flowers there. After ten years I still have days when I yearn to have my healthy eye back with me. This is a sadness only they that have experienced it will understand. We are all individuals, thank heavens, and you will move through the grief at your own pace. Courage is just a word until it is challenged. If I can help anyone out there please let me listen. Let me help the student with her assignment. Good luck to all my new friends.—*Rosalie*

I am associated with an Ocularist in the New York area and I am often asked by our patients where they can find a support group of other patients to meet with and share their experiences. In searching for such groups I have discovered they are not so easily found. I can find nothing of this sort on the internet, and while your site is the closest thing I have found, and a very informative site indeed, it isn't the same thing I seek. Message forums are helpful too, but there are some patients who are not comfortable with the internet or simply prefer a face to face encounter. For some, they feel the social stigma of their condition can best be understood by other patients. Would you have any information on such a group or how to find such a group? Is the need for such a group addressed anywhere on the internet, or by any organization? Thank you for your time and effort in helping us answer this question.—*Stuart*

MESSAGE THREADS

Hello! I lost my left eye last summer. I had a childhood injury that left me almost blind, and my eye very unattractive. About four years ago, I developed severe glaucoma. After 8 surgeries and four years of extreme pain, I finally got a doctor to take my eye. The initial month afterwards was hard, but nor I am doing great. Most people cannot tell that I have a fake eye. But, best of all I am out of pain. I am 31 years old with two young children and I can live my life again. Like Jay has said living with one eye is really no different than living with two! If anyone has any questions about the surgery, recovery, or transition, please feel free to email me!—*Mindy*

First off, congratulations on your great attitude towards the 180 you pulled in your life. But, there are still some of us who hate having one eye. in my case my lawn mower shot me in the left eye with a rock. I now have a coral implant and a small prosthetic shell. It sucks. There is no way that it is anywhere near the same as having both eyes. Just noticing people looking in my fake eye makes me never want to leave my house. It has only been 8 months since my accident but I don't think ill ever get used to it. Oh well.—*Willy*

Don't take this wrong, but maybe professional counseling will help you. Most people don't know that your eye is a "fake" but will assume that you just have a "lazy eye" like so many people have. I mean, unless you take it out and bounce it on the table, how will they know unless the prosthesis is a really bad one. Do whatever it takes to get a positive attitude back. Probably most of us are cancer survivors, and we're just damned glad to be alive, two eyes, one eye, or none.—*Anon*

◆ ◆ ◆

I lost my left eye in Feb. 2001 to cancer. Unfortunately, I had a doctor that had poor bedside minor, and simply told me to follow up with my family doctor for further screening. I had no resources, or support at all. It wasn't until last August (2002) that I found out I was supposed to be seeing an Oncologist for my cancer. I felt alone and left to deal with it by myself. I'm a single dad and I've raised my son alone since he was 4 months old when his mom left. My cancer claimed my career and I'm struggling to re-learn my life. I'm 45 and my son is 7, and he really helps me to focus on what is really important, and not dwell on things I can't change. I'm thankful that I stumbled onto this site, and for a chance to vent and realize that I'm not the only one in the world going through this.—*Dawgs*

Hi! I lost my vision in my right eye due to treatment of a large choroidal melanoma. This is recent, so some days I'm very positive and others aren't so well. I now have glaucoma in my good eye. I have young children and I'm an artist. Everything I love to do is with my eyes and I'm a very visual person. I found out recently that my cancer is a more aggressive version (Epitheliod sp?) not the spindle variety. My goal is to see my young children grow up and finish high school. I've had wonderful medical care in the form of treatment, but no compassion what so ever. I am now in the process of finding a more compassionate doctor.

On the trivial side, I lost all my eyelashes on the treated eye and being a woman it has made me feel shy. I'm pushing forward and trying really hard to be optimistic, but I've had my days. This week a lump showed up on my spine and I have x-rays next week. It appeared almost over night, so I really feel it is due to a back injury I had years ago. I wonder and just keep telling myself that this will be o.k. too. My vision loss hasn't effected my work and for the most part, life is totally normal. More emotional, but normal. I've learned to cherish everyday and even to embrace the yucky stuff we all have to go through. Thanks for letting me vent. I truly needed to tonight. Hugs,—*Sherri*

I am a 35 year old mom with two young daughters. Choroidal melanoma was my diagnosis with a 10mm epitheliod tumor. After researching further, the outlook was not real great, but so far I am still healthy(with 1 prosthetic eye that doesn't look half bad). My husband doesn't talk about this with me because he wants to think that the cancer thing is fixed and over now. He thinks I am a worrier, I think I am a planner. Some days when I am dwelling on what has happened, I try to ensure that I have things in order in case I metastasize. My youngest is 3 and I want to see her grow up. I am glad the website is here because sometimes I feel alone. The best advice is not to focus on what might happen in one or two or five years, but to do fun things that you enjoy. I often tell myself this advice because I do not have a great support network around me. Take care everyone. Also, Jay is an inspiration to me because he seems to have great strength, and I admire that.—*Mary*

◆ ◆ ◆

The other day somebody asked me in a friendly-enough sort of way, "How's your eye doing, the one with the cancer?" Without thinking about it, I responded, "I don't know, it's in a jar at UCLA. Call and ask them." He didn't think it was too funny, but I thought it was funnier-than-hell, and the more I thought about it the funnier it got.—*Jay*

It's GREAT that you have a sense of humor about it! I'd probably be upset that they mentioned the cancer, and that they reminded you about your eye. You seem to have a great attitude! BTW, do you have to go back for checkups to make sure the cancer is gone? I don't know anything about that, since I lost my eye due to an accident.—*Chris*

When I first lost my eye, (I still had on the patch) I went up to the local Wal-Mart with my wife to get some household items. When we were checking out the stupid kid at the counter said, "What's the deal with the patch? you got an eye out for somebody." I then pulled up my patch to show him and he did not think it was too funny then and tried to apologize. My wife and I just walked out and laughed about it. The majority of the public are idiots.—*Jim*

◆ ◆ ◆

Hello everyone, just found this site and thought it was nice to be able to share things with others that can empathize. I wanted to start off by saying that I was born with no vision in my right eye and have been wearing a prosthetic since I can remember. However, for some reason, I've become more self conscious of my prosthetic in recent years. (I'm 23) I often avoid eye contact. Especially since I had a new prosthetic made just a few days ago, and I'm not too comfortable with it yet. I was just wondering, do most people you know, notice the prosthetic. I've told close friends about it and have asked if they ever noticed anything wrong with my eye. Most have said no, some mentioned that they thought I was a little cross eyed. In any case, this post is getting lengthy. Just wanted to know what others thought. Thanks.—*Anon*

Hey Chris, thanks for the reply. I'm a 23 yr old, male I think the main reason I started feeling self conscious was on a recent date.(I'm a shy guy and don't really date much) In any case, I found myself avoiding eye contact during dinner. I tried not to do it that much, but I couldn't help it. I also had to excuse myself to go to the bathroom to put eye drops on my prosthetic because it gets a little bit dirty, especially when the weather is dry. You said that you have a wife and kids, so its great that you were successful in your personal life. Don't mean to pry but I was just wondering, if your wife when you two were dating, did she notice it or did you just tell her? Thanks for your response.—*Andrew*

Andrew, I realized that *I* didn't say if I was male or female either! Duh! I'm female—sorry! To answer your questions. dating was quite a while ago-23 years ago was when I met my future husband. When we first met, we were friends, and I was going through some surgeries, so I had a patch on my eye for a while. He knew the story right away, and nope, I never felt uncomfortable with him, although relaying the "story" was tough. He's been there with me through many years, and many surgeries, although we really don't discuss the self-conscious part of it.—*Chris*

When you're dating, just remember that anyone worth your time won't be weird about it. And if you do tell them, and their heart breaks a little for you, and then they move the conversation on to any one of the three million things about you that are 'way more interesting than you eye, you may have a "keeper" on your hands. Love and big hugs to all,—*Alicia*

I'd like to thank you ladies for your inspirational stories. I really appreciate your advice. I'm glad I found this forum because its hard for other people to understand. Thanks again,—*Andrew*

Also just found this site. I'm 22, from Liverpool in England. I lost my Right eye when I was 2, ran in front of a swing. Thank God I am too young to remember it. Had mine since I was 7, but I totally rejected it and only started to accept it when I was a teenager of about 14 or so. Growing up was really hard to do, everyone made fun of me through school and it was only when I left and began to meet new people. I built up my confidence slowly. Even now I feel terribly self confident sometimes—people don't seem to understand that it's not something that goes away. Of course people you decide to tell say they can't tell, but in the back of your mind you are always thinking that maybe they and everyone else can. I've always struggled getting close to people because of this, not wanting to get into relationships because eventually I know I would have to tell that person.

How hard is that? lol I guess I'm just looking for someone who understands.—*Tracy*

Believe me, when you meet the right person, you won't feel uncomfortable. You're right: The insecurity is something that doesn't go away (30 years and counting), but you'll feel COMFORTABLE enough when you meet someone special.—*Chris*

Hello Chris, I am 28 years old girl/women. I am assertive person but I have to say that because of my prosthesis I don't feel 100% self confident. When I have my new prosthesis I feel like everyone is looking at me. This feeling is stronger than logic. Thanks God I've got very supportive sister and my boyfriend who is telling me that I am a beautiful women. I think all of us need to hear that we are pretty as probably majority of us lost self confidence after having eye removed. It doesn't have o be like that. It's up to us. I know that many people doesn't know that I do not have my right eye, that I have the prosthesis. The most important thing is to feel comfortable with your prosthesis and to know that it doesn't make any difference for other people. At the end I would like to say that I feel much better and prettier with my prosthesis than with my eye which was—thanks God—removed 13 years ago.—*Anna*

Anna, you're right—it's important for us to hear that we're attractive, especially when we don't feel too confident at times. It's hard to remember that we're more than just the way we appear. We want to be accepted and hope that no one dwells on any difference between our eyes. It's good that you have a loving sister and a boyfriend who are supportive. Stay healthy!—*Chris*

Found this site when doing a paper for my college class. Writing about the feelings I had when I lost my eye when I was a kid. Neat to know other people do have the same concerns I had then and now. Hope and pray for anyone that has to accept the loss of an eye that it does not slow them down. I hunt, play softball and anything else I can get away with. I will check in and offer any support I can.—*Chil*

◆   ◆   ◆

How do you find it best to refer to having one eye or to wearing a prosthesis. Over the years I know I've done it wrong. When I had to get time off work for an operation to fit a secondary implant and my boss asked exactly what eye operation I was having, I took it for granted she recognized it as an artificial eye and I heard later that she had been shocked and offended when I referred to it as "a glass eye". Another time I explained to someone "I have an artificial eye" and the response was "I can SEE that". What experiences have you had?—*Chil*

Hi Chil, I had a very similar experience. Mostly people are shocked when I am telling them that one of my eye is not real. I feel really good when people can not notice that. In my opinion generally people do not know. but I have to say that once I had a dinner with my friends and there was an older man which whispered to the other guy "does she have an artificial eye?" He did not know that I heard that. I felt terrible and now I know that I should have been say something but I didn't. I wanted to say something like "Oh, that is amazing that you are still alive, you look so old". I know it is bad to say things like that even to think like that. But really, sometimes it hurts and you want to say: "Why don't those people think!"

But re: your question it is very actual situation to myself because I am having an surgery in 2 weeks and I am thinking what should I say to my colleagues at work and I think I will say that I had a really bad infection and that's why I am wearing an eye-patch. If they will be more interesting what happened I will tell that I want to become a Terminator and the first stage of that process is to put an implant, a red laser point into my eye Why not? Do you think they will believe? Cheers,—*Anna*

Hi Chil, it's Anna again. I am after my surgery. It's been a week. I am wearing an eye patch at the moment/no an artificial eye and I have to tell you that it's difficult, I think more difficult to explain people what's wrong. Everyone is asking what happened? It's funny because when I had my prosthesis no one was asking that question. The most bizarre thing is people who are asking this question are stranger. My reply is: "well, nothing special." That end a conversation, everyone knows that I do not want to talk about it. I am not sure it helps but that's just what is happening with me at the moment. Cheers.—*Anna*

◆ ◆ ◆

Hey Guys, I've finally met someone. YAY! I met him at work and he is sooo lovely, I really get good feelings about him. One problem: He is like the only person in work who doesn't know about my eye (thanks to my manager—who told just about everyone else. Grrrrr). I have such strong feelings for him and I want him to know but I'm not sure how to tell him. I'd like to call on some of the older more experienced guys. HELP—*Tracy*

Tracy, glad to hear that things are going so well for you. I guess I'm in the "experienced" category, since I'm 42 and have dealt with this for over 30 years.

I'm just trying to think back to how I told my "story" to my many boyfriends, friends and then husband. When the time is right, and you are comfortable enough, sit him down and tell him, "There's something I want you to know. It's difficult for me to talk about, but since we've gotten so close, I want you to know." and then I'd proceed to tell him your story—how and what proceeded your enucleation and basically that you have a prosthesis. I don't think I offered many details to begin with, but over time it all came out.

Funny, just recently I've begun to open up about this. I met a dear friend 2 years ago and have told her things that I've never mentioned or realized before. It was freeing. So, don't hold back if you feel comfortable enough, but tell him only what you want to tell! Good luck and let us know how it goes!—*Chris*

◆ ◆ ◆

I think my ocularist did a great job and all, and I've got glasses that have just a slight tint so that it is difficult for people to notice that I've got a prosthesis, but nonetheless sometimes I feel somewhat uncomfortable talking to people who are only a foot or two away, and having to look directly at them.

But on the other hand, I was somewhat uncomfortable with that before I lost my eye too. I was never much of a "hugs" person anyway; more of a Western "keep yer distance pardner" type. Sometimes, I'll wear sunglasses to meetings, which you can often do in Southern California without people thinking much of it, and then of course I don't get those feelings. Thoughts?—*Jay*

Jay, I *am* a hugs kind of person, and I think that I only resent people coming close to me, staring me in the eyes since I lost my eye. The whole time you're trying to look back and them, wishing they'd back up, and hoping that they're not noticing your prosthesis, right? I don't much care for those "close talkers" anyway—makes anyone uncomfortable!

I, too, have my dark blue tinted prescription sunglasses and they help a lot when I'm uncomfortable. They also help when I have a headache and I'm out in public. My "normal" eyeglasses have a light grey tint, and that helps too, but when I get to know people, I feel comfortable enough even if I have NO glasses on. Either they accept me or they don't! I had a close friend who casually mentioned my eye to her two young kids (they were 11 and 8 at the time) and they asked, "IS there something wrong with her eye? We didn't know!". Amazing! So, even when you think people are looking, staring and figuring it out, chances are they aren't noticing. At least that's what I hope!—*Chris*

Jay, I have felt the same as you, but more so after I first lost my eye. You know the old adage, "the eyes are the window to the soul." Well, I couldn't get that out of my head! I'm one of those people that likes to look someone in the eye when I'm speaking to them, and I guess I expect others to be like me, so I felt everyone was staring at me and could tell. And I finally realized that they weren't staring, and that they couldn't tell. I also wear glasses, but I don't have any tinting. One thing I do find myself doing, though, is trying to keep whoever I'm speaking to within a certain range so that I don't have to turn my eyes too far to see them. Although I have fantastic movement with my prosthesis because I have a peg, there are still limits to it's range!—*Nancy*

Jay, I feel kind of weird with close contact too. Sometimes I don't think about it as much, but I do find myself looking at peoples forehead or neck when I talk to them now instead of in their eyes. Recently I was at a family party, and there was a distant nephew I hadn't seen in awhile, and he asked me to point out the lady with the glass eye for him. I just smiled and said that she couldn't make it after all. So maybe they really can't tell.—*Cathy*

◆   ◆   ◆

Hi, I just found this website and found it's got a lot of good info. I'm a 19 yr. old college student, I lost my eye several weeks ago. I haven't had to tell anyone about it yet since I've only seen the family since then. Vacation is over and I'm back to college next week, my question is how or what do I tell my friends about what happened. I'm still stuck with wearing an eye patch till I get a prosthesis, so it's not like it's something I can avoid telling people about. I'm freaked out how they will react and stuff. Any insight is appreciated, Thanks,—*Keith*

Hi Keith, losing an eye is not a nice experience. It is good to have a family around you and forum like this one and friends of course. The question you asked is a difficult one. From my experience I can tell you that I did not tell my friends what happened to me. When people were asking me what happened I was telling that I had an eye-muscle surgery. I was not telling the truth only because talking about a lost of my eye was very painful for me. Is it better to tell the truth? I do not know. What I know is that some people do not know that this is not your natural eye, they just think you've got a small eye problem, something wrong with your muscle or eyelid. Personally I prefer not to tell unless someone who knows how the prosthesis looks like. There is no point of hiding it. Keith, do whatever is the best for you. Good luck. Cheers.—*Anna*

Hi Keith—People are curious, My family/friends are my support and know the whole story, but frequently strangers would ask me when I had my eye covered "what happened to your eye?" I just say, "I had eye surgery." That was the truth and they would be satisfied, normally it would end there, if they pursued the questioning, I just answer, I had a tumor and they removed it." Sometimes, I would get, "the tumor or the eye?" I would just tell them, "the eye." It would be quite shocking but they asked. I don't really care who knows, you can be an example of handling the situation that was given to you in a very positive way. As a hint—what really helped me—I wore an eye band aid—they are normally used for the lazy eye syndrome that kids have but it's a really nice cover over the whole eye and flesh colored—you can get them about 24 in a box at the drug store. They are great in that there is no chance of it falling to the side like a patch and they are very comfortable, you will be able to play sports or anything confidently. Be sure also to get your safety glasses for the other eye. I picked out a cute stylish pair and you will be able to do whatever you did before.—*Loralsar*

Keith, you may be surprised how people will react. Most people won't notice or care. Your friends will be concerned and understanding. Be positive and know that everything will be fine. That will put those around you at ease. You may have only one eye but you are still the same person. I agree with Loralsar.

I was fortunate to a point. I prepared everyone around me of my impending loss. They knew first hand what I was going through. When I returned to work after some time off, I wore no eye patch nor anything to cover my loss. I was lucky. Everyone noticed and asked questions and I felt that God wanted me to educate these people. I work in purchasing and deal directly (in person) with around 60 people. At times I felt self conscious but I reminded myself that I was not the center of the universe and people were not staring at me. Remain positive. You've just experienced a slight bump in the road. God bless you.—*Rich*

Hi, what happened to cause you to lose your eye? I'm a college student to. I was born clinically blind in my left eye. I'm 23 now, and have never had it operated on. I'm sure losing your eye all at once can be a shock though. Don't worry, just tell everyone the truth about what happened, and asked for prayer and support. The support of family and friends can help tremendously in time of trial. I feel a little out of place being a one-eyed college student sometimes at times; but if people don't like me for who I am, then they can bite my butt! Good luck with your situation!—*Tab*

◆ ◆ ◆

Hi, I am new to this forum. I had a Macular hole sugary done on my right eye last June and the sugary failed. The macular hole still open and the vision is very poor. Basically I am like many of you can use only one eye. My good eye has many floaters and the blind spot is bigger than normal person. Although I am back to work as Software Engineer. I am still depressed. I have tried a few anti-depressed medicine, Paxil seems like helps some but the hunger side effect that I could not stand. Now I am totally off anti-depression medicines. I tried a Psychological Therapy for 10 sessions and don't feel much help, may be the Doctor is not expert on depression with eye disorders. Does any one have ideas or suggestions on self help or professional helps on handling depressions caused by eye diseases? Thanks in advance.—*Chuck*

Dear Chuck, I am sorry you are so down and I know from experience that there is not a lot people can say to you. I lost my eye 2 years ago because of cancer so I know what you are going through. I know this is a very good site and you will get some very good help on it. If ever you need to talk don't hesitate to get in touch because just talking and even moaning about it will help. Hope to speak to you soon,—*Anne*

Chuck, first of all, welcome to the board! I think you will find a lot of people willing to help you with your questions and concerns. I, too, suffered from depression after losing my eye. Or maybe the more correct way of putting it is that it worsened something that was already there. Anyway, I went to a psychologist for several months and got limited relief. After about 6 months, he put me on antidepressant medication, and it worked. I was fortunate that the first one we tried did the trick, but my point is that there are several such drugs available and you may have to try a couple before you find one that works for you. I would encourage you to pursue this with your doctor. Good luck, and best wishes for you,—*Nancy*

Hi Chuck. You know, losing any eye is a depressing thing, and it is normal to be depressed, and I know that isn't what you want to hear, but it's true. I have went without my right eye since I was 16, I am now 23, and I'm depressed everyday! I have a prosthetic eye, and I have gotten over that lack of sight from my right eye, which still sucks, but I can cope with it, but the fact that I have hardly any movement is what depresses me. If you still have your original eye, I'm sure it moves just fine, and I'm sure you look perfectly normal. I have never seen you, but I feel I'm accurate, if I'm not, feel free to correct me, and I apologize if I'm wrong. Count that fact you still have your moving eye as a blessing my friend, trust me, I wish I still had a moving eye. About your other eye with the floaters, there are surgeries that can be performed to help remove them, so I see some positives in your future friend, though I do realize the negatives and I feel for you, I really do, but I know you can overcome them! I hope I have helped you.—*Jarrod*

Hi Chuck! Sorry to hear you're feeling down. I am a 23 yr old, married female, from southwest, VA. I was born clinically blind in my left eye, due to a childhood cataract called Posterior Lenticonus. Because surgery is risky, I never had the eye fixed. I only see well with my right eye. I have always led a normal life w/this, and you can too. I got my driver's license, I graduated high school, became a beautician, married, had a child, and am going to college again. I have never let it slow me down. And we should all be thankful if we can see at all.

I saw a story on the news about 2 months ago, about a guy who was about 23 yrs old, and was blinded instantly when a potato gun he was shooting back fired and blew up in his eyes! He was completely blinded in both eyes. I felt so sorry for him, and thought, thank you God that I can see at all. There are so many other people in the world who are worse off. I hope this comforts you some. Take care, and it will all work out, you'll get used to the change with time. Bye!—*Tabitha*

◆ ◆ ◆

Chris, I also have noticed through your posts that you seem to be a very positive and thoughtful person. I am sorry that you get your feelings hurt by insensitive jerks. When I get my feelings hurt, I usually will respond meanly to whoever did this. It is wrong, and I am 36 years old, and should know better, but it is just reflex. If I had been in your shoes I would have said something like "But instead of worrying about my eye, why don't you worry about why you're so.?", (If she had a noticeable flaw, I would bring it up). If she didn't, I would just make up something that I would think would shut her up).

It is a tough world out there (sometimes). Don't give somebody who is unthoughtful, unfeeling, or just rude the satisfaction of ruining one minute of your day. I know my post sounds mean and probably would help nobody. But my intentions are good. I do feel your pain, and wish I could boost you back up to a happy level again.—*Mary*

Chris, keep in mind, this was a 12 year old. When a person cuts another down, ESPECIALLY for something they cannot control/change, it speaks volumes about the person. Mean-spirited comments like these usually come from the mouth of an insecure person. In this case, a 12 year old who is 1) at the age where she isn't sure if she's a woman/child, and 2) likely very torn up about her parents' divorce. I'm not making excuses for her, but sometimes you need to be their bigger person and realize where the comments come from. This sounds like a very insecure child. I feel sorry for her.—*Anon*

Hi Chris, I think most of us would face a situation like yours. I would have acted the way you did if I were you. don't like to confront others who have "big mouth" and out to hurt people's feeling. I would keep quiet especially with my parents around. Don't want them to be hurt as well. For children I would forgive and forget since they are too young to be sensitive to our feeling. But for adults, I would forgive but never forget. Be happy and don't let people like them affect you.—*Anon*

Chris, it's not just the young kids. After a meeting last night, a man I know from the community—probably 60-ish—yelled out to me (OK, said it to my face, but loud enough for anyone w/in a 10 foot radius to hear) "How is that eye doing?" Maybe because I had a stroke, people think the vision will come back. Anyway, I said "no change". He looked at me and said "It looks a lot more normal when you are inside. Last summer when I saw you (outside on the golf course) it looked REALLY weird. Just looks a little off in this light". It didn't upset me, but I thought of you. I guess wisdom doesn't always come with age!—*Jessie*

Jessie, WOW! That amazes me! First of all, do these people think that we don't know how we look? We need for THEM to tell us in detail what they think? How rude! It's hurtful and cruel to even discuss it. Was his comment supposed to be a compliment, as though you looked "bad" outside on a golf course, but you only look somewhat bad indoors in different light? What an ignorant jerk! Sorry, but we know that we don't look perfect and we don't need anyone reminding us! I'm sorry that you had to endure his rude comments! If I were there, I'd have stuck up for you and told him that it's rude and unnecessary to even make those kinds of comments!—*Chris*

I think it is terrible for anyone to point out differences in anybody, no matter what it is! It is not like we are not aware of it! It's like, someone says, hey man, one of your eyes doesn't move! Are you supposed to run to a mirror somewhere and be like, Oh my God, I didn't know I have a prosthetic eye that doesn't move, thanks for pointing that out to me! I would just do my best to try and forget this event, because, no matter what her parents due to her, she will still have the same opinion of your eye, no matter how wrong of an opinion it is! If she wasn't a child, I would not be so kind.

I found that wearing dark glasses, not to dark, helps ward off comments, and matter of factly, no one says anything to me about my eye, cause it is hard to see. And what you can see of it, it is obscured by the darkness. I had prescription glasses tinted, and that way I can say, they are prescription and I had them tinted cause either I have problems with dilation, or I think regular glasses look nerdy, which I don't, but it's an excuse.—*Jarrod*

◆ ◆ ◆

I am a 24 yr old female from Virginia with Posterior Lenticonus in my left eye (childhood cataract). I am clinically blind in that eye, and have been my whole life—surgery is risky. Anyway, I was thinking about my grandmother today, and figured I'd post a message of encouragement for all the "one eyed" people like me in the world.

My grandmother (dad's mom) has had one eye her whole life. I think she has the same condition I have in her right eye, but she's old and tells a story that she fell out of a bed and hit her head when she was young. She says a knot came up on her head and she went blind in her right eye a few days later. Well, honestly, I think she has the same disease as I and I inherited it. She gets confused sometimes. But anyway, she has led a normal life. She had 9 children and raised them well! She has gardened, cooked, and cleaned her house every day for 50 years and she's 76 years old! She has only had one eye her whole life, and has been fine. She said that later in life the blind eye did cause her some discomfort, but she never let it get her down. So no matter what kind of disability we have in life, we can do whatever we want if we put our minds to it. Take care all, and feel free to email me anytime.—*Tabitha*

◆ ◆ ◆

I'm so sick of this life! I got my new eye yesterday, and I hate it! And here is why: 1. It doesn't move! 2. It doesn't move! 3. It doesn't move! 4. It doesn't move! 5. It doesn't move!

Last night, I got so angry, I set my eye outside, and blew it to pieces with a 16 gauge shot gun! There, I confess! I will never wear another glass eye again! I would rather go around with no eye, than looking cross eyed or cock eyed or whatever! I refuse! If I don't get an eye that moves by the end of this year, I'm going to end everything, I mean it too! If by after new years, I'm not on here any more, you all will know what has happened. I'm so sorry everyone, I'm just sick of living, I want to be who I used to be! Or at least closer! It's bad enough I can only see out of one eye, I should at least have the fake one to move! Is that to much to ask? I'm going to do everything I can to get what I want, and if I can't I give up for good.—*Jarrod*

Jarrod, I'm SO sorry! Did the ocularist and/or doctor say it needs time to heal? BTW, I have ZERO movement and I cannot close my eye, and I'm living okay. PLEASE don't let this get you down. Seriously, when I'm looking dead-on, people have NO idea that I have a prosthesis. I've learned to move my head more and I wear slightly tinted glasses.

Your eye isn't the sum of you. If you feel okay, and you're healthy, you're ahead of the game. Please don't give up on anything! We ARE here to support you!—*Chris*

Dear Jarrod, you are a dear and valued member of this, our community. You have given strength and encouragement, even in the depths of your own despair. No matter how much anger you vent, no matter how horrible you feel, we'll be here for you. The depth of your disappointment is immeasurable. You must dedicate yourself to making your life, no matter how hard it is. And it can be very, very hard. Those of us who matter here love you and care for you.—*Alicia*

I just got an artificial eye also, and it doesn't have much movement either, so I know how you feel. I am having a very hard time adjusting too, I am going to get new glasses with a tint, I think that may work some.

You need to go on with your life, and stop feeling sorry for yourself. You CAN see, can't you? We all have problems with our eyes, but you have to be strong, and move ahead. Maybe you should see a doctor for awhile to help you deal with it. But, please do something constructive, don't just give up. You will be OK, if you start looking ahead to the good times that are coming.—*Anon*

Dear Jarrod, I would just like to add that my eye has no movement at all and I can't close it either. I know how you feel about this. My only consolation is people really don't notice and I'm not just saying this to make you feel better. They don't, as I've found out from experience. It is only 2 years since I lost my eye and I had to wait a year before I got my artificial one but every day gets better.—*Anne*

Gosh, how you can compare the lost of a loved one to the lost of an eye? I had to deal with the lost of my eye, and not much movement either. My family used tough love on me and it worked. I feel very lucky to be able to see, and wake up in the morning to this wonderful world we live in. So, I know that losing an eye is terrible and very traumatic, but life must go on. Good luck to everyone reading this.—*Anon*

First of all I'd like to say to Jarrod, please don't give up. Yes, it is very hard to adjust and yes it is depressing sometimes. However, life, although different from how it used to be, will go on and doesn't have to be bad. We all spend a lot of time on the issue of our eye (or lack thereof), but the reality is that there is SO much more to life. You mentioned that you like to exercise and body build. I encourage you to keep doing those things and to use them to relieve some of your stress and pain. I know it's not as simple as that. But you know you are loved and I hope that you believe that. Hang in there!—*Marsey*

Alicia, kudos to you for writing what you did! We all feel the same way! It *is* a loss, whether or not we realize it when it happens, or 30 years down the road when we need a new implant. It's not easy, and this board is a wonderful place to share fears, ideas, questions and support.

As for Jarrod, I hope he's holding out okay. It's a good sign that he was in contact with us and he was honest with his feelings. I just hope we hear from him again soon. He got some advice here that hopefully he took to heart. Thanks to MANY of you here, he did have support, and we did the best we could.—*Chris*

I thought Tough Love was supposed to be for unruly or rebelling youths? I mean come on, what were you thinking? Losing and eye as anyone on here will agree was very traumatic! And everyone is different and grieves in different ways. I know myself I have not fully dealt with my loss. I had so many other things that happened to me during the last 5 years that I just seem to suppress it and when I least expect it I feel down! I mean after I lost my eye, I felt ugly and insecure. My husband assured me he loved me and would be by me no matter what. Well a couple of years after the fact he left me and my life has never been the same since!

Believe me there are days I just feel like ending it, but somehow I just hang on! I would not say my life is anywhere near happy or content but I firmly believe that one day my turn will come and things will look sunshiny and wonderful again! So take care, be strong and if you ever need a friend just remember we are all here for you! I love this site and every time I meet someone like me (monovision) I suggest they check out this site! Take Care!—*Ski*

I have been away from this board for way too long! Jarrod, I'm so sorry to hear of everything you are going through and I hope you don't leave us for good. I know how depressing lack of movement can be and I'm sure at some point we have all thought that we can't go on. You have to look deep inside yourself and find the strength to carry on. If you ever need to talk everyone here will always be here to be support you.—*Tracy*

Hello Jarrod. I was wondering how are you going? I am a 29 year old woman and do not have a full movement in my eye. I know you can imagine how I feel about it but you know what. I think I will be OK. and it is because I've got friends on this board. You guys give me so much, every single one member of that forum is great and I want to thank you all guys for being here. Cheers guys.—*Anna*

◆   ◆   ◆

Hi, I lost the vision in my left eye after an accident while playing hockey which caused a detached retina which the doctors never could fixed. This was almost 20 years ago, I'm 27 now. I adjusted well to living with one eye, the only thing that bothered me really was the that the eye muscles in the blind eye wasn't 100% functional which caused my eye to wander to the left when looking in certain directions. Otherwise I haven't thought so much about my handicap.

But the last couples of months I've been worrying a lot about my healthy eye, thoughts like what if something happens to my only eye and I become blind? I see no really meaning in life if you are going to live in total darkness. These thoughts started after I got an inflammation in my heart muscle that was pretty serious, I've been in and out from hospital the last months but hopefully it's over now. I guess this have made me realize that there is no guarantee that my only eye will be healthy during my life, I worry about getting a serious eye disease like cancer or a stroke that will make me blind, diseases that there is no cure against. Even if this will not be the case now when I'm young, what will happen when I'm older I guess the risk of eye diseases are bigger then.

So my question is, how big is the risk to develop incurable eye diseases like cancer in the eye and other serious eye diseases that will make you blind?—*Daniel*

Hi Daniel, I think we all understand what you are going through. I used to worry all the time about becoming blind. But as I got older, I just don't worry about it anymore. I will be 63 this month, and have had sight in one eye since I was 6 months. So you see Daniel I still have sight in my good eye, that's a long time. The only thing you can do is be careful with your eye. God Bless you, and please don't let it take over your life. You will be ok.—*Anon*

Hi Daniel, Honestly, my deep feeling is you are going to be okay. A lot of people live all their life with one good eye and never go blind! Just take care of it, use common sense and everything is going to be fine. Don't be obsess over it. I went through this stage as well (I was born with one good eye) when younger my good eye has been patched in order to improve the vision in the bad eye. Not only my vision (or the lack of it!) didn't improve, but I was "artificially" blind for a few months. It totally scared me at the time that by only covering my good eye

I was blind! But it also had positive effects, I had to face my fear and today, I don't think about it much. Good luck!—*Zhu*

Hi Daniel, I've been monocular for 30 years, and I don't worry too often about the possibility of going totally blind. This was just mentioned in another thread, but I only worry when I accidentally hurt my "good" eye! Guess we all should protect the vision that we have left, but it rarely crosses my mind! I DO need prescription glasses, but I don't usually have them on when I'm at home—I SHOULD—they'd be some sort of protection!

Anyway, this may be a good reminder to all of us to protect our good eye. Try not to worry about remote possibilities of disease or anything else taking your vision away, and just try to be as careful as you can! Welcome to the board, btw!—*Anon*

◆ ◆ ◆

So after all these years I finally find a web site with a message board, where I can talk to people in the same boat as me. I lost sight in my left eye 14 years ago and had it removed 9 years ago. I feel depressed, I get feelings of terror for nothing and doom! I HATE IT. I feel like I am getting closer to being a paranoid recluse and I am only 31. What do we do?—*Kevster*

HI, I am sorry you lost your eye. But, you are right, we are all in the same boat. You have to try to get on with your life. Try not let the lost of one of your eyes take over your life. I know that is hard to do, but you have to do it. You are more than just your eyes. Just take one day at a time, things will get better. I hate having one eye, but there is nothing I can do about it. I am just happy I can see with my other eye. Thank God, He gave us 2 eyes. God Bless you and everyone on this board.—*Anon*

Hi there. As the mother of a now 3 year old who lost his eye last year I am sorry for your loss. Noah suffers in pain everyday from headaches, pressure and mild seizures. This has not slowed him down a bit. Rather he seems to shrug it off as a mild inconvenience to his mischief making. I hope that you can do that also. I am in awe of his coping skills and how it does not slow him down. I pray that you can find the same resolve and my heart goes out to you.—*Niccole*

◆ ◆ ◆

Hi everyone. I am new to this forum. I was recently a crime victim, and lost my left eye. It's been hard getting used to the new world I have been thrust into.

I am actually looking for support and help getting used to this situation. It's been pretty hard dealing with the loss and the post traumatic shock. But I see I am not alone dealing with this. I'm not happy for anyone who has to endure this, but I have felt for the past few months that I was alone. I'm glad I have found people to actually talk to about it. My doctor hasn't been too much help in trying to explain the difficulties surrounding this. I hope I can learn from some of your life stories. Regards,—*Michael*

Welcome Michael, sorry to hear your loss was so traumatic, hopefully some of the stories here will help! Good luck,—*Tommy*

Hi, Michael. I'm very sorry you've joined these ranks. I hope your recovery and adjustments are moving along in a way that is working for you. Finding this amazing group of people has helped me in too many ways to count. Please don't feel alone. There is great love and care here. Take care—*Alicia*

Thanks for the sincere and kind words. I really do appreciate it. I know that you guys have been going through this longer than me, but my question is: Do you really get used to it? Everyone, including my doctor and ocularist say you do. I just don't see the light at the end of the tunnel. I have explained strange circumstances to my doctor. Sometimes I think I see light on that side. It causes glare to my good eye. I don't know if my mind is playing tricks on me. It's like my good eye is pasting a picture that it sees on the other side. This causes me to have some kind of double vision. I know this is all in my head. When I go to the ocularist, and I'm sitting under the bright light, I see grey. When I cover that side, it goes away. I know this in fact can't be, because there is nothing in there to focus with.

I was just wondering if I'm the only one who has this. My doctor calls it some kind of syndrome, and just starts writing it down when I tell him. Like he is writing some kind of book. His bedside manner needs a lot of work. Anyways. I'm sorry for running on like this. I guess my anxiety gets the best of me. But thanks again for the warm welcome. I look forward to posting about my experiences as well. I just can't go into detail right now about it, because this has become a high profile case. I can't wait for it all to be over with. Tomorrow I go to my Ocularist for my 5th and final visit. I receive tomorrow what I will be calling my eye. Than I guess I will be able to make peace with myself. Regards,—*Michael*

Yes. I am seeing a therapist. It's really not doing any good. I hate rehashing the incident all over. I just want to put it behind me. Everyone means well, but no one can heal how I feel inside. My grieving period is passing. I am more in the anger stage at this time. I guess when this is all over and the perpetrator is put in jail, I will feel better. Right now he is free to walk the streets and do harm to another person. I am trying to do more as the weeks go by. It's just hard to get back into a normal routine at this time. I don't go out much. I have the feeling of fear and vulnerability. I'm sure most of you can relate to this. Not seeing from the side you are blind. Not seeing or knowing who is coming up to you. I think I've scared quite a few people already. I blame myself for not being more aware the day of the incident. My problem is I trust people too much. You also find out who your friends are during a tragedy. I found out the hard way.—*Michael*

◆ ◆ ◆

Did you ever talk with your girlfriend/boyfriend about your eye? I did and it didn't go very well.—*Ivan*

Hi Ivan, I had to respond to your post because I just did this. A very special man has just come into my life. I've known him for a while, but about a month ago, the relationship took a very serious turn. We have really connected on a very deep level. Because of that, I felt comfortable telling him about my eye. I knew it was something I had to do, so during one of our late night talkfests, I told him. He was so alright with it. He was more concerned that I had had cancer and have been healthy since losing my eye. I couldn't have asked for it to go better.

I'm sorry your girlfriend didn't take it well. All I can say is that the fact you have only one eye is only a small part of who you are, and if your girlfriend can't see that, then maybe you need a new girlfriend. I don't mean to sound harsh, but life is too short and you need people in your life who love and support you. Best wishes to you,—*Nancy*

Hi Ivan, if you partner really cares about you, it should be OK for your her and should be accepted. There is nothing wrong with us and don't let anyone to tell you that. Maybe you should talk again about it to your girlfriend? If you don't mind asking, what was the reaction? You don't have to answer. Cheers,—*Anna*

Hi Ivan, good for you. She was obviously not worthy of you. No one should judge you for this. Hugs,—*Willeke*

Dump her. Wait, you already have. Congrats bro.—*Pete*

Do you not find that people will notice that you have something amiss with your eye almost as soon as you meet them? When I was wearing the occlusive contact lens, I went into an office for something, and the receptionist had to take me through the secure door to the department I needed. On the way there in the lift she said "Wow, I love what you've done with your eye. I've always thought about those cool tinted lenses, its even cooler that you've just put it into one eye" Well as you can imagine I had a bit of a laugh, and she was quite red faced when

I told her actually it was a medical device to cover my wonky eye! So I would imagine if it was a boyfriend or someone you were getting to know quite well. They would more than likely have worked it out from the start!

Because the lens that was put into my eye doesn't totally get rid of my double vision, I have to put Pilocarpine (Glaucoma medication) into my eye to make the pupil small, and keep out peripheral light. This causes my pupil to become like a pinprick. And attracts the weirdest of looks, from everyone, even cashiers at the store, and at the moment its really getting to me.—*Elizabeth*

Hi Ivan. I'm really sorry it didn't go well for you. I told the guy I'm seeing about my eye. Much to my surprise and horror, he told me that he had noticed something different about my eyes (this was the first time anyone had said that). He then went on to explain that he worked in the optical field for a number of years before his current job, so he notices things about people's eyes. He asked a lot of questions (and still asks some questions that I guess he was afraid to ask at first). As with my family and all of my close friends, we joke about it. Marc is forever telling me that he'll "keep an eye out" for me and, with it being so cold lately here in New Jersey, I recently joked with him and said that if I stay outside in the cold too long, my artificial eye turns into an "eyesicle." Ok, so the jokes are bad, but they make people more comfortable and I found that if the people I care about most in life can also make jokes about my eye to me, then it's proof that they are comfortable with my only having one eye.

I've also found that those who really care about me will often ask me which eye it is because they forget that I have an artificial eye.—*Danielle*

◆ ◆ ◆

I try not to point any attention to my eye in front of my friends. Seems when I do, they get disgusted, and I don't hear from them for a few weeks. Also. I was watching a movie for the first time. Pirates of the Caribbean with Johnny Depp. There was a disturbing scene when one of the pirates eye popped out, and he was chasing it on the floor. Then he proceeded to pop it back in, and it swiveled around in his socket. I turned it off right there. I know it's only in fun, but I'm still not at the point to accept it.—*Michael*

I was at a MOPS meeting, moms have a time to get together while the kids go to class for a Bible lesson, craft, etc. so, I dropped Jacob off and didn't mention to the teacher his eye. Why should I? He hasn't taken it out in a classroom situation yet. No biggie. I was in my meeting for about 15 minutes when out she came with him and his eye. The teacher handled it well, the 7th grader who was assisted said it freaked him out at first, but then was very kind about it. I hope this "take out your eye at every opportunity" phase is over before he heads to preschool in the fall *sigh*.—*Bethy*

◆ ◆ ◆

I have been struggled with depression and anxiety for 2 years since lost vision of my right eye. I am lucky have a nature eye. I am also in the mid life crisis—lose interest in my job and feel stress at work. Also considering take long term disability. Probably I should not think myself disabled. But the life is quite boring staying at home alone with my dog. I have been told to develop some hobby. Any suggestion or idea are welcome.—*Chuck*

Hey Chuck, It sounds like your having a rough time at the moment! You need to sit back and take it easy. Don't make any rash decisions re: your work right away, but ask yourself: Is this profession fulfilling my goals? Can I progress any further? Are there any avenues I could take to enhance my career prospects? Is there something I always wanted to do but haven't? Then start about making decisions.

As for hobbies, the same would sort of be applicable. Have you got any sporting interests? Are there any pastimes you would enjoy? (Take a look at Jay. Flying has been good for him!) Are there any groups/organizations near you that you could join? How about volunteering, with a local Club/Charity?

Start off slow, and don't be too ambitious, go easy on yourself until you find something suitable and that you enjoy. I really hope you get sorted soon and that you find something which is rewarding and helps you get up out of your feelings at the moment. Remember, its good to talk about how your feeling, and if there is no one at home you feel you can share with, then that's what here is for! Let us know how you get on, Take Care,—*Elizabeth*

Dear Chuck, just like you, we all wish we could turn back the hands of time but unfortunately, that may never come to pass. Reading through your letter, I could almost see a picture of my life being painted by another person. if only people weren't so shallow minded and obsessed with physical beauty, I'm sure that the world would have been a happy place to live in. Take it easy and always remember that you are not lone. we are here with you.—*JM*

Hi, This is Chuck. I started to take short term disability and likely to retire from now. I am 50, it does a big dent to my family's finance. Lately my wife found a benign tumor in here big leg bone. The doctor still wants to remove since so far still inconclusive if it is benign. It adds to my depression and anxiety.

By post here give me some comforts. I wish my eye can be normal again which is unlikely in 5 years with the Science today. How to accept the reality and face it?—*Chuck*

[Follow-Up Message] This is Chuck. I have been feeling so low after taking the disability leave. I am 50 and was a software engineer which I feel burned out. I have been sitting or lying at home. Plus my wife has a bone tumor which will be removed in a week that will put her on crutches for 3-6 weeks. I have count on her drive in the past 2 years after my right eye is legally blind. This aggravates my depression and anxiety. One thing is I don't have thing to occupy me. Are there any job or resources, support group for low vision, vision impaired people near San Diego area?—*Chuck*

Hi, Chuck. I'm sorry you're going through such a rough time! I've dealt with depression off and on for years, and it is certainly no fun at all. Please don't hesitate to ask someone for help if you need it. If you have tried yourself and just can't pull yourself out of it, call your doctor and explain what's going on. It's not admitting defeat or weakness, it's just getting help for a problem.

As for activities or organizations, I don't know much about your area, but try contacting your state's vocational rehab office if you haven't already. I know that in my state there is a division of voc. rehab dedicated solely to helping individuals who are blind/have low vision. I am blind in my left eye and legally blind in my right, but thanks to their support and assistive technology, I have a degree in fine art and work as a graphic designer.

An organization like this will also likely be able to put you in touch with support groups and community organizations in your area. I know how hard it can be not to be able to get out and do things. It's very stressful for me at times, though I've never had any different, so I would imagine that in some ways for you it's even worse because you've known that freedom, so to speak. Hang in there and take care of yourself, and I hope that both you and your wife are doing much better in short order!—*Kelli*

◆ ◆ ◆

Hi, I just wanted to know if anybody else feels awkward bringing up the fact that you have one eye. At work, some people who don't know about my situation come into my office and say "Wow—how come YOU get to have such a big computer screen?" Or if I am going to some school function with my kids and we arrive all wet because it's raining out, how do I say "Well, I can't drive at night because I'm blind in one eye!" I don't want to make others feel uncomfortable and I also don't want to go into the whole story. I am still adjusting, but have a hard time asking for help (asking for rides, etc.). I wish there was some easy way to explain!—*JYS*

I feel the same. I lost my left eye when I was 5 and now I'm 20 and I've never told a soul. I just can't. There have been times in my life when I've gotten so close to a girlfriend, and I would sense that she'd wonder why I don't make as much eye contact as all our friends do with her. Sometimes they'd ask "why don't you look into my eyes when you talk to me?" To which id just panic and move the conversation on.

In 15 years of having this, I've never told ONE person. I just run and hide because I'm that self-conscious. I have hair to my chin which I keep constantly over my face so no one can notice. It felt good getting that out, even if it only was to a monitor.—*Steven*

Steven, I think you really need to think this through. No matter how much people will tell you that "Wow I couldn't tell the difference!" or "You only have one eye? Really? Ahh Come on!" I know lots of people with one eye, and the only one who I never knew had one until he told me was a guy from Kenya who has tar like black skin and beautiful dark brown eyes! LOL (One of which the ocularist did and excellent job on!).—*Anon*

I received more questions when I was a child because I had a congenital Cataract. "What is that white thing in your eye?" Kids were not nice. But as I got older I could joke about it, "Never drove with a person blind in one eye, eh?"—*Christine*

Gee, I just read this. I can't believe that you don't drive at night! I do everything that a normal 2-eyed person does. Really I do. I would not let a slight handicap interfere with any of my daily routines. Life is too short. Start enjoying it. Don't set any limitations on yourself. People will love you for who you are.—*Brenda*

I used to ride a motorbike but found that not being able to look behind over my shoulder was dangerous so I gave it up. Better travel by bus than be killed by an unthinking car driver. I still enjoy my life though. LOL.—*Marmalade*

◆   ◆   ◆

Does everything get better? I had my enucleation in august 3 days after giving birth to my son. I am suffering still not as bad from migraines, but I think I am depressed I am scared I will get cancer again and no matter what if you haven't experienced this no one understands. Any comments or help I would appreciate. Thanks.—*Nicole*

Nicole, things do get better. Allow time to pass. Surround yourself with positive people. Keep busy. Seek professional help if necessary. Only those who have lost an eye truly understand what we all go through.—*Rich*

◆ ◆ ◆

I can't seem to make eye contact with other people without them robbing their eyes or blinking constantly. Does any one experience this? Or has anyone experienced this in the past? And what is the cause of it.—*Jiddy*

This is really interesting. You may be being hypersensitive of course. In my experience people can make eye contact perfectly well but a very few people make it obvious that they find it difficult. I even had one friend assure me that she was alright talking to me now as she'd worked out where to look. As long as your prosthetic has been made and fitted correctly so that it looks in the same direction as the other people should jolly well be able to cope. It may be more difficult if the eye doesn't close or doesn't blink. Checkout how many people with two eyes don't have a matching pair!—*Chil*

I've noticed folks staring at my wonky eye and then quickly scanning back to the good one and so on. Then usually half way through the conversation they will settle on one or the other (usually the good one) and carry on from there. It is like they have to work out what is wrong with the picture they are seeing! Chill, I've also had that comment about "Its ok now, I've worked out which one is the blind one!" LOL.—*Elizabeth*

People will always be a little scared of things they don't know. I once had someone tell me that when we first started working together, he couldn't look directly at me because my artificial eye made him nervous. There is very little you can do to make someone feel better about accepting your situation. However, if you don't make a big deal about your eye, then soon it will just become a part of you and they won't even notice. I am a business consultant and have found that when people initially meet me, they stare at my eye and wonder what is wrong. However, once we begin working together, they forget about it.—*MC*

◆ ◆ ◆

I am feeling depressed tonight because every time I looked in the mirror today I felt like my eye looked so odd. I hate days like this. These are the days when I torture myself remembering hurtful things that people have said to me over the years about my eye. I always try to tell myself to not make such a big deal of it.just laugh and move on. I mean it really doesn't take much to get me going. Someone can just stare too long at my eye and I get all freaked out. I guess that is why I like to have my hair covering my left side. I have tried to deal with this in different ways. I tried for awhile to push my hair back and just deal with it.

My friends constantly tell me that they can't tell that I have a fake eye. They say sometimes that it just looks like I have a sleepy eye. Either way, I look in the mirror and my fake eye just stands out. I just don't want to be self-conscious about it anymore. Overall my life is good but I'm tired of feeling insecure all the time. I have a lot of anxiety in social situations and I'm sick of it.

I have thought about talking to my doctor about surgery to push up my eyelid. I have thought about it for years. I guess its just hard for me to even talk about it. I haven't been to the ocularist in over 5 years. I'm going to make an appointment next week. Is there anyone who has had surgery on there eyelid? My problem is my fake eye looks smaller because of my drooping lid and I do have a scar on the side of my eye that doesn't help either. Any ideas?—*Lisa*

Go see your ocularist. Remember, you are not the only person to ever experience these feelings, or these conditions. Your ocularist sees many people with similar situations, and should be able to provide some direction. As I said, remember that you are not alone in feeling this way. Best of luck. Let us know how things go.—*Navig8r*

Hi Lisa, I realize being depressed about this stuff can really be draining but you might consider seeing an ocular plastic surgeon when you are finished with the ocularist. They both have helped me with eyelid issues. Please let us know what the ocularist tells you. I'm hopeful for you,—*Amy*

Hey, Lisa! I got my prosthesis in March of 2004 and I have the drooping eyelid problem on and off as well. Some days it seems okay, but others it looks like the eyelid went dead. My ocularist told me that if it was still bothering me on my next visit, he could "build up" the eye. He says by making it thicker, it would hold up the eyelid better. If that doesn't work, my surgeon said she would be able to do a lid lift for me. However, she also said that she'd rather not do a lid lift because it might make the prosthesis less comfortable. Since my eye is so comfortable right now, I figure that I'll try to overlook the droopiness. I guess I'd rather be a little self-conscious sometimes than mess around with what's mostly working. However, if the situation is really making you miserable, then check out every option. I'm sure either your ocularist or surgeon will be able to make some kind of improvement. Good luck and keep us updated!—*Adeline*

23

Children's Issues

Sadly, each year many children will be born without sight in one eye, or will lose an eye to accident or disease. Depending on their age, they may not realize the consequences of only having sight in one eye, but as they mature these issues may hit them harder than they do adults who are already emotionally experienced. Parents need to spend particular attention to the problems and needs of children who grow up with only one eye.

In addition to the emotional issues, there are other issues as well, such as fitting the child with an implant and prosthesis. This is strange enough for an adult, and must be terrifying to a child. Fortunately, there are good ocularists available who have experience in fitting children with prosthesis and know how to work with them so that the process is not too unpleasant.

A child may also require repeated surgeries to make sure that the implant fills the orbit sufficiently to provide for normal development. Then there are the practical issues of protecting the prosthesis from loss (younger children like to take their prosthesis out and hide it from their parents) or damage, as well as making sure that special precautions are taken to protect the good eye.

Notwithstanding these issues, as the letters and messages below show, most children will go through their childhood and adolescence more-or-less normally, and will engage in most of the activities that the other children engage in. Indeed, one of the difficulties is in striking a balance between protecting the child's good eye and yet letting them participate with other children such that they feel normal and fit in with others without being considered special.

LETTERS AND E-MAILS

My daughter hurt her left eye on February 23rd. She was in surgery for over 12 hours while doctors tried to save her eye. They "put it back together", but several weeks after the surgery the eye (not open) looked as though it were sinking in. My husband and I took her to every eye clinic we could find. My daughter had her eye removed on July 17th. She had to wait until October to have her artificial eye made. She began the school year with no left eye. It did not bother her at all. She does wear glassed with polycarbonate lenses to protect her good eye. Her vision was perfect and still is in her remaining eye.

Everyone at school has been very supportive of her. She has been fortunate to have such a wonderful school environment. The new guidance counselor this year happened to lose his right eye at the age of 4 and he talked to my daughter about his artificial eye and helped her (she accepted the loss very easily, it was the making of the artificial eye that she did not like) prepare for the fitting of the eye.

Her new eye looks wonderful. She does have a scar from the inside of her eyebrow down around and out towards her cheek. Her safety glasses cover most of it and she is scheduled for laser surgery for the scar in October. That way, summer will be over and the surgery should be more effective (not out in the sun so much).

I believe she has accepted and adjusted to her eye loss a lot better than I have. I am sure it has to do with her age. My main concern is her interest in sports. I bought her some safety goggles (Rec Specs) and allowed her to play basketball. Now she wants to play soccer. I asked her guidance counselor what he thought about her playing soccer. He said I should let her lead a normal life and not limit her. He said he participated in every sport he liked and I should let her do the same. I worry, especially with soccer, about her getting hurt. She won't be able to see anyone coming up from the left side. I really don't think soccer is a sport she should play, but I don't want her to feel like she should limit herself due to her eye loss. Do you have an opinion on this?—*Anon*

Dear Jay : My son, now almost 16 years old, lost his vision when he was 14 due to a BB through the right eye. He just received his learner's permit and seems to be doing well driving, and is really rather calm about the whole thing. I have been sitting in the right passenger seat verbally instructing him and wildly waving my arms around to indicate which direction he should go. While I was driving today I closed my right eye and noticed that I could not see anything going on in the passenger seat and realized that therefore my son could also not see any of my frantic motions—which explains his calm confidence while driving. So, there you have it, one more one-eyed advantage! I am going to tell him about this web site and I hope he accesses it at some time, you have a lot of useful, encouraging information there. He has a scleral shell but refuses to wear it because he says it is painful. We have been back to the ocularist about 4 times but he still says it hurts. He still has his natural eye but it is smaller than the other eye and pretty unsightly at this point. Do you have any advice re this? Thanks for a great site!—*Joyce*

Hi, my son lost one eye, almost one year ago and he plays baseball in Mexico City and he is the best player, he makes homeruns. He is a twins and 7 years old. Sorry for my English.—*Victor*

Looking for anybody who has a child in their teen years who has lost an eye due to melanoma. My daughter is 11 and just lost her eye. I think hearing from other kids especially s would be very helpful to her. Thank You.—*Linda*

My son, Kiel, lost his eye sight in one eye more than two years ago. He is a high school junior. In his first two years he had trouble adjusting and his grades were terrible. He is now doing much better and looking forward to college. I am seeking advice on how to properly position his application and scholarship information.

He was classified as gifted and took the SAT tests as a 7 grade student. Almost 1200 combined as a 7th grader, the next two years were mostly D's and C's. He is now back in the honors program and doing great but his GPA is still low. Any information sources? Thanks—*Kevin*

Thank you very much for your web site. My grandson who is two months old is blind in one eye. The information provided by your experience and your research has been invaluable to my entire family. Thank you again,—*Bob*

Hi Jay, I've been following your site now for over a year. I have appreciated its perspective. On Saturday, my 5 year old Son was at a new friends house visiting after their first baseball game of the season. The boys were alone in the garage and got into the golf clubs. My son stepped into a back swing and traumatized his left eye ball. After several surgeries and no chance of ever being able to see out of it, the decision came to enucleate the eye, fill with an orbit, and build a prosthetic. Also, we wanted no chance of sympathetic eye. Our Doctor has been wonderful and my son, now 7, is the bravest person I know. He moved on immediately, is very contentious of protecting his eye [Glasses, Goggles, etc.], and continues to be very active in baseball, soccer, and swimming. He now wants to wrestle and take Karate lessons. This makes me nervous, but the Doctor says OK as long as he protects his eye. His optic nerve is in tact, and earlier this year I've heard of new developments in seeing through improved technology. Hopefully he'll be able to have his sight back when he is older. I proud of him and worry about him every day. Thanks for your page! Sincerely,—*Rob*

Wonderful site! My daughter lost vision in her left eye September when she was 15 due to idiopathic optic neuritis leading to optic nerve atrophy. It was a very difficult time for her and us, but she has handled herself so well. She earned her driver's license without any problems and is now a typical 17 year old. Living with one eye is a challenge and reading the message boards help me understand what she is living with. I have recently started searching the web for any info on scholarships that may be available to someone with this impairment. Thanks.—*Janet*

Hello Jay, 25 years ago, a lense of my eyeglasses shattered resulting in my losing an eye. Make sure everyone know that they should be wearing polycarbonate lenses for safety. They are actually lighter then normal lenses and everyone should wear them, especially CHILDREN. They are more expensive, but necessary.—*AS*

I am a 12 year old who lost my sight to my left eye. I had a bottle thrown at me. I've had 4 surgeries within a month. I am scared and would like to know how to cope with this being that I am only 12. please if any one can help thanks.—*Jon*

My teenage daughter is learning to drive. She has severe amblimyopia in one eye (legally blind in this eye) She doesn't seem very confident about turns into traffic. I am thinking just a lot more practice. Any suggestions?—*Michelle*

Hi my daughter who is only 16th years old lost the sight in one eye due to an accident. It has been hard for all of us. Please give some tips so we can heal. Thank you.—*Esther*

Hi, my name is Jamie and I am 13 with one eye. I've had 22 operations, but still no change whatsoever. However, nobody I know in my town also has one eye, and everyone I meet says "Were you born like that?" and I say that my eye did not grow while in my mom's womb.—*Jamie*

Thank you so much for your website. My daughter lost her right eye to a headgear accident 3 years ago. The facebow snapped out of her fingers and both metal prongs punctured her eyes. Her right eye also suffered an eye infection. Her left eye has 2 corneal scars and without glasses is 20/70. Thankfully with her glasses, she is 20/25.

Of course as her mother, I worry about what life will have in store for her. We're told that in the future she will need to have a prosthetic eye. She is now 15 and wants a contact lens in the worst way but we feel that her glasses are her insurance policy against any type of injury she may sustain. I am so fearful that something will happen to the good eye (which isn't so good, but at least she can see!). Thank you again for helping me get through this. This is a wonderful resource for support.—*Wendy*

Hello, we are considering adopting a little girl from China who was born without an eye. Does a child have to be a certain age before they can be fitted for a prosthetic eye? How often would they need a new eye made? Because this little girl was born with this, are there other conditions or syndromes associated with this that we need to be aware of? I have found lot of information about adults losing an eye to an accident, but very little information on congenital eye deformations. Any help would be greatly appreciated. Thanks.—*LeeAnn*

My seven year old daughter lost the vision in her left eye after an accident last month. She was sledding in the snow, lost control of her sled and crashed face first into the back of a brick cabin. Her vision loss was instant, and despite several days in the hospital, treatment was unsuccessful. The fluid build-up on her optic nerve caused it to atrophy and die. I would sincerely appreciate hearing from any other parents whose children are blind in one eye, or people who lost vision in one eye as a child. Thanks you.—*Bridget*

I have a 3 year old son who lost his eye this summer after an accident while visiting my in-laws. It has been a long few months, but he has adjusted well. He had his left eye eviscerated and now wears an ocular prosthetic.

I am looking for other parents who have dealt with the problems associated with a small child in this situation. He has had the prosthetic since September, but in the past few weeks has taken to removing it regularly. Since I don't know what its like to wear a prosthetic, its hard to determine what might be bothering him or becoming uncomfortable. He often has it out by morning, losing it during the night.

I'd love any ideas those of you with a child who wears a prosthetic or adults who do might have. Thanks!—*Beth*

I was wondering if you have a lost eye support group for kids? I have a ten year old who lost his eye in an accident and thinks he's alone. Help.—*Shannon*

My 16 yr old son lost one eye in an accident from another child 2 years ago. After many surgeries, his left eye is not normal looking and will not ever get sight. He is devastated. School, life, responsibility, god are non-caring issues to him. Any advise, sites or other teenage successes in life you can share? Thanks,—*Steve*

I am the mother of a 7 year old who has lost the sight in his right eye due to having a pencil poked in it at school. I came across your website by accident and it has given me a lot of hope. My son who is also named Jay is coping remarkably well and never complains. As yet he hasn't had his eye removed and I have been told that they won't do this unless it is deemed necessary. I enjoyed reading the letters in the forum. Thanks from a grateful mum.—*Stephanie*

Hi there, I'm just surfing the net trying to find info on secondary cancer in RB survivors. Please forward this to anyone you may know who can help me. My son, now 9 yrs old was diagnosed with unilateral Retinoblastoma in January 1997, then 2 yrs 9 months old. His left eye was enucleated, bone marrow and LP were negative, no family history. No other treatment was needed or recommended. He had thorough follow-up that gradually stretched to yearly checks. We were seen in January of this year, my boy was the picture of health and vitality, until suddenly in late March of this year, the gaze of his prosthetic eye changed, he started looking bulgy and had headaches, we had an MRI right away, and he had a large mass in his sinuses. Long story short, rhabdomyosarcoma, sinuses, stage 3, parameningeal. This is our worst nightmare come true, after years of fearing something like this to happen, it did.

My message is dual purposed. #1, Is there anyone out there who has had this same/similar outcome? We are told he must have a germ-line mutation, but we have never had testing, this diagnosis supports this deduction. After going thru the trauma of RB with our precious boy, we truly felt we had paid our dues, if we are able to escape this with only losing an eye [considering I originally thought he may need glasses, how quickly our priorities change], then certainly God will let him live his life and bring to the world all the great things he is here to do). #2, If anyone has any worries, do not let them be talked away by reason, because logically, it doesn't make sense. The likelihood is, you're child is fine. The reality is logic, likelihood and percentages mean nothing if it is happening to you. Put your foot down., insist on tests, it's ok if they think you are an out of control parent. The reality is you are very much in control and don't need to relinquish it! Thanks so much, I hope no one else is living our nightmare, but I want everyone else to learn from our nightmare!—*Tammy*

Congratulations on getting your pilot's license! I like your site. My 6 yr old daughter lost her right eye to retinoblastoma when she was 2. She loves flying with me (pilot since '80) in my decathlon. Regards,—*Ken*

I have several questions in regard to my 15 yr old daughter. My questions specifically are in regard to the types of mirrors used to assist in driving; (yes, she's 15!), and you mentioned on your site "new technology" coming in regard to implants. She is scheduled to have her implant procedure done in November 2005, and I have heard nothing concerning new procedures from her opthamologist or ocularist. Thanks for taking the time to read this, and I certainly appreciate your site. I just recently discovered it, and my daughter and myself have learned a lot! Thanks again.—*Buzz*

Thank you so much for this website. I am 13 years-old and I just got my eye removed. About a week and a half ago I found out that I would have to get my eye removed. It was really hard for me to face the fact that I would have to get my eye removed at such a young age. But I had a chance of that since I was 6 years old.

When I was 5 I was diagnosed with something called VHL. VHL is known as Von Hipple Lindale. This was passed from my mother to me. Well when I was 5 we noticed that my left eye was floating to the side.

My family and I went to a highly recommended hospital. When we were there the doctors said that I had a tumor on my optic nerve. So to take care of the matter I had to get surgery that dried up the fluid and the surgery would make me go blind.

Well about 8 years later which is this year I started having problems with really high pressure in my eye. To relieve the pain I would have to get my eye removed. The doctors said it wouldn't be a really big deal with me cuz I couldn't see out of it anyway but they don't really understand how hard just the thought of it is.

I know to all of you reading this getting your eye removed sounds really scary but in the end it is really the best thing. After reading through this website I am not scared anymore I now know what to expect. I know that I will be able to drive when the time comes and I will be able to do all the things I have been able to do.

I had the worst pain I could imagine before the surgery but now it feels better then ever and I still have about 5 weeks of recovery left.

This website has helped me more then ever and I hope that my letter can help all of you who just got your eye removed or is about to. It really isn't hard dealing with it. You really just have to face your fears and this website helps you with that.

Thanks so much to Jay for providing this website because now I know that you all have been thru this before and now I know what to expect. Thanks,—*Alex*

MESSAGE THREADS

I'd just like to say a big hi to everyone here. its so nice to find a website full of people that understand how I feel. I lost my eye when I was two and now wear a prosthetic. Although I have great friends who are really understanding, it's nice to know that I'm not the only one who feels self conscience at time. I'd like to hear from you all. what a great place.—*Tracy*

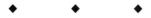

Hi everyone I have a special favor to ask you all. My nurse at hospital is looking for a site to help parents of young children with an artificial eye. A lot of these kids are really struggling to come to terms with this problem. any replies would be much appreciated and I could pass any information on. Thanking you all in advance.—*Anne*

Hey Anne, this site is the best place to help anyone come to terms with whets going on. I myself am only 22 and lost my eye when I was two, I'm always here to offer any advice and support to anyone as I'm sure everyone else is. We've all found it hard to come to terms with. but thanks to all the support I've had I'm happy with who I am and what I look like. if I can help e-mail me).—*Tracy*

Hi! I would be happy to help the parents in any way possible. I lost my left eye when I was 5 due to congenital glaucoma. Actually, since the eye was enlarged and painful, I was relieved to be rid of it. I remember that I asked what they did with it. My parents told me that they would use it to study, so that maybe another little girl would not lose her eye, or go blind. I was happy with that answer, and it may well have been true since I was a patient at a teaching hospital. Food for thought: Orthodox Jews bury all parts of the body. I think this is a nice custom. Loss of the eye did not affect my reading development, though I probably saw very little out of it anyway. In fact, I excelled in school and in art and music (I played the flute). As for sports, I figure-skated in high school, and enjoy swimming and biking, as well as skating, today. I was not very good at ball sports, but then I had little interest in them, and did not practice. I think I could have been decent at basketball if I had tried.

I work as an elementary school teacher and am getting a Master's in Education. I drive, including interstates. I don't like to search for new locations, and get good directions with good landmarks. As far as I know, the children did not know that I had any problem worse than glasses. I needed to sit close to the board due to a small focusing problem with my good eye, and sometimes the other students would resent that I always got the front of the room whereas everyone else had to alternate. "Why can't you see?" they asked. "You've got glasses!" There is a new implant that is better than what I had originally-hydroxyapatite, and the more muscles are attached, the better the eye movement. However, these are difficult to remove. My old silicon implant was too small as an adult. Parents may want to investigate the type and size of implant their child receives. Most adults have an 18mm implant.—*Vivacemist*

◆ ◆ ◆

Hi there! I am new to all this so please bare with me. Our 2 year old son, Noah, lost his eye this summer. He lost his balance and fell on a 3/8 inch metal rod while with my in-laws. The doctors tried all summer to save his eye (a scleral buckle) not sure how that is spelled, but finally it was determined that it had to be removed after 4 surgeries. He just received his prosthetic eye 3 days ago. We have been told that he may need a new eye within anywhere from 3 months to a year and half due to his age. Because of his age this is all cosmetic (according to medical provider). He has a silicone oil ball 85% the size his eye will be when he is 20. Can you please give me guidance and a little help on what to expect. I am new at this and as a mom looking in from the outside I am terrified and uninformed. Sincerely,—*Niccole*

I also suffered a trauma to the eye similar to Noah's four year ago. The doctors tried as hard as they could to save my eye. I too had a vitrectomy. That is when they remove (my leaked out) the natural fluid in the eye and fill the eye with a silicone gel in lieu of the natural fluid. This procedure ensures that the eye will not collapse. (Sometimes when the eye suffers trauma the eye pressure becomes very low and that can cause collapse if it is not filled with the silicone jell) It sort of works on the same principle as a water balloon. The scleral buckle which is placed on the outside of the eye (around it) acts to hold the eye from the outside. Sort of like a rubber band but without the elasticity. The prosthetic that he is now wearing DOES NOT HURT. When I had my scleral shell (prosthetic) made, there was a little girl in the office (about 4 years-old) she was like any other 4 year old playing in the waiting room waiting for her turn to see the ocularist but all of a sudden she went over to her mother, popped her eye out and said "here mommy" as if it was the most natural thing in the world! Kids are wonderful and they are very adaptable. It is important to keep the prosthetic clean—her mother just took out a case and placed the eye in the case and they continued to chat as if nothing had happened.—*Heidi*

◆ ◆ ◆

Hiya all! I wanted to let everyone know that Noah is doing great. Our church has been amazing and after talking to various hospitals, we found an organization through the Children's miracle network that has paid for all of his medical bills.

I have a question. When Noah doesn't have his prosthesis in he doesn't open his eye lid. Is that normal for everyone. Thank you for your valuable insight and answering my ignorant questions. Sincerely,—*Niccole*

Niccole, you are not asking silly questions we all asked these sort of questions. My specialist told me that my lid didn't open without my false eye in as it is the eyeball which holds the lid open and the muscles which close it. So it is perfectly normal for Noah to be like this. Hope this has been of help to you,—*Anne*

Niccole, first of all, congratulations on Noah doing so well. That's great! It must also be a relief to know that the medical bills are taken care of! Good for you! My lid stays closed without the prosthesis in there too. I think it works that way for everybody. The prosthesis is what holds it open. Hope Noah has continued success. Sounds like you're all doing well!—*Chris*

Hi Niccole, my eyelid is closed without my prosthesis. Seems like everything is going well with Noah! Ask as many questions as you need. In my opinion we are here to share our experience, ask questions and answer them. Take care.—*Anna*

◆ ◆ ◆

Hello everyone. I just started checking out this site. To make a long story short.my 3 week old daughter just had her left eye removed Tuesday due to PHPV and possible Retinal Blastoma. I was just curious if there was anyone I can talk to that went through the same thing. Thanks in advance,—*Lauren*

Lauren, I lost my right eye to retinoblastoma when I was one year old. Currently, I'm 20 years old. If I can help you in any way, you know. Greetings,—*Santiago*

◆ ◆ ◆

Hello Noah is fine except for the fact that his nose has started to grow towards the injured side of his face. His right side of his mouth is also starting to slant. I was told that he had a bigger silicone ball implanted so that his face would grow somewhat the same. He seems to be slurring his words a little more and I just so need to know if anyone else has gone through this and what to expect. I am back to not knowing anything. Plastic surgery isn't going to be an option for many years. any help you can give me would be greatly appreciated. Sincerely,—*Niccole*

Niccole, my recommendation is to go to 2-3 doctors, or better ocularists and ask them for their opinion. I think it is very important to do it now while Noah is still very young and his bones and muscles are flexible. I would strongly recommend to go to another specialists, maybe they will say the same but at least this is more than 1 opinion. All the best.—*Anna*

◆ ◆ ◆

My daughters left eye was removed last week. I have so many questions about conformers, prosthetic eyes, just everything. This is all new to me. Thanks so much.—*Lauren*

Hello Lauren and welcome to the forum. My now 3 year old son lost his eye last year and many questions doesn't even begin to cover it. If there is anything I can do to help or just be here to listen and support. Good luck I know for me, this last year has been my testimony that what doesn't kill you, makes you stronger.—*Niccole*

Hi, Lauren, I'm sorry you and your family is going through this. It will be ok. It will. It's just very hard sometimes. You've found a wonderful place. Please ask away—someone here will have the information you need or will help you find it. Love to you,—*Alicia*

Lauren, my 3 year old lost his eye in July. I just discovered this site but have done a ton of reading about eyes, conformers, prosthesis, etc. I assume by now your child is probably through that part of the process but I am now learning that there are some "parenting" type things that I'd love to brainstorm with other parents who have a child with a prosthesis.—*Bethy*

◆ ◆ ◆

My little girl had her eye removed back in August. Anyway she is doing good but every time she wakes up from a nap (she is 4 months old) her "eye" is crusted shut. I know the Ocularist told us there would be some drainage, but does this always happen? Sometimes it is really bad! Thanks and sorry if it's a dumb question.—*Lauren*

Hi, Lauren, I've had my eye since I was seven and I remember lots of crusted-over time when I first got it. Warm washcloth was and is still often my best friend! Since having my socket rebuilt in the summer of 03, I've gone through more frequent periods of the gooey eye thing. Over the years, it is the worst when I have a cold and everything is runny, and when I go from climate extremes—from cold cold outside to very warm inside, or hot days with air conditioning inside. So glad you've found this site. Jay has given us a huge gift. Love,—*Alicia*

Hi Lauren, I have trouble with the same thing occasionally but like said by the others it is just from time to time. When I have a cold it gets a little worse. I remember seeing your daughter's picture a while back. She's adorable, you must be so proud of her. I wish you and your little girl all the best. Hugs,—*Willeke*

Thank you all for replying. I guess it's just something that we will deal with! You guys have been great on here! And thank you Willeke for the nice comment on my Isabelle Hope you all have a great day!—*Lauren*

◆ ◆ ◆

Hi guys it has been awhile since we have posted anything. This is because we have been waiting to hear about Noah's last ct scan. He has developed a blood clot between the silicone ball and the severed nerve endings, where the scar tissue is. He will be going on a regiment of a medication called Lovenoxx and then will undergo a 4 day medicated coma to go in and try to get rid of the clot. Rather scary. He is still doing great and his 4th birthday is coming up. Anyone that sees this please just pray hard. Thank you and hope everyone else is doing great and we keep everyone in our prayers.—*Niccole*

Niccole, when does Noah go in for this treatment? He is such a little trooper, and has really been through the mill! I will remember him (and you!) in my prayers daily, keep us posted, God Bless.—*Elizabeth*

Thank you first and foremost for the prayers. He is slated for another CT scan on March 1st, to start the Lovenoxx on March 3rd, and the surgery March 28th. We still cannot find a medical company that will touch him and the home owners' insurance has still refused to pay so we are having a fund raiser on Feb. 26th to try and off-set the cost of this. The Lovenoxx is a medication they give stroke victims and has the same components as rat poison from what I understand. It is to try and make it slippery back where the blood clot is, so that the surgery will have a better chance of success and so this doesn't happen again.—*Niccole*

Hi guys. As you guys may remember the doctors put an oversized silicone ball in Noah's socket to help his face grow somewhat conformed (didn't work, his nose is slanting towards left side of face and he started slurring his words), anyhow, apparently the scar tissue has formed a blood clot. His seizures started getting worse and so were his sensitivity to anything. When we go in for his next CT scan, I am going to bring up about the silicone beads. Have you had any rejections since that was done?—*Niccole*

It really isn't the implant that seems to be the problem. It seems that the severed nerve endings had quite a bit of scar tissue and that is what caused a net that started the blood clot, that and the oversized implant. The oversized implant didn't seem to work as well as we had hoped. His nose is growing slightly to the right side of his face and he slurs his words more and more. I know this is sort of off topic but Noah refuses to have bowel movements. He holds it in and we have to give him a natural remedy with prunes in it (boy does this recipe work too). I believe it is due to the pressure in there, but not able to have real candid conversations with Noah so not sure.

The other thing I believe is that this is the one thing in his body that he has control over that no one is poking or prodding and so he holds tight to this as his last form of control, we just got him potty trained again 2 months ago, but this continues to be a problem. Now with his upcoming surgery and medication, I am so worried he will regress. It took us a year to get him to come out from under a blanket. (He looked like the US flag with skinny white legs walking around). He is the littlest of 4 boys and he is the rowdiest. We try and even out our time and yet every time we think things are about to get back to semi-normal it seems that Noah has a set back. Boy is it crazy in our household. Sorry guys kind of just letting it out and rambling thanks to anyone that is reading this. Any suggestions on any of this is helpful. By the way I noticed that I put that his nose slants to the left earlier and it doesn't, it slants towards the right. Sorry for any confusion.—*Niccole*

◆ ◆ ◆

My 3 year old son who lost his eye this summer after an accident while visiting my in-laws. It has been a long few months, but he has adjusted well. He had his left eye Eviscerated and now wears an ocular prosthetic.

I am looking for other parents who have dealt with the problems associated with a small child in this situation. He has had the prosthetic since September, but in the past few weeks has taken to removing it regularly. Since I don't know what its like to wear a prosthetic, its hard to determine what might be bothering him or becoming uncomfortable. He often has it out by morning, losing it during the night. I'd love any ideas those of you with a child who wears a prosthetic or adults who do might have.—*Bethy*

Hi Lauren! My 3 1/2 year old had his eye removed in August. He has not had the problem with crusting except in the beginning, I think he was still using the conformer and maybe his early days with the prosthetic. We would offer him a warm wash cloth, but I didn't work really hard at "cleaning it" because I didn't want to distress him more than he already was. When did your daughter receive her prosthetic?

I just discovered this board, but it's nice to find other parents who are dealing with small children in this situation.—*Bethy*

Hi Beth, I am a 23 year old who had her eye enucleated this summer. I received my prosthesis in September as well. Perhaps as the eye healed, it is now rubbing against the shell and causing your child discomfort? Also, before I had the enucleation I had had another surgery done in which my eye was still present in the socket and I wore a shell over it. my eye was too sick to tolerate the shell and I never had any form of comfort so I had to resort to having the whole eye removed. I'm sure that this isn't the case for your child, but maybe their eye cant tolerate the prosthesis and needs to be removed completely? My suggestion to you would be to contact your ocularist or another one. I live in NY and I know that my ocularist deals with children all of the time and she would definitely have some suggestions to give to parents. Hope that everything works out. feel free to private message me anytime. Love,—*Jodi*

Thanks Jodi for your reply! Jacob fell from the couch towards the end table. Unfortunately, there was a glass drinking glass sitting on the coaster which shattered cutting his face and eye. He had surgery early in the morning to "repair" his ruptured globe. A few weeks later, he saw the retina specialist who determined vision was a total loss. It was at that time we decided to have the eye enucleated due to the risk of sympathetic opthamalia and pain. He has an implant inside of his sclera which is covered by the conjunctiva. (I'm assuming this is similar to what you have?!). I am planning on calling his ocularist in the morning. He usually takes it out and says "my eye is dirty". We offer the wetting drops each night too. It's certainly possible it's rubbing, he's such a trooper and has put up with so much, it's so hard to communicate. If you don't ask the questions right, he'll start inventing things from the questions if you know what I mean!

I'm sorry to hear about your loss, I have been awed by the amazing power of God to heal and how incredibly resilient my son has been. To see him running and playing with his friends, you'd have no idea he only has one eye.—*Bethy*

Wow you blew me away. I have a 3 yr old son that lost his right eye as a result of an injury sustained at my in-laws as well. He is about to undergo another surgery soon and if you ever need to talk. Well you are in good company.—*Niccole*

Dear Beth, perhaps the artificial eye is bothering him because there is little lubrication and is rubbing the socket tissues. Wetting drops are not sufficient for an anophthalmic socket. Buy some Refresh PM or similar lubricant from your local pharmacy, such as Walgreen's. There is no prescription required. It comes in a tube and should contain mineral oil and petrolatum. Next soak the eye in a little Johnson's baby shampoo to remove tear film buildup. Rinse thoroughly, apply a little ointment to the back of the ocular and reinsert it. It should feel a lot better to the child. It may be a good idea to let the ocularist know about the dryness problem.—*Lisa*

Lisa, thank you for your information. I will try to get some of that ointment. We've even gone so far as to consider a whole house humidifier but, that won't help him when he's away at school and such.

The ocularist suggested some drops that are actually rewetting drops for hard contact lenses. Not just a saline drop, it has some lubricative properties but doesn't seem to last very long. They are by Boston, but I can't recall the name. We're also having difficulty (I think there's another post about this) with his eyelid getting 'stuck' open. Any ideas? or could that be the same lubrication problem?—*Bethy*

Dear Beth, I think that the child's eye socket may be dry, causing the eyelid to get stuck open. Eye ointment is far more lubricative than "re-wetting drops". It is nonprescription too, and it can be found under the name, Refresh PM, or Hypotears Ointment, or a similar name. Just look on the label to see that it has mineral oil and petrolatum in it, not wax. It comes in a small tube. A person wearing a prosthesis needs a much heavier lubricant than someone without one. Also, the tear glands are not as efficient at coating the prosthesis because of the size of an average ocular. So you need lubricant.

Do you see discharge from the eye socket? Is the ocular shape very rounded? Sometimes the shape can be causing the eyelid to stick open, but I think it would be a good start to try the ointment first. When was the last visit to the ocularist? It may be time for a polish or even reshaping it to be more flat anteriorly, just a guess. If there is discharge, what color is it? If it is clear or white it is irritation, dryness. If it is yellow or green it is infection and he may need an antibiotic ointment from the eye doctor. I would take the eye out, soak it in dilute Johnson's baby shampoo, rinse thoroughly, apply the ointment to the back and put it back in. Good luck!—*Lisa*

Hello there. Do you use erythromycin ointment every time you put your child's eye in? We use the ointment and then 3 times a day we have been told to put the refresh gel in. It seems to make it easier for him. We take the eye out at night (if we don't it, it becomes a treasure hunt in the morning). This allows the skin to breathe a little. PS: Has your little one discovered there is no feeling in the eye socket? Noah has and a few times I have seen him touching the inner eye and even poking at it.—*Niccole*

No need to use erythromycin ointment every time, just when there is an infection. You can use Refresh PM ointment or similar (which contains no antibiotic, unlike erythromycin) perhaps at most, once per day. If you put on too much it will congeal in the back of the eye, and build up there, trapping debris. There is some sensitivity in the eye socket, but there should never be pain.—*Lisa*

I was told by the eye surgeon to only use the Ciproflaxin ointment when their is an infection. Using it all the time is not good,—*Michael*

Hmm I understand what you are saying. However for us, we were told by Noah's ocularist to put the antibiotic ointment every time as young children are prone to staph infections. This is why every time that eye is put back the ointment goes on and this has been going on for almost 2 years. This is after he stopped with the atropine, prednisone and another antibiotic.—*Niccole*

Well, it would be best to ask the doctor when to use the antibiotic, not an ocularist. The ocularist should have told you to check with the doctor who can do cultures and testing. We do not prescribe medications, nor direct how to use them. There are now strains of antibiotic resistant staphylococcus aureus because of the overuse of antibiotics. In fact, my brother called me tonight to help out as they will be attending a funeral tomorrow. One of their friends had passed away unexpectedly. She was 49 years old. She died of staph A infection. It was resistant to antibiotics.

So, when you take the eye out, just wash it with baby shampoo, put a little ointment on it and even a drop of mineral oil, and barring any discolored discharge from the eye, replace back into the socket. It should be fine.—*Lisa*

Everything we do is in conjunction with Noah's MD's. In fact it was the doctor that removed his eye and put in the ball who prescribed the meds. But if it might cause him problems I am all for backing off use.—*Niccole*

Phew, the information is so confusing! I guess there are no standardized guidelines, which as a parent is incredibly frustrating!

Lisa, you keep mentioning baby shampoo. I asked at our last visit if it mattered what I washed it with and was told any soap was fine as long as it wasn't abrasive. There are times when I just rinse it and rub it off really good without using soap at all.—Jacob does not appear to have any discharge from his socket, but I'm curious what the sign of an infection would be? Unfortunately, at this time not taking it out and handling it is not an option we have. I trust he will be outgrowing this stage, sooner would be nice. As a parent, I try not to make a big deal about it or talk to him about it too much. I have a little guy's self-esteem to worry about too.—*Bethy*

◆　◆　◆

My son, courtesy of a moron with a pellet gun, permanently lost the vision in his left eye in 2004. Our doctor performed surgery upon his eye, but there was too much internal damage, and as a result he is looking at one day, being enucleated.

Our question is this: At what point, does enucleation become a medical necessity? For now, due to a fluke with scar tissue plugging the drain (so to speak), his eye is holding pressure, although it is a little low. His eye is droopy and visibly smaller, although the only folks that really notice it are those that know him, and there are kids he goes to school with that are unaware of his problem. His pupil is for practical purposes, closed, but unless you get close, and are specifically looking for something, you won't notice there is any thing wrong with his eye.

He is not at all self conscious about his appearance, and of course, like his parents, is not at all looking forward to the finality of having his eye removed. Any ideas at "what point" enucleation will become a medical necessity?—*John*

If the eye is not bothering him, and there is no penetration of the uveal tract (that can lead to sympathetic ophthamia), no pain, nor chance of cancer etc, then enucleation may never become a necessity for him. I hope he never has to have it removed, but ask your doctor what are his reasons for it. If it is for a better prosthetic result, it may be better to keep the eye and do an evisceration. Even leaving the eye alone, doing neither enucleation nor evisceration, he can still be fitted for an artificial eye if his eye becomes too shrunken.—*Lisa*

◆　◆　◆

We are parents of a young boy who has just lost his eye to Retinoblastoma. We have all been through the mill over the last month but the stories I have read here are really an inspiration. Like 99% of the population we had never heard of Retinoblastoma, now it is a huge part of all our lives and a great shock to us all.

He has just had his prosthetic eye fitted. He is obviously very scared of anyone coming near his eye and it was a horrible experience trying to fit his scleral shell. He was very pleased to have a new eye but there doesn't seem to be much movement. It is not the final one we will be fitting, but he is too scared (3 years old) and not mature enough for the ocularist to take a mould of his eye. My question is, when a proper shell is fitted, how much movement will there be in eye?—*Vince*

I'm not sure how much help I will be but here is our story. The short version: Our daughter was born and they thought it could be Retinoblastoma.the only way to know was to remove it. She was 3 weeks when they did surgery. She got her fist "eye" at 3 months. There was no movement. We were upset, but 3 months later when she got a "build-up" we noticed movement. It was very minimal but there was some. Then she went back again4 months later for another "build-up" and again we noticed more movement. She now goes again next month and we are excited to see how that one goes. Our Ocularist told us that through the years we should start seeing more movement. Then again everyone is different.

There are a few other parents on this board that have children your son's age, so maybe they will be more help. My understanding is that the muscles need to build up and that's how you'll get more movement (I could be wrong). I wish you and your son luck. Just remember that it takes time.—*Lauren*

Thanks for your replies. I feel with my sons enucleation we have become part of a much wider family of people who have gone through the same thing. This forum is a real help.

My son now has his new eye and it is very convincing. It is a little on the large side and his top lid doesn't come down as far as the OK eye but I'm sure this is because he hasn't had a 'made to measure' eye so to speak. Just for the record, the classic sign of Retinoblastoma is that when the child has a picture taken of them, instead of classic 'red eye' reflection, you get a 'white eye'. This is because the retina is detached and there is now retina for the light to bounce off of. Of course on reflection (no pun intended!), all his photos had this symptom but of course we put it down to a dodgy camera. Thanks again for you info.—*Vince*

◆   ◆   ◆

Hello! Any thoughts or tips on teaching my daughter how to operate a car? She's had a prosthesis since the age of 6 months, so is well adjusted to lack of peripheral vision. Any special mirrors (as mentioned on the home page), techniques, etc.? Any help would be greatly appreciated.—*Buz*

Hello and welcome, Buzz. I also lost my left eye at a very early age. I have to turn my head around further than normal to see if a car is coming and be extra careful when changing lanes on the interstate. Instead of relying on my side mirrors, I also look to be sure there isn't a car in my blind spot. Other than that, I can't really think of anything else. Doesn't sound as if your daughter has a problem with depth perception. She will do just fine, although dad may need to pop a nerve pill. LOL—*Brenda*

I've never had vision in my right eye. no problems driving. Just remember that you see things "differently" than she does. If you try to drive with one eye covered, it isn't the same.—*Navig8r*

Welcome. If your daughter has gone for 15 years with monocular vision, then she's used to it. She just has to take extra care when driving—turning her head more to accommodate her vision, but I'm SURE that it'll come naturally to her. No one had to tell me those things!

Just a side note: I've always been a little leery of driving in major cities. I'm comfortable doing slower paced driving on more open roads. Might just be a fear of *mine*, but I'm pretty cautious when driving. Kudos to you for going through the driving thing with your daughter. We're going through it with our daughter (she's 17) and it's nerve-wracking!—*Chris*

◆   ◆   ◆

Dear All, sorry if this is long—but I need your advice, encouragement. My name is Alvin and my son's name is David. We were involved in a car accident and our son took the brunt of the accident. He had a ruptured globe, torn retina and the lens is no where to be found. There was a lot of vitreous fluid loss as well. He had surgery and all of the eye docs state that the best interest is to remove the eye—enucleation.

Here is my dilemma—we visited the ocular plastics surgeon today and I frankly asked him if that was his son, what he would do—he hesitated a bit and told us that would be a tough decision to make. He looked at his bad eye again (he will never see again on his R eye) and stated that his bad eye has good movement and told me to come back next Wednesday. It kind of gives us hope. My son is on Homatropine twice a day and the plastics Doc added Pred Forte 1% every two hours.

Our doctors concurred that it would be best to remove his eye since it will not be useful and to prevent systematic opthamlia (sorry if its written wrong)—when the body fights the bad eye and the good eye. We were told that this was a 1 in 1000 or 1 in 2000 chance of this happening. Please help—this a tough decision for us to make. Regards,—*Al*

My son does not have systematic olthamia, but we were warned about it due to it possibly damaging the real eye and cause total blindness. May I ask, how did you lose your sight in one eye? My son's eye was ruptured and I don't think it is full size. Thanks again.—*Al*

Al, first of all welcome to LostEye. I'm only sorry that its under such circumstances! However, everyone here has had some form of sight loss in one eye, with a lot of folks having had an enucleation. And so you have really come to the right place for info and support. I still have my blind eye, but I know a few others who have been faced with the Sympathetic Ophthalmia issue and have eventually opted for a full enucleation.

Sympathetic Ophthalmia is a condition where the fellow, previously unaffected eye becomes inflamed (uveitis) to the point where sight is threatened. It usually occurs when the Uveal Tissue of the injured eye is affected (as would be the case with your son). I know that Sympathetic Ophthalmia is a rare complication, but it is a very real one also, and for that reason I wouldn't hesitate in having the eye removed. The only reason someone would want to keep a blind eye would be for cosmetics, but from the sound of your sons injury (globe rupture etc) it sounds like if he kept his eye he would need a scleral shell anyway, so the issue of having the appearance of a prosthesis will remain which ever decision you make.

I've had lots of eye surgery, to the point where I had almost become complacent about the warnings and possible side effect issues that the doctors must go over before every surgery. Then last year I developed Uveitis after what was essentially a cataract procedure (quite rare) and a month later Scleritis. which is very rare! Reason I tell you this is that although the risk may be 1 in 1000 that still means that there is a risk, and as all of us are testament to. Your son will be perfectly able to function normally with monocular vision after a period of re-adjustment.

To be honest I don't know of anyone who has ever "looked back" (excuse the phrase!) after the enucleation of a blind eye with no potential, due to trauma. Yes it takes some adjusting to, i.e. the visual and self image issues, but with support most people get over these problems relatively quickly. What age is your son? At the end of the day it is your decision, and I don't want to sound as if I'm pushing you one way or the other, but I'm just coming straight up about it, because that's the way Id want it if it were me, or my child. I hope that helped. Do keep us informed of how David is getting on,—*Elizabeth*

Liz, my son is 9 years old. Thank you for your words—the eye removal is probably going to be our course of action. I'll keep you updated. He also complains about pain in the eye at nights and I know that is a good reason to proceed with the procedure. Thanks again,—*Al*

Al, I'm really sorry for what happened to your son. Despite I have no vision in it, I still have my eye, so I wouldn't know about the whole procedure you're going through. I just wanted to stress that despites it's a tough time for you and David, living with one eye is really not a big deal. I'm 22 now, but I had pretty much the same age as David when I had my good eye patched (to try to improve the other one), then had surgery etc. From all those experience, I don't even have bad memories. Children are actually very adaptable and pretty tolerant with each other. When I look back, I'm like "oh my good, how did I even make it?" (especially when looking at old picture with eye patch and all). But my old friends barely remember me as "the one eye girl". And as for everyday life, I've never had any problem. This is the first time my eye bothering me: I just got my drivers license and I'm still scared to drive (but after all, you can blame it on me being a chicken). Sorry this post isn't too helpful about the issue you're facing now, but I'm sure David will do great.—*Jul*

Thanks, I guess you had a "lazy eye" when a kid? My wife too. She actually monocular vision too. Which is something my son will have to adjust to too. My biggest fear is two fold—if I decide to leave his eye, what happens if he is the 1 out of 1000 that will get sympathetic Opthalmia? He may not recover and I could never deal with him not seeing at all! I spoke to the original eye doc and stated that I might want to leave his eye and he said NO—Please don't do that! This doc also told me he could not remove his eye if he had to so he said "if this was my son, I would take him to UMDNJ in Newark, NJ" He was candid and honest with me and showed emotion as well. So I have to assume he has my son in mind. A lot of eye docs can be callous—I mean they do this all the time and sometimes when they have too many accolades and degrees etc.—well I am sure you know what I mean.

On the other hand, what if I remove the eye and ten years from now with stem cell research and all there is something that can be done! I have spoken to several doctors and they just tell me that it would be foolish to keep his eye and risk the disease. I am just venting and I am sorry if I repeat myself.

As far as him living with one eye—my son has surprised me. Today I convinced him to go to the soccer practice only to see the team practice. Even though his eye is shut and still swollen from the accident, he made the effort after me prodding him to come—I am an assistant coach and I wanted to see my other soccer kids too. His response to me floored me—he said "Daddy, if I get a glass eye and I get hit with the ball, it may shatter and I would have to go to the hospital again". I responded to him that there are no more glass eyes and that it would be a composite and he said "ooh yeah". He has more will power than I.

Regardless, I may have to opt to remove his eye based on the fact that, if I don't, there may be a slight chance that the disease can get him, and then my wife and I could never live with that decision. Thanks for listening.—*Al*

Hi, Al, my heart goes out to you and your wife and son. I had my right eye removed when I was fifteen after a failed corneal transplant. My parents were also faced with a similar decision because of a risk of septicemia. Looking back now, I think I coped much better being young than I would now if I was faced with the same prospect. The loss of my eye didn't really strike me as a huge deal and I adapted to it very quickly.

The first prosthesis I got was really good and moved very well (not sure how much your son would have removed but if its just the eyeball itself he will probably still have very good movement) Nobody could tell which was the false eye. (I use the past tense because my situation is different now due to other complication related to my disease) So basically my point is that the artificial eye will in all likelihood look very natural and move with the real eye. I know my mother worried about what the future might hold with advances in medical science as you mentioned but I think the reality is that the kind of advancement we would need is a long way off. I can quite honestly tell you that the loss of my eye never bothered a lot and I never even think about the blindness in my right eye. I learned to drive with one eye when I was 17 and never felt it impeded me in any way. I played various sports and never felt it affected me there either.

Its so unfortunate that this has happened to your son but I really believe that kids cope and adapt to these things better than adults would. Wishing you the best,—*Valerie*

Hi, Al, I'm glad you found us. My mother and father were faced with this choice after I was injured in a gun accident when I was seven. The doctors tried to save my damaged right eye for four weeks, then posed the question to my parents about trying to keep the damaged eye in place to provide a base for a prosthetic or some kind or to remove it completely. There was a possibility of the undamaged eye getting sick, so they decided do have the right one removed.

I never questioned their decision, ever. When I went through my implant rebuild two summers ago, everything came back to me and I know my mother was going through all kinds of stuff, too. It was important for me to let her know that I never, ever questioned or blamed her for her decision. My heart broke for her, a young mother just post-divorce, having to make such a horrifying choice. We'd never talked about it much before those surgeries, I know that my dad, who died in 88 and was the shooter in the gun accident carried huge guilt for the accident. When he was mentally unwell not long before he died, he asked me to forgive him. I told him that I never was mad at him for what happened. He asked did I hate him. it was so sad—we had a very close relationship, no fights, no stress or trauma and the thought that he'd been carrying all that since 1969 just made me so sad.

I guess I'm writing this kind of from your future—no one can go back to question or second guess the decisions made by traumatized parents. I'm glad they decided what they did—which was essentially to ensure the sight and safety of my left eye. I'm very sorry for your sad situation. Please take care and trust yourselves. With love,—*Alicia*

Thank you for your kind words. Our emotions are on a roller coaster ride since the accident. Your words "I'm glad they decided what they did—which was essentially to ensure the sight and safety of my left eye." made me tear—but thank you so much. It makes our decision more palatable. Thanks,—*Al*

[Follow-Up Message] Hi everybody, we went to the Ocular Plastics Surgeon yesterday and he gave us hope in two ways. One that we should consider leaving his eye in and monitoring it closely at three months intervals. The other was that David did see light! He recommended that we see his wife a retinal surgeon—we are going to see her today—wish us luck! Thank you all,—*Al*

[Follow-Up Message] Hi everyone, David is going in to surgery this Tuesday to see what they can do. Our surgeon can't really say, but she needs to see how badly the eye is damaged. They tried an ultra sound but there was too much blood and could not see into the eye/retina etc. The retina is very fragile, but by going in the eye she can see what else they can do. Wish him luck. Will keep you all posted.—*Al*

Hi everyone, David was operated on Tuesday and the retina was re-attached. We had the post-op visit on Wednesday. David still has light vision which he might have lost. He does not have any shadow vision, docs don't think so, but you never know! We are still hopeful. We have our next visit on next Thursday. Take care all,—*Al*

Al, glad to hear the surgery went well, Great news about the retina, that's super! Give David our love and tell him to hang in there. Keep us posted,—*Elizabeth*

Hi everyone, David has been a bit depressed and in pain the last two weeks. The initial surgery to repair the ruptured globe was only about ten stitches—the retina repair (May 17th 2005), I am not sure how many stitches, but the medical folder shows over 30. He is hanging in there and he is a boy.

We see the retina doc tomorrow, to see how the retina is holding up. He still sees light, but the best the doc's think he will see is shadows if there is a miracle. I would like to thank all of you that have responded and have given us encouragement. Thank you all so much,—*Al*

Hi, we visited the Cornea specialist. They said that his eye is healing very well. He had a eye pressure check and measured 6. I have been told that 15 is normal. The Doc stated that if he continues to heal like he is healing, depending what the retina specialist says, we may be able to improve his vision with a contact lens. This shocked us and was vary good news. It wasn't so long ago that we were thinking to remove the eye.

His eye is much smaller, we are camping now and family friends kids noticed it. You know kids—kids say the truth. David was questioning about his eye and trying to get a real good look at he eye. Anyway, until next time when hopefully we will have better news.—*Al*

Hi Al, great to hear about David's progress. About the pressure, 6 is a little bit low, but mine sits at about 5 or 6 all the time so its livable! The range is about 10 to 21 (15 being in the middle, so a pretty good guide). Take care,—*Elizabeth*

Thanks Liz, funny that you mentioned pressure—this was the first time his pressure was ever checked. I guess the eye was too fragile to test before. Will the pressure ever get higher? I was under the assumption that once the vitreous fluid was lost, there was nothing that can be done. But after the retina was attached they said they filled the eye with oil. Does the eye normally fill this overtime? Thanks again for your support.—*Al*

Hi all. The traumatic summer has come to an end. David is coping with his loss very well. The only thing I notice is when he pours himself a drink as it is funny how a simple task can be a bit difficult with one eye. Our last visit with the cornea specialist, shocked me—I had no idea that the stitches in his eye had to be removed! I thought that they would dissolve. He is a very scared—he wants to be asleep—I guess its because he knows if he goes under, there is no pain. He will have them removed in December.

He is back in school and playing traveling soccer and our last game (we won), he saved a penalty kick! I will keep you updated as time goes on—once again thank you all for your support.—*Al*

◆ ◆ ◆

Hi there guys. We have decided to go camping this weekend and I was wondering if there are any extra precautions to be aware of. He will be wearing his conformer and I have packed his ointments to keep it wet and a bottle of saline. As the one that has to put Noah's prosthetic eye in and his conformer, I am a bit squeamish as well. He hates it and fights me. At the end of this he is crying and I am walk away hoping the next time will be better. He has learned to pop it out from the bottom and has even gone as far as taking it out and hiding it. Any ideas? Please help frazzled mom!—*Niccole*

Greetings Niccole. The very first thing that comes to my mind, are safety glasses! This should be worn most of the time, I had mine made of that indestructible material, and they are the flex frame, and look just like a pair of eye glasses! If Noah is camping, I would really look into getting some safety glasses, cause those little limbs, sticks and bugs can go right into you eye! I hope this helps.—*Jarrod*

◆ ◆ ◆

Glad to have found this site. My son, Alan is 12 yrs old, and so far, has been a successful BMX (bicycle moto-cross) Racer. On May 8th of this year, he was shot in the left eye with a pellet gun. He watched a month of racing get away from him, as he laid face down in bed waiting for surgery to heal, but the damage was too intensive, and we found out this past Thursday, that his eye is shrinking, and he is going to lose it. Yes, he initially cried, as this is truly an unfair situation, and he knows that it means he will live life with one eye. BUT, he also knows that it could have been a real gun, and that there are kids out there worse off than him. He has looked thru your website a little bit, and was encouraged to find a place that was solely dedicated to persons in his same position. Our first visit to the plastic surgeon will be on the 15th of July, and he is already compiling a list of questions.—*John*

John, I'm glad that you and your son found this website. It's informative and supportive. I'm sorry about what happened to your son. The SAME thing happened to me 30 years ago. I was the same age as your son. It was my "best friend" who "accidentally" shot me in the eye with a bb gun. The results were immediate and devastating. They tried to remove the bb, but it got pushed further near my brain, where it's stayed for 30 years. They did an enucleation (removal of the eye) right away. Being a girl at that age, it was very traumatic for me, but I handled it fine.

As far as your son goes, he'll need time to physically heal. A lot depends on his particular case—how he'll handle each surgery. My case was pretty bad because my body rejected implants and I was allergic to many medications, etc. But if you read here, lots of people had it much better. Your son WILL get back to being a healthy, active boy. Having "one eye" (I *hate* that terminology!) didn't slow me down at all. As soon as I healed, I was back to being a healthy, active person. I played sports and had a normal life. He will too. We DO have to take some precautions, but other than that, it won't slow him down. I'd reassure him of that fact. Good luck with the surgery. If you have questions or if either of you need support, we're all here to do that. Take care!—*Chris*

It has been awhile since I have posted any progress reports, and quite frankly, that is in a way a good thing. Alan has not had to be enucleated yet, although it is still an eventuality. For now, simply due to a fluke involving drainage within his eye, his eye is actually building pressure slowly. SO, his physical appearance is actually better than it was a couple months back. His eye is a bit larger, so his lid doesn't look so droopy, and doesn't draw much attn. Of course, it is still a quiet, blind eye, but he is adjusting well. Surgery will probably be done later this winter, but for now is not a medical necessity.—*John*

◆   ◆   ◆

Hi guys! Thank you so much for all of your support, it's wonderful to have a group to turn to for help with my son. It's so hard to know how it feels and how to help when something is amiss. Jacob is having problems with the eyelid getting "stuck" to his prosthesis. He'll try to blink and it's stuck. It doesn't really seem to bother him, but as he's ready for preschool next year I'd like to help him be aware of it and correct it. I am praying that kids are more tolerant now than they were when I was a child, but I know better.

SO, any thoughts? why would it get stuck? We've been to see the ocularist and had it polished just recently, although the 'getting stuck' problem seems to be new in the past few weeks. (Yes, it's winter here and can be quite dry). Thank you,—*Bethy*

I've noticed the sticking as well. The cold seems to freeze whatever tears are in the eye, and my lids either get stuck open or closed. No one can tell because I still wear sunglasses everywhere. I can surely tell. What a strange feeling.—*Michael*

Maybe a patch that you can call an Eye Warmer, worn in the spirit of earmuffs as Ear Warmers? When he goes to school, talk to his teachers about his eye and stash some supplies with them—eye drops, a patch, something to put the eye in if it comes out and they can't get it back in. If you have a great teacher, s/he may even be able to learn how to take it out and put it in, just in case. A good teacher can even see when his eye is sticking and be able to get an eye drop in there without making it a big thing. Just my thinking. Love,—*Alicia*

I would definitely talk to the teachers/resource personnel and administration at the school your son will be attending. I know at our schools, teaching staff are not allowed to assist with an ocular prosthesis, taking it out, putting it in or putting drops in are considered "medical procedures" and the teaching staff are not allowed by contract to perform these. I know of a young student with an ocular prosthesis and it is hard on his parents. Any time there is even the slightest problem with it, the school calls home and the parents must come to the school to deal with it immediately. Talk about centering the child out. I hope you have much better luck with your child's school. Perhaps if the school has educational assistants they may be able to help with any prosthesis issues, as e.a.'s are often allowed to perform simple "medical procedures". Best of luck.—*Star*

◆ ◆ ◆

Jacob, my 3 1/2 year old son, fell today in Sunday School. He started crying and his dad saw blood coming from each side of his prosthesis. It was not a LOT of blood, but nevertheless it was concerning. I talked to the Ophthalmologist who suggested examining the socket and advised that she'd see him if we were still concerned.

Everything looks good, and there doesn't appear to be any visible injury but I was wondering if this has ever happened to anyone else? He was wearing his glasses and it looks like they pushed into his face pretty good so I don't know if the nose piece got him or what.—*Bethy*

Oh, that day is coming. I have no doubt! His 3 1/2 year old friend was over playing one day and came out of his room and handed me Jacob's eye. I just roll with it, I hope the school doesn't make a big deal about it all the time.

At what age were you able to start reinserting it yourself? The biggest problem I see at this point is that if it comes out I'm going to have drive up to school to put it back in. I don't want some school nurse trying to do it.—*Bethy*

◆ ◆ ◆

Hello Everyone! My daughter is now 10 months old and we are taking her to the beach next week for the first time. My question is.should I take her eye out or leave it in? The reason I ask is b/c she keeps "popping" it out. Several times it took us a bit to find it. I'm just afraid if she looses it in the sand or ocean.it's gone. I do plan on taking a squirt bottle with clean water in it, b/c I know she's get sand there no matter what, but if the eye is out, would the sand irritate the socket? Any input would be appreciated! Thanks!—*Lauren*

Leave it in. Make leaving it in the default.—*Chil*

They do have goggles made for kids, I would recommend that when in the water. All the best,—*Bill*

Lauren, I have gotten sand in my socket and it hurts! I was never bright enough to remember to bring my eye drops with me! That would be a great idea (that and some cotton balls).

I'd keep the prosthesis in. With it out, she could get MUCH more sand and debris in her socket! Don't ever leave it out, if you can help it! Guess it'll be a pain, but you really have to keep after her to try and keep it in her socket. She'll eventually get used to it. Good luck!—*Chris*

◆ ◆ ◆

I lost my eye when I was 5; and society made me self-contained, angry and lonely. I never had a girlfriend, I don't even try to get one. Don't get me wrong, I tried to get along with society but I got rejected.—*Nick*

Nick, Just out of curiosity, how old are you now? As you get older, it shouldn't matter as much to you what other people think. There are lots of different people in this great big world, many of which are great people. Don't give up on society. You must have just run into some bad apples in your life. I'm sure there are many people who would love you for who you are, eye problems or no eye problems. You've just got to go out there and keep trying, no matter what! Good luck!—*Renee*

978-0-595-39264
0-595-39264-4

CPSIA information can be obtained at www.ICGtesting.com
Printed in the USA
LVOW11s1042091016

508017LV00002B/482/P